Psychological Assessment of Surgical Candidates

In this volume, two of the world's foremost experts on presurgical psychological assessment provide a thorough review of the literature and specific, evidence-based guidelines for work in clinical settings. Chapters are helpfully organized around patient groups, such as those being considered for bariatric, spine, gender embodiment, breast cancer, gynecological, and solid organ surgery. Chapters on psychometrics and ethics offer up-to-date best practice summaries. Each chapter weaves contemporary science with helpful clinical recommendations. This book is a must-have for any professional interested in presurgical psychological assessments.

—Christopher J. Hopwood, PhD, Professor of Personality Psychology, University of Zurich, Zurich, Switzerland

This up-to-date book presents an excellent general approach to presurgical assessments, including good arguments for the inclusion of psychological testing conducted prior to the patient interview, the role of these evaluations in interdisciplinary team processes, and ethical concerns for practices that benefit the patient and are conducted within systems that continue to display and perpetuate significant health disparities. The text includes current coverage of telehealth practice now common since the start of the COVID-19 pandemic. Rich chapters by respected experts on the growing variety of specialty areas that rely on the contributions of psychologists clarify the importance of baseline medical knowledge and continuing education in medicine and surgery as well as psychology to provide the most useful input to patient-care teams. So many good reasons to understand that the days of psychologists "winging it" when requested to provide one of these assessments need to be over.

—Mary Ellen Olbrisch, PhD, ABPP, Board Certified in Clinical Health Psychology, Professor Emeritus of Psychiatry, Virginia Commonwealth University, Richmond, VA, United States

Marek and Block have assembled the leading experts in presurgical psychological assessments, who provide comprehensive, up-to-date, empirically supported guidance and identify best practices for conducting these evaluations. Seasoned practitioners and trainees alike will find integrative research reviews and valuable clinical insights in chapters covering the broad spectrum of presurgical psychological assessments.

—Yossef S. Ben-Porath, PhD, ABPP (Clinical), Kent State University, Kent, OH, United States

Psychological Assessment of Surgical Candidates

Evidence-Based Procedures and Practices

Ryan J. Marek
Andrew R. Block
Editors

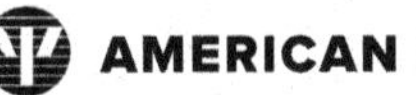
AMERICAN PSYCHOLOGICAL ASSOCIATION

Published by
American Psychological Association
750 First Street, NE
Washington, DC 20002
https://www.apa.org

Order Department
https://www.apa.org/pubs/books
order@apa.org

In the U.K., Europe, Africa, and the Middle East, copies may be ordered from Eurospan
https://www.eurospanbookstore.com/apa
info@eurospangroup.com

Typeset in Charter and Interstate by Circle Graphics, Inc., Reisterstown, MD

Printer: Gasch Printing, Odenton, MD
Cover Designer: Anthony Paular Design, Newbury Park, CA

Library of Congress Cataloging-in-Publication Data

CIP Data has been applied for.
Library of Congress Control Number: 2023931210

https://doi.org/10.1037/0000346-000

Printed in the United States of America

10 9 8 7 6 5 4 3 2 1

To my wife, Dr. Jaime Anderson, and our daughter, Alice.

—RYAN J. MAREK, PhD

For Michele—and for the grands: Adam, Nora, Stella, and Alice.

—ANDREW R. BLOCK, PhD, ABPP

Contents

Contributors

Wendy Balliet, PhD, Medical University of South Carolina, Charleston, SC, United States

Andrew R. Block, PhD, ABPP, Texas Back Institute, Plano, TX, United States

Andrea Bradford, PhD, Baylor College of Medicine, Houston, TX, United States

Shane S. Bush, PhD, ABPP, Long Island Neuropsychology, Lake Ronkonkoma, NY; University of Alabama, Tuscaloosa, AL; and VA New York Harbor Healthcare System, Brooklyn, NY, United States

Lillian Christon, PhD, Medical University of South Carolina, Charleston, SC, United States

Emily Cockle, PhD, The Alfred Hospital, Melbourne, Australia; Monash University, Melbourne, Australia

Honor Coleman, PhD, The University of Melbourne, Melbourne, Australia; The Alfred Hospital, Melbourne, Australia; Monash University, Melbourne, Australia

M. Scott DeBerard, PhD, Utah State University, Logan, UT, United States

Allyson Diggins, PhD, Cleveland Clinic Bariatric & Metabolic Institute, Cleveland, OH, United States

Jennifer A. Foley, BSc (Hons), DClinPsychol, CPsychol, National Hospital of Neurology and Neurosurgery, Queen Square, London, England; Queen Square Institute of Neurology, University College London, London, England

D. Brian Haver, PsyD, Medical University of South Carolina, Charleston, SC, United States

Zo Amaro Jimenez (they), PsyD, Lyon-Martin Health Services, San Francisco, CA, United States

Christine D. Liff, PhD, Michigan Neurology Associates and Pain Consultants, St. Clair Shores, MI, United States

Charles Malpas, PhD, The University of Melbourne, Melbourne, Australia; Royal Melbourne Hospital, Melbourne, Australia

Ryan J. Marek, PhD, Sam Houston State University, Conroe, TX, United States

Stacey Maurer, PhD, Medical University of South Carolina, Charleston, SC, United States

Julie Murray, MS, Utah State University, Logan, UT, United States

Andrew Neal, PhD, The Alfred Hospital, Melbourne, Australia; Monash University, Melbourne, Australia

Ninoska Peterson, PhD, Cleveland Clinic Bariatric & Metabolic Institute, Cleveland, OH, United States

Genevieve Rayner, PhD, The University of Melbourne, Melbourne, Australia; Austin Health, Heidelberg, Australia; The Alfred Hospital, Melbourne, Australia; Monash University, Melbourne, Australia

Colt St. Amand (he/they), PhD, MD, Mayo Clinic, Rochester, MN; University of Houston, Houston, TX; Baylor College of Medicine, Houston, TX, United States

Jayme S. Warner, BS, Utah State University, Logan, UT, United States

Psychological Assessment of Surgical Candidates

INTRODUCTION

Presurgical Psychological Assessments—Historical Perspectives and Current Status

RYAN J. MAREK AND ANDREW R. BLOCK

Presurgical psychological assessments (PPAs), a practice that includes thoroughly evaluating psychosocial factors that may affect (positively or negatively) postsurgical outcomes (Block & Marek, 2020), are becoming increasingly common across the United States and in other countries. One may ask, "Where does psychology fit into surgery?" To help answer this question, let's briefly discuss a few cases.

Case 1: A 53-year-old woman presented at the clinic for a spinal cord stimulator assessment. She had two previous spine surgeries that she stated "did not go well." During her visit, she reported only being able to stand for 15 minutes, she was unable to walk, and she slept in a recliner chair. She also reported taking a high dose of hydrocodone six times per day. She stated she is unable to go back to work because of her back pain and is currently receiving disability benefits. She shared that her husband is her primary caretaker but that he is severely diabetic and has a great deal of difficulty walking as a result of neuropathy in his feet.

The patient had undergone a spinal cord stimulator trial before the evaluation and reported about a 50% reduction in her pain. Even though she

https://doi.org/10.1037/0000346-001
Psychological Assessment of Surgical Candidates: Evidence-Based Procedures and Practices, R. J. Marek and A. R. Block (Editors)

expressed to the surgeon that she was uncertain about stimulator, the surgeon convinced her to undergo the permanent implant. Despite working with the manufacturer's representative to obtain a beneficial stimulation pattern, she reported limited pain change and dissatisfaction with the permanent implant. Several months later, she had the stimulator explanted.

Case 2: A 42-year-old woman presented at the clinic to be evaluated for bariatric surgery. Her body mass index was 66 kg/m^2, and she had numerous medical comorbidities, including Type 2 diabetes, obstructive sleep apnea, and hypertension. Her medical chart documented numerous instances of non-adherence, including not adhering to use of her CPAP (continuous positive airway pressure), not checking her blood sugar, and not attempting to make dietary changes. During a presurgical visit, she did not understand the post-operative regimen of a Roux-en-Y gastric bypass and thought she would "just be able to eat less." She reported a number of symptoms related to depression, such as depressed mood, anhedonia, lethargy, death ideation, and worthlessness, despite being on antidepressants. The surgical team felt her uncontrolled medical comorbidities needed to be addressed quickly and expedited her for surgery.

At her 3-month postoperative appointment, the patient's weight trajectory demonstrated a fair amount of weight loss, and her hemoglobin A1c levels returned to normal; however, she was quite tearful at her appointment. She reported she was in the emergency department because of dehydration; reported numbing from her waist down following surgery; was picking and nibbling on sweets, leading to multiple instances of *dumping syndrome*, a constellation of symptoms, such as diarrhea, nausea, light-headedness, and/or fatigue after a meal, that is caused by rapid gastric emptying; and reported that her depression had gotten worse. She said she regretted having bariatric surgery.

Case 3: A 59-year-old man reported to the clinic to be considered for a liver transplant. The patient was a high-profile business leader with a history of alcohol use disorder that led to cirrhosis. He would drink five to six scotches at a business outing or at home, and he drank these excessive amounts almost daily. He reported he often drank to cope and to socialize with some of his business partners. He insisted he was "not crazy" and was "not an alcoholic anymore." He stated he had not had many drinks since his liver started to fail, and he denied using other substances, including nicotine. His toxicology screen demonstrated positive results for tobacco and marijuana use.

During a follow-up session, he insisted that his friend, who had driven him to the appointment, had been smoking both cigarettes and marijuana, and thus he had inhaled both. He was referred for substance use treatment but insisted he was sober and did not need to go. He eventually received a new liver. Three years following his liver transplant, he returned to the clinic to be considered for another liver transplant. He indicated that he lapsed back into drinking when he had returned to work but stated that he would "do better this time."

These three cases highlight complex, although not uncommon, scenarios seen in surgical settings. In all instances, the surgical procedures were done correctly. The surgeons attended to the patients' medical problems but minimized the significance of psychosocial functioning. In each case, the consequences were detrimental. The patients did not fully benefit from the procedure and even experienced worsening of symptoms. They experienced increased emotional distress and became dissatisfied in the level of care provided. Unfortunately, in such situations of failed surgical procedures, patients may become angry or feel they were victims of negligence, sometimes even threatening lawsuits for unsuccessful surgical results. Often, additional surgical interventions may be required, costing insurance providers tens of thousands of dollars.

Although all three cases had chronic and severe medical comorbidities, psychosocial factors were prevalent and likely contributed to their poor outcomes. In Case 1, the patient's primary caregiver was also disabled, contributing to and exacerbating the patient's pain behaviors. The patient reported quite a bit of stress and hesitancy about the spinal cord stimulator and was on a heavy dose of opioids. Further, after multiple spine surgeries, she was still experiencing debilitating pain.

The patient in Case 2 had severe medical comorbidities that have been well documented to improve after bariatric surgery (Syn et al., 2021), but she also had numerous psychosocial concerns. For instance, her depression was not alleviated by her current psychotropic regimen, and the way antidepressants are absorbed after bariatric surgery (Roerig et al., 2012) is a cause for concern because antidepressants are not well absorbed following a procedure like the Roux-en-Y gastric bypass. Further, many patients continue to report a sense of loss of control of their eating, and they overeat after surgery (Conceição et al., 2015). Had these issues been addressed before surgery, it is possible the patient's quality of life would have been improved.

Case 3 demonstrates how important psychology can be for a transplant team. The patient was being considered for a liver transplant and insisted to all his providers that he had stopped drinking. However, his toxicology screen demonstrated that he had nicotine and marijuana in his system. Despite the recommendation to have substance use treatment, he opted not to adhere to that recommendation. He eventually had a liver transplant but was back in the hospital a few years later with problems related to alcohol and his liver. This case demonstrates the importance of addressing underlying psychosocial functioning. In addition, having psychological testing that incorporates methods of detecting underreported behaviors could have benefited this patient and the care team. Greater focus on psychosocial factors, such as untreated substance abuse, may have prevented the failure of his transplanted liver.

BENEFITS OF PRESURGICAL PSYCHOLOGICAL ASSESSMENT

All three cases could have benefited from having a PPA. Indeed, the practice is becoming more common in the United States, and some insurance providers now require PPAs to be conducted before covering elective surgical procedures. These PPAs can be thought of as a risk assessment to protect all stakeholders: the patient from having a poor outcome, the surgeon from liability for failed outcomes, the hospital's reputation, and the insurance provider from the expense of additional hospital visits or revisions of surgery.

An example of the values of PPA can be seen in the case of spine surgery. Approximately 10% to 40% of elective spine surgery patients report suboptimal outcomes to some degree, such as reporting limited pain relief, ongoing functional impairment, and emotional dysfunction (Atlas et al., 2000; Marek et al., 2021; Turner et al., 1992, 2004). As a result, many of these patients become medication dependent or are unable to return to work (Armaghani et al., 2014; Khan et al., 2019). In cases of failed spine surgery, insurance providers incur significant costs with no benefit and with ongoing obligations to cover subsequent treatment costs (Elsamadicy et al., 2017), and surgeons often have to deal with dissatisfied patients (Soroceanu et al., 2012).

THE CHANGING ROLE OF MENTAL HEALTH IN WORKING WITH SURGICAL CANDIDATES

The past 50 years have seen a paradigm shift in the role of mental health in medical settings. Initially, surgical teams would call on psychologists and other behavioral health specialists to determine if a patient had the capacity to understand informed consent. In some cases, psychologists and other behavioral health specialists simply would provide psychoeducation to groups of patients before they had surgery to help them cope with possible postoperative difficulties. As time moved forward, research on psychosocial factors and their ability to predict outcome began to accumulate. In some instances, psychosocial factors accounted for more variance in outcomes than medical risk factors (Block et al., 2001). Surgical teams began consulting psychologists and other behavioral health specialists to evaluate patients before surgery to help identify risk factors that could impede surgical outcomes.

The overall goal of PPA is to provide recommendations to both the surgical team and the patient regarding a prognosis of how psychosocial factors may affect surgical outcomes. If adverse factors are identified, psychologists work with the patient and the medical team to develop presurgical treatment interventions and recommendations, recommend postsurgical follow-ups, or discuss whether surgery is the best treatment option at that time.

Despite a growing number of clinical health psychologists who conduct a presurgical assessment, methods of conducting the assessment vary widely among practices. For instance, a survey of presurgical bariatric assessment practices suggested that only around a third of providers use some form of psychological test or symptom inventory in their practice (Bauchowitz et al., 2005). Of those, 55% of psychologists use a few symptom measures, notably the Beck Depression Inventory–II (Beck et al., 1996) and the Beck Anxiety Inventory (Beck & Steer, 1993), whereas only approximately 30% use a broadband test that includes validity scales and broader assessment of psychosocial factors, such as the Minnesota Multiphasic Personality Inventory–2 (Butcher et al., 1989), as part of their assessment (Bauchowitz et al., 2005). Some medical societies, such as the American Society for Metabolic and Bariatric Surgery, have provided recommendations on the type of information that should be gathered as part of a presurgical psychological assessment (Sogg et al., 2016), whereas other surgical areas have offered no formal recommendations.

Perhaps a major reason for the limited use of PPA is that many physicians view surgical success as limited to correction of the patient's medical problem. In the case of spine surgery: Did the bones fuse properly? In the case of bariatric surgery: Was the gastric bypass successfully completed? However, in almost all of the surgeries reviewed in this book, patients expect a great deal more. Depending on the type of surgery, patients may envision improvement in their overall function and health, reduction in their physical pain, or elimination of medications. They may expect great improvement in lifestyle and the ability to return to work. For many whose physical conditions have created greater emotional upheaval, reduction in depression and anxiety as well as improved relations with family and friends may be desired. Even, as in the case of gender embodiment, patients may see the surgery as the means to recovering their identities. And certainly, no surgical candidate is counting on worsening physical, mental, or emotional functioning. It is unfortunate that one of the most underrecognized values of PPA is the ability of this process to determine the full range of patient outcome expectations, discuss the plausibility of these expectations, and anticipate how psychosocial factors may influence events so that reasonable expectations can best come to fruition.

This book comes at a time when PPAs have become more routine and are being required in surgical practices. A surge in examining psychosocial factors and their relations to postoperative outcomes has occurred in the empirical literature. The overall goal of this text is to provide a foundation for the development of empirically based methods for conducting PPA. We anticipate that readers who are licensed behavioral health professionals or trainees in the area of clinical health psychology who are aiming to begin the process of PPA will be in the best position to apply and build on the methods presented in this book. In addition, we believe readers who are already well versed in PPA practice will also benefit from this book because many of the chapter authors are the experts leading the research in their respective areas. Further many of these authors present updated empirical work in their areas that can serve as good updates for the reader's practice.

ORGANIZATION OF THE BOOK

Chapter 1 presents a flexible model—we call it the *risk identification and mitigation model*—for the conduct of PPA across a broad range of medical conditions. Chapter 2 reviews psychometric considerations for both the clinical interview and psychological testing, including considerations for telehealth-based evaluations. Chapter 3 illustrates the importance of PPAs' ethical and legal foundation, including the increased movement toward assessment practices via telehealth.

Chapters 4 through 11 focus on empirical foundations and the review of psychosocial factors in specific surgical areas in which PPAs are routinely conducted. Chapter 4 examines psychopathology that is commonly assessed among bariatric surgery patients and how these factors are associated with poorer outcomes. The authors also review recommendations to mitigate risk factors.

Chapter 5 reviews the best available research evidence for the use of PPA in spine surgery interventions. It also provides a rubric of PPA best practices for psychologists.

Chapter 6 discusses and critiques the history of mental health evaluations for gender care surgeries, identifies and discusses multiple surgery options for gender care, and reviews affirming practices. The chapter includes sample assessment letters for insurance coverage and coordination of care with surgeons.

Chapter 7 provides common psychological outcomes following breast surgery in the setting of cancer treatment or prevention. The author also reviews assessment domains and procedures that are relevant to the psychosocial care of this population.

Chapter 8 examines the psychosocial, behavioral, psychiatric, and cognitive factors related to transplant outcomes and posttransplant quality of life. The authors review guidelines for using evidence-based practices in assessing these factors, conceptualizing the patient experience, and implementing effective treatments to assist mental health and medical transplant providers in optimizing transplant candidate selection and postoperative outcomes.

Chapter 9 discusses how to assess and select patients for deep brain stimulation (DBS) surgery, focusing on cognition, behavior, mood, and expectations. The authors review outcomes of DBS not only in terms of targeted functions but also in terms of cognition and patients' lived experience.

Chapter 10 takes a close look at the psychological outcomes and risk factors associated with commonly performed gynecologic surgeries, such as hysterectomy, and those of less common but more radical procedures for life-threatening conditions, including gynecologic cancer. The chapter briefly covers emerging procedures, such as uterine transplantation.

Chapter 11 provides a road map for understanding the evolution of postoperative patient outcomes for temporal lobectomy over time—over and above static measures of success, such as seizure freedom or recurrence. It offers guidelines for evaluating and counselling patients around these issues.

The concluding chapter, Chapter 12, offers practical tips for conducting PPA and provides information on future directions in the field of psychosocial evaluations of patients facing surgeries or other treatment for acute or chronic medical conditions.

It is our hope that this book provides a comprehensive overview of the current state of PPA. We also hope it points to areas in which further research should be conducted to solidify the empirical basis of PPA within specific types of surgery.

REFERENCES

Armaghani, S. J., Lee, D. S., Bible, J. E., Archer, K. R., Shau, D. N., Kay, H., Zhang, C., McGirt, M. J., & Devin, C. J. (2014). Preoperative opioid use and its association with perioperative opioid demand and postoperative opioid independence in patients undergoing spine surgery. *Spine, 39*(25), E1524–E1530. https://doi.org/10.1097/BRS.0000000000000622

Atlas, S. J., Keller, R. B., Robson, D., Deyo, R. A., & Singer, D. E. (2000). Surgical and nonsurgical management of lumbar spinal stenosis: Four-year outcomes from the Maine lumbar spine study. *Spine, 25*(5), 556–562. https://doi.org/10.1097/00007632-200003010-00005

Bauchowitz, A. U., Gonder-Frederick, L. A., Olbrisch, M. E., Azarbad, L., Ryee, M. Y., Woodson, M., Miller, A., & Schirmer, B. (2005). Psychosocial evaluation of bariatric surgery candidates: A survey of present practices. *Psychosomatic Medicine, 67*(5), 825–832. https://doi.org/10.1097/01.psy.0000174173.32271.01

Beck, A. T., & Steer, R. A. (1993). *Beck Anxiety Inventory*. Psychological Corporation.

Beck, A. T., Steer, R. A., & Brown, G. K. (1996). *Manual for the Beck Depression Inventory–II*. Psychological Corporation.

Block, A. R., & Marek, R. J. (2020). Presurgical psychological evaluation: Risk factor identification and mitigation. *Journal of Clinical Psychology in Medical Settings, 27*(2), 396–405. https://doi.org/10.1007/s10880-019-09660-0

Block, A. R., Ohnmeiss, D. D., Guyer, R. D., Rashbaum, R. F., & Hochschuler, S. H. (2001). The use of presurgical psychological screening to predict the outcome of spine surgery. *The Spine Journal, 1*(4), 274–282. https://doi.org/10.1016/S1529-9430(01)00054-7

Butcher, J. N., Dahlstrom, W. G., Graham, J. R., Tellegen, A., & Kaemmer, B. (1989). *The Minnesota Multiphasic Personality Inventory–2 (MMPI-2): Manual for administration and scoring*. University of Minneapolis Press.

Conceição, E. M., Utzinger, L. M., & Pisetsky, E. M. (2015). Eating disorders and problematic eating behaviours before and after bariatric surgery: Characterization, assessment and association with treatment outcomes. *European Eating Disorders Review, 23*(6), 417–425. https://doi.org/10.1002/erv.2397

Elsamadicy, A. A., Farber, S. H., Yang, S., Hussaini, S. M. Q., Murphy, K. R., Sergesketter, A., Suryadevara, C. M., Pagadala, P., Parente, B., Xie, J., & Lad, S. P. (2017). Impact of insurance provider on overall costs in failed back surgery syndrome: A cost study of 122,827 patients. *Neuromodulation, 20*(4), 354–360. https://doi.org/10.1111/ner.12584

Khan, I., Bydon, M., Archer, K. R., Sivaganesan, A., Asher, A. M., Alvi, M. A., Kerezoudis, P., Knightly, J. J., Foley, K. T., Bisson, E. F., Shaffrey, C., Asher, A. L., Spengler, D. M., & Devin, C. J. (2019). Impact of occupational characteristics on return to work for employed patients after elective lumbar spine surgery. *The Spine Journal, 19*(12), 1969–1976. https://doi.org/10.1016/j.spinee.2019.08.007

Marek, R. J., Lieberman, I., Derman, P., Nghiem, D. M., & Block, A. R. (2021). Validity of a pre-surgical algorithm to predict pain, functional disability, and emotional functioning 1 year after spine surgery. *Psychological Assessment, 33*(6), 541–551. Advance online publication. https://doi.org/10.1037/pas0001008

Roerig, J. L., Steffen, K., Zimmerman, C., Mitchell, J. E., Crosby, R. D., & Cao, L. (2012). Preliminary comparison of sertraline levels in postbariatric surgery patients versus matched nonsurgical cohort. *Surgery for Obesity and Related Diseases, 8*(1), 62–66. https://doi.org/10.1016/j.soard.2010.12.003

Sogg, S., Lauretti, J., & West-Smith, L. (2016). Recommendations for the presurgical psychosocial evaluation of bariatric surgery patients. *Surgery for Obesity and Related Diseases, 12*(4), 731–749. https://doi.org/10.1016/j.soard.2016.02.008

Soroceanu, A., Ching, A., Abdu, W., & McGuire, K. (2012). Relationship between preoperative expectations, satisfaction, and functional outcomes in patients undergoing lumbar and cervical spine surgery: A multicenter study. *Spine*, *37*(2), E103–E108. https://doi.org/10.1097/BRS.0b013e3182245c1f

Syn, N. L., Cummings, D. E., Wang, L. Z., Lin, D. J., Zhao, J. J., Loh, M., Koh, Z. J., Chew, C. A., Loo, Y. E., Tai, B. C., Kim, G., So, J. B., Kaplan, L. M., Dixon, J. B., & Shabbir, A. (2021). Association of metabolic-bariatric surgery with long-term survival in adults with and without diabetes: A one-stage meta-analysis of matched cohort and prospective controlled studies with 174 772 participants. *The Lancet*, *397*(10287), 1830–1841. https://doi.org/10.1016/S0140-6736(21)00591-2

Turner, J. A., Ersek, M., Herron, L., & Deyo, R. (1992). Surgery for lumbar spinal stenosis. Attempted meta-analysis of the literature. *Spine*, *17*(1), 1–8. https://doi.org/10.1097/00007632-199201000-00001

Turner, J. A., Loeser, J. D., Deyo, R. A., & Sanders, S. B. (2004). Spinal cord stimulation for patients with failed back surgery syndrome or complex regional pain syndrome: A systematic review of effectiveness and complications. *Pain*, *108*(1), 137–147. https://doi.org/10.1016/j.pain.2003.12.016

1 THE RISK IDENTIFICATION AND MITIGATION MODEL FOR PRESURGICAL PSYCHOLOGICAL ASSESSMENTS

RYAN J. MAREK AND ANDREW R. BLOCK

For the conclusions reached in presurgical psychological assessments (PPA) to be valid and effective across the spectrum of medical problems, many conditions must be met. The PPA process requires a strong empirical foundation as well as flexibility with regard to the types of testing implemented and the types of adverse psychosocial factors assessed during the clinical interview. Further, psychological factors that have been demonstrated to have positive effects on surgical outcomes—mitigating factors—should be assessed. Mitigating factors in this context are good prognostic indicators that would lessen the effect of risk factors, such as evidence of sustained health behavior changes, self-efficacy, and resilience. Standardized methods of integrating data need to be developed, and the range of recommendations should be considered.

Recently, we developed a general framework for PPA, the risk identification and mitigation (RIM) model (Block & Marek, 2020; see Figure 1.1), that is designed to be the basis for assessments that are empirically based and systematic. RIM is a five-step process: (a) identification of risk factors via psychological testing; (b) clinical interviewing and medical records review;

https://doi.org/10.1037/0000346-002
Psychological Assessment of Surgical Candidates: Evidence-Based Procedures and Practices, R. J. Marek and A. R. Block (Editors)

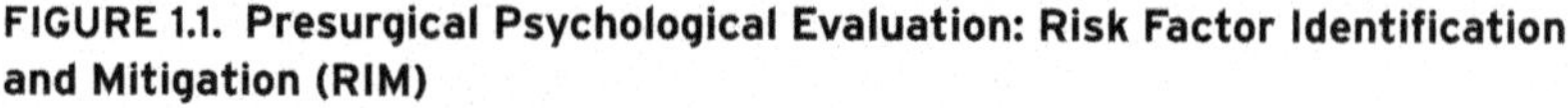
FIGURE 1.1. Presurgical Psychological Evaluation: Risk Factor Identification and Mitigation (RIM)

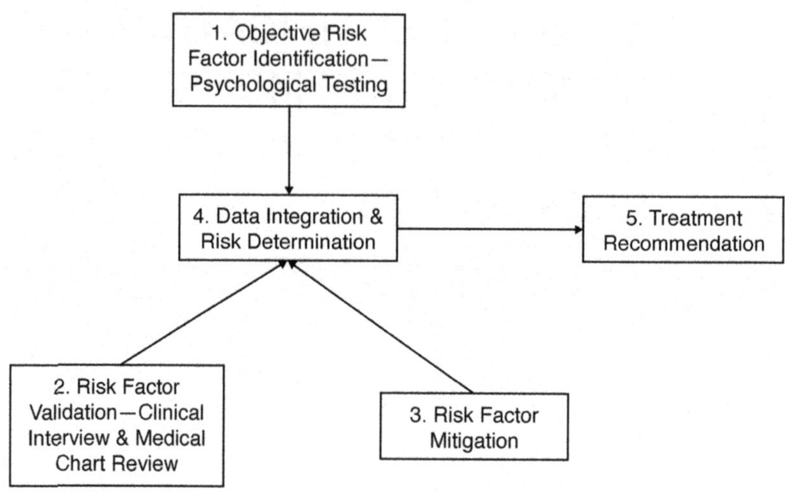

Note. From "Presurgical Psychological Evaluation: Risk Factor Identification and Mitigation," by A. R. Block and R. J. Marek, 2020, *Journal of Clinical Psychology in Medical Settings*, *27*(2), p. 397 (https://doi.org/10.1007/s10880-019-09660-0). Copyright 2019 by Springer Science+Business Media, LLC, part of Springer Nature. Reprinted with permission.

(c) identification of risk-mitigating factors; (d) integration of data gathered, including determination of overall risk; and (e) treatment recommendations (Block & Marek, 2020). This model of conducting PPA is meant to be comprehensive (e.g., bariatric surgery, organ transplant, spinal surgery, deep brain stimulation, and more are covered in this text) while also allowing for flexibility regarding the types of methods used to gather data (e.g., structured vs. unstructured interviews, type of psychological tests that are integrated), risk factors assessed, and mitigation factors considered.

OBTAIN EVIDENCE OF PSYCHOSOCIAL RISK FACTORS

The first step in the RIM model is to use a method to obtain objective evidence of psychosocial risk factors. The method that most effectively provides such evidence is psychometric testing, preferably measures with embedded validity scales that assess a broad array of psychopathology (termed *broadband testing*). Indeed, we recommend the use of psychological testing, when able, especially because psychological testing helps psychologists and mental health professionals capture aspects of the patient they may not otherwise have gathered via an interview, allows them to assess the severity of various constructs of interest, and may allow the patient to disclose things they may not readily feel comfortable disclosing in person. Although traditional psychological assessment practice often uses testing following the clinical interview, for PPA, it is preferable to complete testing before the interview. In many cases of PPA, because the psychologist/mental health professional has only one opportunity to speak with the surgical candidate, testing before the interview ensures that risk factors emerging from testing can be fully explored. This also ensures that the patient does not need to return in the event additional or conflicting information emerges during testing that was not readily apparent during the clinical interview.

Psychometric testing can be divided into two different categories: (a) broadband and (b) narrowband. *Broadband measures* provide a comprehensive assessment of psychopathology and behavior within one test. Examples of broadband tests include the Minnesota Multiphasic Personality Inventory–3 (Ben-Porath & Tellegen, 2020a, 2020b), the Personality Assessment Inventory (Morey, 1991) and Personality Assessment Inventory Plus (Morey, 2020), Millon Behavioral Medicine Diagnostic (Millon & Antoni, 2006), the Battery for Health Improvement 2 (Disorbio & Bruns, 2002), and Symptom Item Checklist-90–Revised (Derogatis, 1996). Many broadband instruments also contain embedded validity scales that detect random/fixed responding, overreporting of symptoms, or underreporting response styles. When possible, it is recommended that a well-validated, broadband measure be used for PPAs.

Broadband testing takes more time to complete, although most broadband tests can be administered in under an hour. Although they assess for a wide array of symptoms, some measures may not contain content specific to risk factors associated with the surgical population. For instance, although the Personality Assessment Inventory and the Personality Assessment Inventory Plus (Morey, 1991, 2020) assess constructs that are relevant to eating disorder pathology, they do not contain specific scales or indices that assess risk for eating pathology that may be relevant to the assessment of patients seeking bariatric surgery.

The other category of testing includes *narrowband measures,* which provide a brief screening of symptom severity that can aid in diagnostic interpretation, elucidate risk factors assessed on broadband measures, and help track symptom changes over time (Tarescavage & Ben-Porath, 2014). Narrowband measures can be used to follow up on risk factors when a broadband test does not adequately cover the domain. They can also be used if the patient will be seen for follow-up visits to track symptom change over time. Many narrowband measures have been developed for conditions specific to the surgical setting. For instance, the Oswestry Disability Index (Fairbank & Pynsent, 2000) is a 10-item questionnaire that is sensitive to detecting functional disability resulting from back pain, and the 16-item Binge Eating Scale (Gormally et al., 1982) is a good proxy for severity associated with binge eating.

Often, psychologists and mental health professionals include at least one broadband measure and an array of narrowband measures specific to the surgical population as part of their PPA battery. More detailed information about how to evaluate a test or measure for your practice is covered in Chapter 2 of this volume.

VALIDATE AND OBTAIN MORE DETAILS ABOUT RISK FACTORS

The second step of the RIM model is to validate and expand on risk factors identified in psychometric testing, both through review of the patients' medical records and the clinical interview. A thorough review of medical records may document many relevant issues; for example, a history of drug or alcohol abuse (including emergency room–related visits that were substance related) may serve as a good proxy for the severity of substance use. Prior surgical history and the follow-up notes can provide insight into how well patients managed prior surgeries that may give rise to concerns about postoperative medication compliance and appointment adherence (Block & Marek, 2020; Dobmeyer, 2018). Examining the history of prescription medications, such as opioids and psychotropic medications, can elucidate how long some issues may have persisted and whether a patient potentially may have abused some medications in the past (e.g., early requests for refills). Medical records can be a good source of information that can contribute to the overall prognosis of the patient with regard to the surgery they are presenting for.

It is not uncommon for patients to feel hesitant about meeting with a psychologist/mental health professional for an assessment. For many, it is their first time seeing a mental health professional. To that end, patients may view the PPA as an obstacle to moving forward with surgery (Block & Sarwer, 2013). As part of the interview, the psychologist/mental health professional should review data from the medical records and testing with the patient.

During the informed consent, it is recommended that the psychologist/mental health professional provide an introduction describing their professional training in the area; the purpose for the psychological assessment; the length of time required for testing and interview; and the manner in which information obtained from the process will be used, including identifying those who will have access to it. Establishing a strong therapeutic alliance is an important aspect to PPAs (Sogg et al., 2016).

The clinical interview is more than a diagnostic interview. In addition to evaluating for psychological diagnoses, a psychologist/mental health professional also needs to assess for knowledge related to the surgical procedure; assess for the motivation for undergoing the procedure; and take a full psychosocial history that includes factors such as abuse, outpatient or inpatient treatments, suicidality, substance use, social or caregiver support, current coping strategies, and current quality of life. In addition, each surgical setting emphasizes specific aspects of the psychological history and current functioning. For instance, understanding patients' history of dieting behaviors (and successes and failures related to dieting), weight loss/regain history, and possible history/current eating disorders are important in bariatric surgery assessments. In contrast, current pain levels, duration of pain, behaviors affected by pain, catastrophizing, and somatization are critical to assess in spine surgery assessments.

A critical aspect of this step involves behavioral observations. Behavioral observations can be informative, notably, if they are not congruent with what the patient has reported. Psychologists and mental health professionals conducting PPAs should include usual components of behavioral observations typically reported in addition to population-specific facets, such as pain behaviors matching with pain severity reports.

ASSESS FACTORS THAT CAN POSITIVELY INFLUENCE SURGICAL OUTCOMES

The third step of the RIM model aims to assess mitigating factors. The first two steps use methods that assess for risk factors that could adversely affect surgical results. This third step examines psychosocial factors that may positively influence surgical outcomes or buffer risk factors (Block & Marek, 2020).

Although understanding mitigating factors is not as well researched as risk factors, extant literature suggests some such mitigating factors, including realistic expectations of surgical outcomes (van Hout et al., 2005); an increase in patient activation regarding involvement in their health care (Block et al., 2019; Hibbard et al., 2004); positive, competent, and proactive social supports (Conceição et al., 2020); self-efficacy (Batsis et al., 2009); and resilience (Huang et al., 2019). To this end, narrowband self-report measures can be embedded into Step 1 and discussed with the patient during the interview. These measures include, but are not limited to, the Expectations Scale (Mahomed et al., 2002; Riddle et al., 2017), the Patient Activation Measure (Hibbard et al., 2004), Social Support (Sarason et al., 1987), New General Self-Efficacy Scale (Chen et al., 2001), and the Brief Resilience Scale (Smith et al., 2008). These indices may help aid in understanding whether factors exist that may reduce the adverse effects of identified psychosocial risk factors (e.g., depression, substance use) and whether the patient has some strengths that will aid in their postsurgical outcome.

SYNTHESIZE DATA TO IDENTIFY FACTORS THAT WILL AFFECT POSTSURGICAL OUTCOMES

The fourth step in the RIM model is the integration of information obtained across the prior three steps to narrate a comprehensive report that identifies psychosocial factors that may negatively and positively affect postsurgical outcomes. For some surgical settings, easy-to-use risk factor models and algorithms have been developed to streamline the integration process.

For spine surgery, an algorithm can be used that integrates all data across methods of assessment, including psychological testing, interview or medical chart review, medical data, and interpersonal interactions. The algorithm yields very good concordance with outcomes as far as 1 year following spine surgery (Marek et al., 2021) and guides the user to one of five categories that predicts prognosis (Excellent, Very Good, Fair, Poor, and Very Poor). The Cleveland Clinic Behavioral Rating System (Heinberg et al., 2010) was designed to integrate 9 domains of psychosocial functioning to derive a dimensional domain associated with prognosis for bariatric surgery. The Transplant Evaluation Rating Scale (Twillman et al., 1993) and the Stanford Integrated Psychosocial Assessment for Transplant (Maldonado et al., 2012) have been developed to aid with data integration to predict prognosis in solid organ transplant evaluations. Neuropsychiatric risk factors have also been identified for deep brain stimulation (Foley et al., 2018) and bone marrow transplant (Austin & Rini, 2013). All can be used as tools to help with clinical judgment and should be guided by data obtained during the psychological assessment of the patient seeking surgery.

CREATE A SET OF RECOMMENDATIONS FOR THE PATIENT AND THE SURGICAL TEAM

The fifth step in the RIM model focuses on recommendations both for the patient and for the surgical team. In this final stage, the psychologist/mental health professional considers different evidence-based interventions that may improve postoperative outcomes for patients. These recommendations fall into three main categories: (a) interventions that enhance surgical results, (b) interventions that increase motivation and compliance, and (c) consideration of alternative medical interventions for those at high risk for having a poor outcome. In the first category, psychologists and mental health professionals recommend and implement interventions that increase patient's ability to better manage their symptoms and have them engage in healthy activities (Block & Marek, 2020). For instance, a psychologist/mental health professional may recommend (or require) patients to complete cognitive behavior therapy for reducing binge eating behaviors before bariatric surgery (Ashton et al., 2009) or cognitive behavior therapy for reducing pain and improving functioning before spinal surgery (Rolving et al., 2015).

In the second category, if psychosocial factors may interact at a more moderate level (e.g., smoking, wound healing), some interventions to improve motivation and adherence are to be recommended. For instance, a psychologist/mental health professional may recommend smoking cessation (Fiore et al., 2008), reduction or abstinence of alcohol use (Fernandez et al., 2015), opioid tapering (Hassamal et al., 2016), weight loss (Sogg et al., 2016), medication management for mood disorders (Roerig & Steffen, 2015), and more intensive motivational enhancement treatment strategies (e.g., motivation interviewing; Rollnick et al., 2008).

The third category focuses on alternative, more conservative medical interventions for those at high psychosocial risk. If a psychologist/mental health professional thinks the patient may not do well after surgery, they discuss other options with members of multidisciplinary treatment programs and whether more conservative treatment approaches might be appropriate before scheduling the patient for the procedure. For those struggling with chronic alcohol or substance use, more intensive inpatient or outpatient services may be suggested before revisiting elective surgery as a treatment option. Those patients with poorly managed, severe psychopathology (e.g., schizophrenia) should be provided with appropriate referrals and demonstrate good adherence and symptom management before surgery (Archid et al., 2019). Surgical intervention can then be reevaluated once sustained adherence or symptom reduction has been documented (Block & Marek, 2020).

CONCLUSION

The RIM model is a standardized, yet flexible model for conducting PPAs. A number of authors in the coming chapters of this book follow procedures outlined in the RIM model, and each discusses important aspects within these steps unique to their surgical areas. The writing of other authors in this book is in more emerging areas of PPAs in which some steps may not necessarily be applicable (e.g., distress screening instead of psychological testing in breast surgery) or are still developing (e.g., understanding which, if any, risk factors predict suboptimal outcomes in gender embodiment).

The authors (e.g., as in Chapters 4, 5, 8) in areas in which PPA procedures are well developed with consistent evidence pointing to how presurgical psychosocial factors predict diminished outcomes have outlined procedures similar to the RIM model. Other areas—such as those outlined in Chapters 6, 7, and 10—are still accumulating outcome data to best understand whether aspects of the RIM model are necessary (e.g., psychological testing) and how best to integrate information to predict outcomes. Continued outcome research linking various presurgical psychosocial factors to various outcomes across these areas are crucial to refining the assessment process for patients seeking surgery.

REFERENCES

Archid, R., Archid, N., Meile, T., Hoffmann, J., Hilbert, J., Wulff, D., Teufel, M., Muthig, M., Quante, M., Königsrainer, A., & Lange, J. (2019). Patients with schizophrenia do not demonstrate worse outcome after sleeve gastrectomy: A short-term cohort study. *Obesity Surgery*, *29*(2), 506–510. https://doi.org/10.1007/s11695-018-3578-0

Ashton, K., Drerup, M., Windover, A., & Heinberg, L. (2009). Brief, four-session group CBT reduces binge eating behaviors among bariatric surgery candidates. *Surgery for Obesity and Related Diseases*, *5*(2), 257–262. https://doi.org/10.1016/j.soard.2009.01.005

Austin, J. E., & Rini, C. (2013). *Bone marrow and stem cell transplant*. American Psychological Association. https://doi.org/10.1037/14035-006

Batsis, J. A., Clark, M. M., Grothe, K., Lopez-Jimenez, F., Collazo-Clavell, M. L., Somers, V. K., & Sarr, M. G. (2009). Self-efficacy after bariatric surgery for obesity. A population-based cohort study. *Appetite*, *52*(3), 637–645. https://doi.org/10.1016/j.appet.2009.02.017

Ben-Porath, Y. S., & Tellegen, A. (2020a). *The Minnesota Multiphasic Personality Inventory–3: Manual for administration, scoring, and interpretation*. University of Minnesota Press.

Ben-Porath, Y. S., & Tellegen, A. (2020b). *The Minnesota Multiphasic Personality Inventory–3: Technical manual*. University of Minnesota Press.

Block, A. R., & Marek, R. J. (2020). Presurgical psychological evaluation: Risk factor identification and mitigation. *Journal of Clinical Psychology in Medical Settings*, *27*(2), 396–405. https://doi.org/10.1007/s10880-019-09660-0

Block, A. R., Marek, R. J., & Ben-Porath, Y. S. (2019). Patient activation mediates the association between psychosocial risk factors and spine surgery results. *Journal of Clinical Psychology in Medical Settings*, *26*(2), 123–130. https://doi.org/10.1007/s10880-018-9571-x

Block, A. R., & Sarwer, D. B. (2013). Introduction. In A. R. Block & D. B. Sarwer (Eds.), *Presurgical psychological screening: Understanding patients, improving outcomes* (pp. 3–24). American Psychological Association. https://doi.org/10.1037/14035-000

Chen, G., Gully, S. M., & Eden, D. (2001). Validation of a New General Self-Efficacy Scale. *Organizational Research Methods*, *4*(1), 62–83. https://doi.org/10.1177/109442810141004

Conceição, E. M., Fernandes, M., de Lourdes, M., Pinto-Bastos, A., Vaz, A. R., & Ramalho, S. (2020). Perceived social support before and after bariatric surgery: Association with depression, problematic eating behaviors, and weight outcomes. *Eating and Weight Disorders*, *25*(3), 679–692. https://doi.org/10.1007/s40519-019-00671-2

Derogatis, L. R. (1996). *SCL-90-R: Symptom Checklist-90-R: Administration, scoring, and procedures manual*. NCS Pearson.

Disorbio, J., & Bruns, D. (2002). *Brief Battery for Health Improvement 2 manual*. Pearson.

Dobmeyer, A. C. (2018). *Psychological treatment of medical patients in integrated primary care*. American Psychological Association. https://doi.org/10.1037/0000051-000

Fairbank, J. C., & Pynsent, P. B. (2000). The Oswestry Disability Index. *Spine*, *25*(22), 2940–2953. https://doi.org/10.1097/00007632-200011150-00017

Fernandez, A., Sturmberg, J., Lukersmith, S., Madden, R., Torkfar, G., Colagiuri, R., & Salvador-Carulla, L. (2015). Evidence-based medicine: Is it a bridge too far? *Health Research Policy and Systems*, *13*(1), Article 66. https://doi.org/10.1186/s12961-015-0057-0

Fiore, M. C., Jaén, C. R., Baker, T. B., Bailey, W. C., Benowitz, N. L., Curry, S. J., Dorfman, S. F., Froelicher, E. S., Goldstein, M. G., & Healton, C. G. (2008). *Treating tobacco use and dependence: 2008 update*. U.S. Department of Health and Human Services.

Foley, J. A., Foltynie, T., Limousin, P., & Cipolotti, L. (2018). Standardised neuropsychological assessment for the selection of patients undergoing DBS for Parkinson's disease. *Parkinson's Disease*, *2018*, Article 4328371. https://doi.org/10.1155/2018/4328371

Gormally, J., Black, S., Daston, S., & Rardin, D. (1982). The assessment of binge eating severity among obese persons. *Addictive Behaviors*, *7*(1), 47–55. https://doi.org/10.1016/0306-4603(82)90024-7

Hassamal, S., Haglund, M., Wittnebel, K., & Danovitch, I. (2016). A preoperative interdisciplinary biopsychosocial opioid reduction program in patients on chronic opioid analgesia prior to spine surgery: A preliminary report and case series. *Scandinavian Journal of Pain*, *13*(1), 27–31. https://doi.org/10.1016/j.sjpain.2016.06.007

Heinberg, L. J., Ashton, K., & Windover, A. (2010). Moving beyond dichotomous psychological evaluation: The Cleveland Clinic Behavioral Rating System for weight loss surgery. *Surgery for Obesity and Related Diseases*, *6*(2), 185–190. https://doi.org/10.1016/j.soard.2009.10.004

Hibbard, J. H., Stockard, J., Mahoney, E. R., & Tusler, M. (2004). Development of the Patient Activation Measure (PAM): Conceptualizing and measuring activation in patients and consumers. *Health Services Research*, *39*(4p1), 1005–1026. https://doi.org/10.1111/j.1475-6773.2004.00269.x

Huang, Y., Huang, Y., Bao, M., Zheng, S., Du, T., & Wu, K. (2019). Psychological resilience of women after breast cancer surgery: A cross-sectional study of associated influencing factors. *Psychology Health & Medicine*, *24*(7), 866–878. https://doi.org/10.1080/13548506.2019.1574353

Mahomed, N. N., Liang, M. H., Cook, E. F., Daltroy, L. H., Fortin, P. R., Fossel, A. H., & Katz, J. N. (2002). The importance of patient expectations in predicting functional outcomes after total joint arthroplasty. *The Journal of Rheumatology*, *29*(6), 1273–1279.

Maldonado, J. R., Dubois, H. C., David, E. E., Sher, Y., Lolak, S., Dyal, J., & Witten, D. (2012). The Stanford Integrated Psychosocial Assessment for Transplantation (SIPAT): A new tool for the psychosocial evaluation of pre-transplant candidates. *Psychosomatics*, *53*(2), 123–132. https://doi.org/10.1016/j.psym.2011.12.012

Marek, R. J., Lieberman, I., Derman, P., Nghiem, D. M., & Block, A. R. (2021). Validity of a pre-surgical algorithm to predict pain, functional disability, and emotional functioning 1 year after spine surgery. *Psychological Assessment*, *33*(6), 541–551. Advance online publication. https://doi.org/10.1037/pas0001008

Millon, T., & Antoni, M. (2006). *MBMD: Millon Behavioral Medicine Diagnostic*. NCS Pearson.

Morey, L. C. (1991). *Personality Assessment Inventory professional manual*. Psychological Assessment Resources.

Morey, L. C. (2020). *Personality Assessment Inventory Plus professional manual*. Psychological Assessment Resources.

Riddle, D. L., Slover, J., Ang, D., Perera, R. A., & Dumenci, L. (2017). Construct validation and correlates of preoperative expectations of postsurgical recovery in persons undergoing knee replacement: Baseline findings from a randomized clinical trial. *Health and Quality of Life Outcomes*, *15*(1), Article 232. https://doi.org/10.1186/s12955-017-0810-x

Roerig, J. L., & Steffen, K. (2015). Psychopharmacology and bariatric surgery. *European Eating Disorders Review*, *23*(6), 463–469. https://doi.org/10.1002/erv.2396

Rollnick, S., Miller, W. R., & Butler, C. (2008). *Motivational interviewing in health care: Helping patients change behavior*. Guilford Press.

Rolving, N., Nielsen, C. V., Christensen, F. B., Holm, R., Bünger, C. E., & Oestergaard, L. G. (2015). Does a preoperative cognitive-behavioral intervention affect disability, pain behavior, pain, and return to work the first year after lumbar spinal fusion surgery? *Spine*, *40*(9), 593–600. https://doi.org/10.1097/BRS.0000000000000843

Sarason, I. G., Sarason, B. R., Shearin, E. N., & Pierce, G. R. (1987). A brief measure of social support: Practical and theoretical implications. *Journal of Social and Personal Relationships*, *4*(4), 497–510. https://doi.org/10.1177/0265407587044007

Smith, B. W., Dalen, J., Wiggins, K., Tooley, E., Christopher, P., & Bernard, J. (2008). The Brief Resilience Scale: Assessing the ability to bounce back. *International Journal of Behavioral Medicine, 15*(3), 194–200. https://doi.org/10.1080/10705500802222972

Sogg, S., Lauretti, J., & West-Smith, L. (2016). Recommendations for the presurgical psychosocial evaluation of bariatric surgery patients. *Surgery for Obesity and Related Diseases, 12*(4), 731–749. https://doi.org/10.1016/j.soard.2016.02.008

Tarescavage, A. M., & Ben-Porath, Y. S. (2014). Psychotherapeutic outcomes measures: A critical review for practitioners. *Journal of Clinical Psychology, 70*(9), 808–830. https://doi.org/10.1002/jclp.22080

Twillman, R. K., Manetto, C., Wellisch, D. K., & Wolcott, D. L. (1993). The Transplant Evaluation Rating Scale: A revision of the psychosocial levels system for evaluating organ transplant candidates. *Psychosomatics, 34*(2), 144–153. https://doi.org/10.1016/S0033-3182(93)71905-2

van Hout, G. C., Verschure, S. K., & van Heck, G. L. (2005). Psychosocial predictors of success following bariatric surgery. *Obesity Surgery, 15*(4), 552–560. https://doi.org/10.1381/0960892053723484

2 SELECTING AND ADMINISTERING PSYCHOLOGICAL MEASURES FOR PRESURGICAL ASSESSMENTS

RYAN J. MAREK

Psychological measures are being constantly developed and published in peer-reviewed journals across disciplines. To that end, the availability of measures that can be incorporated into a presurgical psychological assessment (PPA) may seem limitless. As delineated in Chapter 1, these measures range from broadband to narrowband, and selection of these instruments and tests is based on the assessment goals. Perhaps a measure focused on binge eating is the measure of choice for a bariatric surgery assessment, but the measure would not bode well in a spine surgery assessment. Moreover, maybe the provider is interested in assessing for more constructs associated with poor outcomes and decides to expand the number of instruments and tests they include in their assessment. Perhaps providers are interested in assessing socially desirable responding or overreporting of problems and would like a measure that assesses validity. Some measures can be administered and scored electronically, and some testing software even creates interpretative reports. The availability of measures to tackle these issues is not the problem; rather, the appropriateness of these measures for PPAs is certainly a matter of discussion. At the end of the day, you want to know: "Is this a good measure or method, and does it make sense for my practice?"

https://doi.org/10.1037/0000346-003
Psychological Assessment of Surgical Candidates: Evidence-Based Procedures and Practices, R. J. Marek and A. R. Block (Editors)

I begin this chapter with a brief refresher on psychometrics—both as they pertain to selecting measures and with regard to clinical interviewing. Rather than focus on math and statistics, I point you to critical topics that I anticipate will make evaluating these methods a bit easier. My goal for this chapter is to outline important factors that you should consider when choosing what psychological measures to incorporate into your assessment of surgical candidates.

BASIC CONSIDERATIONS

It is encouraged that psychological testing be incorporated into the PPA, and some medical subspecialty societies directly recommend using psychological testing. Indeed, data obtained from psychological tests and measures generally add to clinical interviews and are oftentimes superior to clinical judgment (Grove & Lloyd, 2006; Grove & Meehl, 1996). Thus, it is important to put time and effort into considering what measures you would like to include. If you have already developed a battery of measures, evaluate it regularly, bearing in mind that no single psychological test or measure will capture everything relevant to the assessment of surgical patients. Common screeners in health psychology, such as the Patient Health Questionnaire–9 (PHQ-9; Kroenke & Spitzer, 2002), may be ideal if depression severity is deemed a construct of interest. However, many patients seeking elective procedures do not present solely with depression if psychopathology is present. When selecting tests and screeners to use in practice, the breadth and scope of the test battery must cover the broad range of psychological domains pertinent to the specific surgical type, with special attention to the psychometric strengths and limitations of your battery.

Another significant concern is context of the test administration. Can the measure be administered electronically? And if so, do you have the equipment needed to both administer and obtain test score information efficiently? Can or should the measures be given ahead of the office visit to expedite the assessment process? If given in person, will the hospital provide a quiet testing space for the patient to accomplish this task? Keep these considerations at the forefront of designing the assessment to protect test integrity and validity of scores obtained.

PSYCHOMETRIC CONSIDERATIONS

This section focuses on various psychometric considerations to evaluate in the context of assessing patients who are seeking surgery. Specifically, I review standardization, reliability, validity, availability of normative/comparison group data, and classification accuracies (e.g., sensitivity, specificity, positive predictive power) in the sections that follow.

Standardization

Standardization, a critical component of psychometric testing, relies on consistency in the conduct of assessment procedures. Standardization should be used across domains of the PPA, including the clinical interview, self-report measures, and behavioral observations. Standardization is important because replication cannot be determined if standard procedures are not readily used. For instance, abundant mixed evidence is available about whether presurgical psychosocial functioning affects bariatric surgery outcomes. To a large extent, differences in measurement (e.g., structured versus unstructured interviews, validated versus self-created self-report measures) likely contribute to inconsistent findings in the area of bariatric surgery (Marek et al., 2016). Standardized methods of assessment will more likely lead to consistent, replicable results. Thus, this process is not only important in the creation and use of self-report measures, but for the entire assessment.

Most instruments, whether structured interview, a behavioral assessment, or self-report measure, have standardized methods for administration, scoring, and interpretation. These instructions must be carefully followed to avoid introducing error that can result in scores that are not replicable or useful. Some measures, such as structured diagnostic interviews, require training and have extensive scoring and interpretation rules, and they can be easily misused. Other lengthy tests are frequently misused by administering only parts of the test (sometimes this is valid if standardized procedures for doing so are published and supported). In some cases, the validity of test interpretations is questionable when they rely on programs that use alternative scoring or make use of personally derived interpretations that do not necessarily align with peer-reviewed empirical findings.

Reliability

Reliability essentially captures the level of consistency in a person's scores on a measure (Wasserman & Bracken, 2013) in a multitude of ways, including internal consistency, interrater reliability, and test–retest reliability. Reliability is an estimate of how much consistent true score variance is present on a measure because variability in a set of scores on a measure reflects a true score in addition to error. For instance, if psychologists and mental health professionals are interested in measuring the construct of "depression," we would develop a set of items and administer them to a group of individuals. We would expect that we are capturing variance in responses that represent the individuals' true score of depression; however, it is likely that variance is being captured that is unrelated to depression. The variance that is not capturing depression is likely either unsystematic or systematic error, or both.

Unsystematic error, also known as "random error," includes things like lighting, noise, individuals' mood at the end of the day versus the start of the day, distractibility, or fatigue. *Systematic error* is not random and can affect the validity of a measure. It includes the items not measuring our construct of depression, reactivity, bias, and more. Thus, the actual scores we receive from our patients reflects their true score plus or minus random and nonrandom error. A measure with good reliability is necessary to evaluate its validity. One common misconception is that once reliability has been reported, it implies that reliability will be unchanged when used in a different sample. Reliability is a characteristic of the scores obtained in specific samples and constantly needs to be evaluated when used across different samples (Rouse, 2007; Vacha-Haase et al., 2002).

A common metric for reliability reported is *internal consistency*, which examines whether all items or elements of a measure contribute to the total score in a consistent manner. *Cronbach's alpha* is a common metric reported; coefficients closer to 1.00 imply better internal consistency. However, Cronbach's alpha can be influenced by the number of items on a measure. For shorter scales, mean interitem correlations (the average correlation of all the correlations between items) may be more appropriate, with coefficients of greater than or equal to .15 to less than or equal to .50 considered to be evidence of good internal consistency (Briggs & Cheek, 1986). Other coefficients, such as *McDonald's omega* (McDonald, 1999; interpreted similarly to Cronbach's alpha, although is derived differently), may be better indicators of reliability. *Interrater reliability* is necessary for measures that are interviewlike in nature, such as structured diagnostic interviews, or are meant to capture observed behaviors. These reliability coefficients, typically estimated with a kappa coefficient (1.00 indicates perfect agreement), reflect the degree to which two raters observe and score the same behaviors or symptoms. And *test–retest reliability* estimates whether the measure obtains a similar score when readministered at a later point. Timing between assessments can be critical, notably, when testing reliability of more traitlike versus more statelike characteristics.

A scale score's reliability is important to establishing validity and should be considered first when evaluating tests and screeners. As just reviewed, Cronbach's alpha is commonly reported metric for internal consistency but is not always the appropriate coefficient to consider. Reliability provides insight as to whether a scale is consistently measuring a construct. However, reliability coefficients alone do not attest to the validity of the scale (i.e., Is the scale actually measuring the construct of interest?). Reliability does, however, set the upper bounds for validity that I describe next.

Validity

Good reliability does not imply validity. One way to think about this is by visualizing a dartboard. A cluster of holes on the board implies consistency of dart throwing, but is it hitting the bull's-eye? If the darts are hitting the bull's-eye (or are getting close to it), one implication is that the player is good at darts (valid). If the cluster of holes is off of the dartboard (i.e., the player misses the target even though the darts consistently hit the same area on the wall), a person would imply that the player is not good at darts but is quite reliable (i.e., the player is good at hitting some other target—in this case, an area of the wall).

The same can be said about the validity of a psychological measure. Let's use the earlier example of the depression measure. Perhaps the measure shows good internal consistency and test–retest reliability in a sample. However, when the measure is pitted against other criteria that also measure depression (perhaps major depressive disorder captured via a structured interview or through other established self-report measures of depression), we may find that it correlates well with those criteria (validity) or does not correlate well with those criteria (lack of validity). Equally important, we want our new depression measure to correlate well with depression criteria but have weaker associations with anxiety and substance use criteria (shows good discrimination). To these ends, we have numerous methods for establishing validity, including content validity, criterion validity, convergent and discriminant validity, and predictive validity.

Content validity essentially captures whether the measure's content covers aspects of the construct(s) of interest. *Criterion validity* implies that the measure's score is consistent with theoretically aligned indicators of interest (e.g., a diagnosis, performance on a task, indicators in medical records). Generally, correlation coefficients are used to establish this kind of validity. *Convergent* and *discriminant validity* aim to establish whether our scale scores are associated with constructs of interests. We want our scores to correlate well with constructs that are similarly targeted with our new measure (convergent), but we want them to be more weakly associated with constructs that are not related to what we are targeting with our new measure (discriminant). Although measures should always be used in conjunction with a good clinical interview, incremental validity is also valuable because it demonstrates that a measure's scores add to the assessment above and beyond other data—such as the clinical interview. Because the goals of PPAs are to predict outcomes for our patients, *predictive validity*, the ability of our scale scores to predict a measured outcome, is especially important. If we are assessing risk or mitigating factors, our methods for assessing those risk factors should, to some degree, correlate with other outcomes across surgical settings. Predictive validity is more difficult to capture, primarily because it is longitudinal in nature.

Overall, those who are conducting PPAs will want to consider not only reliability but also validity. Measures that yield good convergent and discriminant validity help build confidence that one is accurately capturing the construct of interest. Because these measures tend to yield dimensional scores, adding validated measures to the assessment help one to assess severity and to track the effect of interventions. Paying particular attention to measures that also yield incremental and predictive validity for PPA will add better precision to assessing how surgical candidates will fare after surgery.

Availability of Normative or Comparison Group Data

For many psychological measures, particularly if one is considered a psychological test, standardization and the establishment of normative data are important. These give rise to how to use a reliable and valid score because they establish a way to interpret scale scores using a reference group, cutoff scores, or both. A person who scored high or low on a measure is relatively meaningless without a reference group with which to compare their scores. For example, consider the Minnesota Multiphasic Personality Inventory–3 (MMPI-3; Ben-Porath & Tellegen, 2020a, 2020b). The test's norms are based on 2020 projected census data and thus are representative of the United States population as they pertain to gender, race/ethnicity, and age. A look at the MMPI-3 technical manual also delineates several comparison groups, including one for the assessment of spine surgery/spinal cord stimulator patients. Thus, a provider who is conducting a PPA for spine surgery can also compare their patient's test scores to those of other patients who have also sought spine surgery.

Many other broadband tests contain data relevant to assessing patients in various health care settings, suggesting that many of these tests are useful for assessing presurgical patients. Other measures may function differently in surgical settings and may require additional comparison group data. For instance, the PHQ-9 (Kroenke & Spitzer, 2002) appears to function differently in bariatric surgery settings. Although a cut score of greater than or equal to

10 yields good sensitivity and specificity in detecting major depressive disorder in primary care settings, a higher cutoff score of greater than or equal to 15 may be more appropriate when assessing patients for bariatric surgery (Cassin et al., 2013) largely because of the number of medical comorbidities (and, thus, overlapping symptoms) in many patients who are seeking bariatric surgery face. Overall, it is important to understand how normative data were derived.

Classification Accuracies

As mentioned earlier, the use of cutoff scores on measures is important. They help with clinical decision making and allow the health care provider to feel confident about their ability to make predictions. Table 2.1 provides an example of a method used to evaluate various cut scores on measures. Two-by-two contingency tables like this one allow for easy calculations of the performance of various cut scores on a continuous measure. This method of evaluating cut scores is ideal when the criterion can be dichotomized (e.g., presence versus absence, diagnosis versus no diagnosis). Calculations for various statistics to evaluate cut scores are listed at the bottom of Table 2.1.

Sensitivity is the proportion of individuals with the risk factor or disorder who were correctly identified with the self-report score cutoff specified. For instance, Grupski et al. (2013) examined the cut score of greater than 17 on the Binge Eating Scale (BES; Gormally et al., 1982) using binge-eating disorder (derived from a clinical interview) as the criterion. Grupski et al. (2013) reported a sensitivity of .94, which represents the proportion of those who were predicted to have binge-eating disorder based on the BES score. *Specificity* is the proportion of individuals without risk factor/disorder who were correctly predicted by the self-report score cutoff to not have the risk factor/diagnosis. Grupski et al. (2013) reported a specificity of .76, which represents the proportion of patients who scored below 17 on the BES and who also did not have binge-eating disorder. Thus, the "optimal" cut score

TABLE 2.1. Classification Accuracy Calculations

	Presence of risk factor/disorder	
Prediction	**Present**	**Absent**
≥ Cut score	True positive (*a*)	False positive (*b*)
< Cut score	False negative (*c*)	True negative (*d*)

Note. Calculations for various statistics to evaluate cut scores are as follows: Base rate = (*a* + *c*) / Sample size; Hit rate = (*a* + *d*) / Sample size; Sensitivity = *a* / (*a* + *c*); Specificity = *d* / (*b* + *d*); Positive predictive power = *a* / (*a* + *b*); Negative predictive power = *d* / (*c* + *d*).

to use on a self-report yields a combination of good sensitivity (values closer to 1.00) and good specificity (values closer to 1.00). A cut score with high sensitivity but low specificity may overpathologize people, whereas low sensitivity and high specificity may continually miss capturing risk factors/diagnoses. Thus, sensitivity and specificity start with the true classification and look to see how well a cut score on a measure did regarding these classifications.

Positive predictive power represents the proportion of patients with scores at or above the cut score on the measure who were correctly identified as having the risk factor/disorder. On the other hand, *negative predictive power* represents the proportion of patients with scores below the cutoff on the self-report measure who were correctly identified as not having the risk factor/diagnosis. Thus, positive predictive power and negative predictive power function similarly to sensitivity and specificity. However, they reference the rows and are reflective of what psychologists and mental health professionals actually do in our practice. Thus, positive predictive power and negative predictive power use the cut score as having or not having the risk factor/disorder and then examine how many individuals actually have the risk factor/disorder.

Although sensitivity and specificity are routinely reported in the literature, positive predictive power and negative predictive power are reported less frequently even though these statistics are more reflective of how we use self-report measures in practice. Fortunately, the calculations for these statistics are included in Table 2.1, and they are easy for psychologists and mental health professionals to use, thus providing a two-by-two contingency table for their report.

Let's consider a few other statistics in two-by-two tables. *Hit rate* is the proportion of correct predictions in the overall sample. *Base rate* can be considered the prevalence statistic that encompasses the percentage of individuals who are "positive" on the criterion (i.e., have the diagnosis or have the risk factor). Base rate typically does not affect the sensitivity and specificity of a measure, but it does affect positive predictive power and negative predictive power because correctly classifying rarer events with a self-report measure becomes increasing difficult to do.

Receiver operating characteristic curves, or ROC curves, are another method used to evaluate cut scores of a measure. A benefit to ROC curves is that they allow one to evaluate a range of cut scores (via sensitivity and specificity) against a criterion simultaneously. True positive rates on a criterion with every cutoff of a measure are plotted against true negative rates on a criterion. ROC curve values between 0 and 1 are then calculated, with .5 indicating that a cut score is as good as chance, whereas 1 would indicates perfect classification of a cut score. The area under the curve is also calculated and references an estimate of predictive efficacy of a measure. Areas under the curve can be used to compare measures on their efficacy against a criterion or with a measure using a criterion in a different population.

TELEHEALTH AND ELECTRONIC ADMINISTRATION AND SCORING

The novel coronavirus (COVID-19) pandemic beginning in 2020 certainly changed the way behavioral health providers practice. Methods for conducting psychological assessments rapidly came to light. For instance, tests like the MMPI-3 (Ben-Porath & Tellegen, 2020a, 2020b) and Millon Behavioral Medicine Diagnostic (Millon & Antoni, 2006) were given telehealth options and can now be administered remotely. Guidance on how to use these various instruments in a telehealth environment is also being published. For instance, Corey and Ben-Porath (2020) reviewed secure methods for administering MMPI instruments via telehealth platforms, such as using video software that is compliant with the Health Insurance Portability and Accountability Act of 1996, also known as HIPAA; having a live proctor present (to protect test security and ensure the patient is indeed the person taking the test); providing informed consent to electronic testing; and documenting in one's report that the measures were administered via telehealth. A more detailed checklist is provided in Table 1 of Corey and Ben-Porath's (2020) review. These methods should be carefully reviewed and applied when using most instruments or measures via a telehealth method.

Block et al. (2020) provided guidance on how to maintain psychometric integrity of PPAs during the COVID-19 pandemic. Some guidance will extend beyond to telehealth assessment of presurgical patients. Notably, behavioral observations are a bit more difficult to reliably assess during a telehealth assessment. Because many electronic devices have cameras that focus on the face of the patient, behaviors (e.g., pain-related behaviors) and other observations, such as the smell of remnants of cigarette or marijuana use, hygiene, use of assistive devices, such as cane, and so on, are not easily observed and can decrease the thoroughness of the assessment. On the other hand, telehealth can allow the practitioner to capture a glimpse of the patient's home environment, which can aid in conceptualization.

Although it is convenient for the patient to not have to travel to the clinic for a presurgical assessment, it is important to protect psychometric integrity when using self-report measures by having a live proctor during testing to protect test security, maintaining standardized administration to the extent possible, and making note of this method in the final report. It is also important to acknowledge limitations of the behavioral observations.

CLINICAL UTILITY

Once the aforementioned data are gathered, one must weigh their clinical utility. Behavioral health providers must consider how long they want their assessment to go. If providers only have 60 minutes to do a clinical interview, using a fully structured diagnostic instrument is likely not a consideration. Likewise, time for psychological testing will dictate what measures to include. Some broadband tests yield shorter administration times when administered electronically than do paper-and-pencil tests, thus allowing for additional narrowband measures specific to the surgical population to also be administered. In contrast, the MMPI-2 (Butcher et al., 1989, 2001), which averages 60 to 90 minutes, is likely out of the scope of practice if 60 minutes is the provider's only window for psychological testing. Cost can also be a factor. Although one can bill for psychological testing and be reimbursed for the time it takes to score and interpret the measures, the reimbursement-to-cost ratio may be a factor (TheraThink, n.d.). It is also critical for one to stay up-to-date with the literature and ensure that the test software is routinely updated so that automated interpretative reports stay reflective of the evidence-based literature. Many organizations require information technology (IT) approval for software updates, and some organizations do not update software unless it is updated for all providers using the system. It is essential that behavioral health specialists who include testing develop a process with their IT departments to ensure smooth, regular updates to testing software for the benefit of their practice.

CONCLUSION

This chapter aimed to review psychometric considerations when developing or updating PPA. From the clinical interview to psychological testing and behavioral observations, one needs to strive to use standardized methods to the extent possible and feasible. Reliable and valid methods are critical, as is the use of instruments that have appropriate normative or comparison group information. Clinical utility, including understanding appropriate cutoff scores for interpretation, cost, and feasibility of administration are also important characteristics to consider.

Although a full discussion of the topic of telehealth assessments is beyond the scope of this chapter, having a live proctor during testing can help maintain test security and allow one to administer instruments in a standardized fashion as closely as possible. Some aspects of the assessment may be hampered by telehealth, such as behavioral observation or a lack of scores having demonstrated validity in a telehealth administration. Overall, though, psychometrically sound instruments provide the foundation for presurgical assessment. It is critical to carefully consider what instruments to include in the assessment and carefully critique their psychometric properties.

REFERENCES

Ben-Porath, Y. S., & Tellegen, A. (2020a). *The Minnesota Multiphasic Personality Inventory–3: Manual for administration, scoring, and interpretation*. University of Minnesota Press.

Ben-Porath, Y. S., & Tellegen, A. (2020b). *The Minnesota Multiphasic Personality Inventory–3: Technical manual*. University of Minnesota Press.

Block, A. R., Bradford, A., Butt, Z., & Marek, R. J. (2020, April 17). *How COVID-19 may affect presurgical psychological evaluations*. American Psychological Association Services. Retrieved July 1, 2021, from https://www.apaservices.org/practice/news/presurgical-psychological-evaluations-covid-19

Briggs, S. R., & Cheek, J. M. (1986). The role of factor analysis in the development and evaluation of personality scales. *Journal of Personality, 54*(1), 106–148. https://doi.org/10.1111/j.1467-6494.1986.tb00391.x

Butcher, J. N., Dahlstrom, W. G., Graham, J. R., Tellegen, A., & Kaemmer, B. (1989). *The Minnesota Multiphasic Personality Inventory–2 (MMPI-2) manual for administration and scoring*. University of Minneapolis Press.

Butcher, J. N., Graham, J. R., Ben-Porath, Y. S., Tellegen, A., & Dahlstrom, W. G. (2001). *Minnesota Multiphasic Personality Inventory–2 (MMPI-2): Manual for administration and scoring* (Rev. ed.). University of Minnesota Press. https://doi.org/10.1016/B0-08-043076-7/01294-8

Cassin, S., Sockalingam, S., Hawa, R., Wnuk, S., Royal, S., Taube-Schiff, M., & Okrainec, A. (2013). Psychometric properties of the Patient Health Questionnaire (PHQ-9) as a depression screening tool for bariatric surgery candidates. *Psychosomatics, 54*(4), 352–358. https://doi.org/10.1016/j.psym.2012.08.010

Corey, D. M., & Ben-Porath, Y. S. (2020). Practical guidance on the use of the MMPI instruments in remote psychological testing. *Professional Psychology: Research and Practice, 51*(3), 199–204. https://doi.org/10.1037/pro0000329

Gormally, J., Black, S., Daston, S., & Rardin, D. (1982). The assessment of binge eating severity among obese persons. *Addictive Behaviors, 7*(1), 47–55. https://doi.org/10.1016/0306-4603(82)90024-7

Grove, W. M., & Lloyd, M. (2006). Meehl's contribution to clinical versus statistical prediction. *Journal of Abnormal Psychology, 115*(2), 192–194. https://doi.org/10.1037/0021-843X.115.2.192

Grove, W. M., & Meehl, P. E. (1996). Comparative efficiency of informal (subjective, impressionistic) and formal (mechanical, algorithmic) prediction procedures: The clinical-statistical controversy. *Psychology, Public Policy, and Law, 2*(2), 293–323. https://doi.org/10.1037/1076-8971.2.2.293

Grupski, A. E., Hood, M. M., Hall, B. J., Azarbad, L., Fitzpatrick, S. L., & Corsica, J. A. (2013). Examining the Binge Eating Scale in screening for binge eating disorder in bariatric surgery candidates. *Obesity Surgery, 23*(1), 1–6. https://doi.org/10.1007/s11695-011-0537-4

Health Insurance Portability and Accountability Act of 1996 (HIPAA), Pub. L. 104–191, 42 U.S.C. § 300gg, 29 U.S.C. §§ 1181–1183, and 42 U.S.C. §§ 1320d–1320d9.

Kroenke, K., & Spitzer, R. L. (2002). The PHQ-9: A new depression diagnostic and severity measure. *Psychiatric Annals, 32*(9), 509–515. https://doi.org/10.3928/0048-5713-20020901-06

Marek, R. J., Ben-Porath, Y. S., & Heinberg, L. J. (2016). Understanding the role of psychopathology in bariatric surgery outcomes. *Obesity Reviews, 17*(2), 126–141. https://doi.org/10.1111/obr.12356

McDonald, R. (1999). *Test theory: A unified treatment*. Lawrence Erlbaum Associates.

Millon, T., & Antoni, M. (2006). *MBMD: Millon Behavioral Medicine Diagnostic*. NCS Pearson.

Rouse, S. V. (2007). Using reliability generalization methods to explore measurement error: An illustration using the MMPI-2 PSY-5 scales. *Journal of Personality Assessment, 88*(3), 264–275. https://doi.org/10.1080/00223890701293908

TheraThink. (n.d.). *Psychological testing reimbursement rates in 2022*. https://therathink.com/psych-testing-reimbursement-rates/

Vacha-Haase, T., Henson, R. K., & Caruso, J. C. (2002). Reliability generalization: Moving toward improved understanding and use of score reliability. *Educational and Psychological Measurement, 62*(4), 562–569. https://doi.org/10.1177/0013164402062004002

Wasserman, J. D., & Bracken, B. A. (2013). Fundamental psychometric considerations in assessment. In J. R. Graham & J. A. Naglieri (Eds.), *Handbook of psychology: Vol. 10. Assessment psychology* (pp. 50–81). John Wiley & Sons.

3 ETHICAL CONSIDERATIONS IN THE ASSESSMENT OF SURGICAL CANDIDATES

CHRISTINE D. LIFF AND SHANE S. BUSH

Surgeries are performed for both medically necessary and elective reasons. Decisions about whether to undergo a surgical procedure require the surgical candidate to (a) have the cognitive capacity to make such decisions and (b) be free of psychopathology that could hamper the outcome of the surgery or recovery or that might contribute to iatrogenic effects. When cognitive capacity is lacking, decisions regarding medically necessary procedures must be made by a surrogate. In the context of elective surgeries, such as cosmetic and bariatric surgeries, questions arise regarding the candidate's emotional state, personality traits, and motivations. Across surgical contexts, questions emerge regarding the candidate's expectations, social supports, substance abuse potential, and other psychosocial issues. In addition, understanding a surgical candidate's strengths and resources that can lead to positive outcomes is important for all involved parties.

To gain a clearer understanding of such psychosocial matters, surgeons and other health care professionals turn to psychologists and mental health professionals for their expertise. Psychologists and mental health professionals, in turn, often use standardized psychometric measures as key components

https://doi.org/10.1037/0000346-004
Psychological Assessment of Surgical Candidates: Evidence-Based Procedures and Practices, R. J. Marek and A. R. Block (Editors)

of the information on which their opinions are based. Each aspect of the assessment process is informed by ethical principles and guidelines as well as the laws of the jurisdiction in which the service is provided. Through this process, psychologists and mental health professionals are well positioned to address the needs of those who are considering undergoing surgery and the surgeons and other treatment team members who are involved in arranging and performing the surgery.

Effective presurgical psychological assessment (PPA) involves appropriate selection and use of assessment procedures and methods. Although some models have been articulated (e.g., the risk identification and mitigation model; Block & Marek, 2020), because of the relative infancy of this specialty and variability across surgical settings, there is limited agreement regarding which procedures and methods are preferred and how to integrate the results of standardized testing with other sources of information to arrive at sound conclusions and helpful recommendations. In addition, in part because the need for PPA seems to outpace the availability of experienced examiners, some practitioners who perform such assessments are unaware of, or neglect, the relevant research related to this area of practice. Professional ethics and relevant laws inform the PPA process, and attention to such guidelines can maximize good surgical decisions and outcomes. This chapter illustrates the importance of this ethical and legal foundation, including the increased movement toward assessment practices via telehealth.

RELEVANT ETHICAL ISSUES

The shared values of health care professionals underlie general bioethical principles, which are often reflected in the ethics codes of specific professions, including psychology. The American Psychological Association (APA, 2017) *Ethical Principles of Psychologists and Code of Conduct* (APA Ethics Code) incorporates the general bioethical principles in its aspirational general principles.

General Bioethical Principles

The ethics of health care include four basic principles on which to base the viability and efficacy of a patient procedure or treatment modality. Specifically, for a procedure or treatment to be considered ethical, it must adhere to the four principles of (a) respect for autonomy, (b) beneficence, (c) nonmaleficence, and (d) justice. These principles and their applications to PPA are covered in this section. See Table 3.1 for a summary of ethical issues and their corresponding representations in the APA Ethics Code.

TABLE 3.1. Common Sources of Ethical Conflict in Presurgical Psychological Assessments With Corresponding APA Ethical Standards

Ethical issue	APA general principle or standard[a]
Beneficence/nonmaleficence	General Principle A: Beneficence and Nonmaleficence
	Standard 3.04 Avoiding Harm
Justice	General Principle D: Justice
Respect for people's rights and dignity	General Principle E: Respect for People's Rights and Dignity
Professional competence	Standard 2.01 Boundaries of Competence
	Standard 2.03 Maintaining Competence
Roles/relationships (dual/multiple)	Standard 3.05 Multiple Relationships
Informed consent/patient autonomy	Standard 3.10 Informed Consent
	Standard 9.03 Informed Consent in Assessments
Confidentiality	Standard 4.01 Maintaining Confidentiality
	Standard 4.02 Discussing the Limits of Confidentiality
	Standard 4.04 Minimizing Intrusions on Privacy
Assessment (methods, norms, interpretation, security)	Standard 9.01 Bases for Assessments
	Standard 9.02 Use of Assessments
	Standard 9.06 Interpreting Assessment Results
	Standard 9.09 Test Scoring and Interpretation Services
	Standard 9.10 Explaining Assessment Results
Test security	Standard 9.11 Maintaining Test Security
Conflicts between ethics and law	Standard 1.02 Conflicts Between Ethics and Law, Regulations, or Other Governing Legal Authority
	Standard 1.03 Conflicts Between Ethics and Organizational Demands

Note. APA = American Psychological Association.
[a]Information in column 2 is from American Psychological Association (2017).

Respect for Autonomy

Competent adults in Western societies have a fundamental right to make the decisions that govern their bodies, including which medical procedures to undergo. This principle is reflected in the APA Ethics Code in General Principle E: Respect for People's Rights and Dignity. For example, it may be strongly recommended that an older adult with advanced gangrene in a lower extremity resulting from uncontrolled diabetes undergo surgical amputation of the extremity to prolong their life. However, despite the pleas of the surgical team or loved ones, a competent adult may elect not to undergo the surgery, aware that death will ensue. When decisional capacity or motivation to avoid surgery is questionable, psychologists and mental health professionals play an important role in assessing the candidate's cognition and emotional state, including their long-held values and potentially misinformed beliefs. Respect for patient autonomy underlies informed consent (APA Ethics Code Standards 3.10, Informed Consent, and 9.03, Informed Consent in Assessments), which is covered in more detail later in this chapter.

Beneficence

Beneficence involves doing or producing good for another. As stated in General Principle A: Beneficence and Nonmaleficence of the APA Ethics Code, "Psychologists strive to benefit those with whom they work" and "seek to safeguard the welfare and rights of those with whom they interact professionally and other affected persons." In the context of PPA, the goal of the surgical team, including the psychologist/mental health professional, is to identify those who are good candidates for a proposed surgery and will benefit from the procedure. Similarly, psychologists and mental health professionals recommend caution when the evidence from an appropriate assessment indicates that the result may be harmful to the person. Conclusions and recommendations that are beneficial to the candidate are not always those that are consistent with the wishes of the candidate. For example, the results of a PPA may indicate that a person is at high risk for poor outcome of bariatric surgery, despite the person's strong desire to undergo the surgery. Despite disappointing the candidate, the recommendation not to go forward with the surgery may nevertheless safeguard the person's welfare.

Nonmaleficence

Nonmaleficence is the obligation for clinicians to "first, do no harm"—primum non nocere. General Principle A: Beneficence and Nonmaleficence of the APA Ethics Code advises psychologists to "take care to do no harm," and Standard 3.04, Avoiding Harm, outlines the need for psychologists to "take reasonable steps to avoid harming their clients/patients, students, supervisees, research participants, organizational clients, and others with whom they work, and to minimize harm where it is foreseeable and unavoidable." Included in this principle is the need to address one's *implicit bias*, or the beliefs and assumptions that can taint or skew a psychologist's ability to help relevant populations. Arriving at inappropriate conclusions about a candidate's suitability for a surgical procedure or their ability to make decisions for themselves about a procedure can result in a harmful outcome for the person. For example, in a PPA for organ transplant, failure to assess the candidate's compliance with current medications and medical appointments would be a significant omission that could lead to an inappropriate decision regarding appropriateness for surgery (Block & Sarwer, 2013). That decision would be harmful for the candidate. Use of psychometric testing can help limit bias on the part of the psychologist or mental health professional.

Justice

Justice is the concept that all persons are entitled to the benefits of psychology, with unbiased distribution of the "processes, procedures, and services" provided by psychologists (see General Principle D: Justice of the APA Ethics Code). Ethical psychologists remain cognizant of, and prevent, any personal biases or professional judgments from unequally affecting their patients or leading to unfair treatment. In PPA contexts, psychologists and mental health professionals may have biases for or against certain procedures in general or for a specific person; those biases can influence the assessment process, the conclusions reached, and the recommendations offered. For example, a psychologist/mental health professional may be opposed to a young woman's undergoing a surgical procedure to harvest and sell her eggs. In such instances, the psychologist/mental health professional should strive to understand the effect of that bias on their professional activities and take steps to eliminate the effect; otherwise, the psychologist/mental health professional should decline to perform the assessment.

Professional Competence

Professional competence is defined in the online Medical Dictionary as "proficiency in the application of the arts and sciences of healing. Such competence requires communication skills, dedication to serving others, empathy, good judgment, and technical knowledge" (Farlex, n.d.). Competence is the foundation for all effective professional services; it is required for the services provided to benefit—and not harm—the surgical candidate. Competence can be conceptualized as consisting of two components (Fouad & Grus, 2014; Health Service Psychology Education Collaborative, 2013; Rodolfa et al., 2005): (a) *foundational competencies,* which include scientific knowledge and methods, evidence-based practices, diversity, ethical and legal issues, and interdisciplinary systems, among others; and (b) *functional competencies,* which have to do with activities that practitioners perform, including assessment, report writing, and intervention.

To perform effective and useful PPAs, psychologists and mental health professionals must obtain the proper knowledge base and skill set, including the ability to conceptualize and formulate appropriate assessment protocols. Professional competence also includes knowing when one has not gained the proficiency necessary to perform a particular service. APA Ethics Code

Standard 2.01(a), Boundaries of Competence, states that psychologists only provide services for populations "within the boundaries of their competence, based on their education, training, supervised experience, consultation, study, or professional experience." Standard 2.01(d) further states that with cases for which competency has not been obtained, the psychologist is to "make a reasonable effort to obtain the competence required" or "make appropriate referrals."

Competence is not a static phenomenon or a milestone to attain. It is ever evolving and depends on self-assessment of one's knowledge and abilities. APA Ethics Code Standard 2.03, Maintaining Competence, addresses the need for psychologists to remain vigilant to new developments in their area of competency and to make "ongoing efforts to develop and maintain their competence." In addition, providers who perform PPAs best serve all involved parties by remaining current with scholarly literature that addresses capacity assessments and the psychological characteristics that typically lead to positive surgical results. For example, the Australian Psychological Society (APS, 2018) published a practice guide that outlines the psychological characteristics that both reduce and improve the likelihood of positive surgical outcomes for patients seeking cosmetic surgery.

There has been growing investment of select professional societies and associations in the development of credentialing systems for specific PPAs. One such system in consideration was suggested by the American Society for Metabolic and Bariatric Surgery. According to Rouleau et al. (2014), that recommendation included "an apprenticeship model where a licensed mental health professional obtains competence through reading [bariatric surgery]-specific content and training under a more experienced mental health specialist" (p. 3). Although certification standards are not yet established, mental health providers can attain competence to assess select medical patients by continuing their education through coursework and seminars, reading relevant articles and research, obtaining peer consultation or supervision, attending the meetings of professional networks and organizations, and abiding by their professional ethical standards. In Canada, an interdisciplinary 40-hour training module for bariatric behavioral health care providers was developed by the Alberta Health Services, culminating in a knowledge-based exam that must be passed (Rouleau et al., 2014). Such efforts are important for promoting professional competence in this practice specialty.

Informed Consent

Surgical candidates, like all persons who receive health care services, have the right to make decisions about whether a proposed procedure is right for them. To make the right decision for themselves, the candidates must be informed of, and understand, the nature of the procedure, including anticipated benefits and risks; this is *informed consent*. Providing this information so that the candidate can make an informed decision is consistent with the principle of respect for patient autonomy. The informed consent process, which is best managed through a discussion and not just a form, ideally concludes with mutually understood goals between candidates and clinicians. Goals should be consistent with the candidates' values and be realistic. Thus, at the outset of the service, health care and mental health professionals must provide surgical candidates with the information needed to make an informed decision about a given procedure and then respect candidates' wishes regarding their decision. Informed consent is needed for the surgical procedure itself and for any tests or procedures that are presurgical requirements, including the PPA. Of course, in the context of elective surgeries, just because a person wants a procedure does not mean it is appropriate for them. The PPA helps shed light on that issue.

According to APA Ethics Code Standard 3.10, Informed Consent, before any psychological service being offered to a patient, the psychologist obtains "the informed consent of the individual or individuals using language that is reasonably understandable to that person or persons" (Standard 3.10[a]) "and appropriately [documents] written or oral consent" (Standard 3.10[d]). Further, Standard 9.03, Informed Consent in Assessments, outlines informed consent as it relates specifically to psychological assessment, including conditions under which the purpose of testing is to assess decisional capacity. Informed consent includes an explanation of the purpose and nature (what the process entails) of the assessment, anticipated benefits and risks, fees, involvement of third parties, and limits of confidentiality. Opportunity is provided for candidates to ask questions and receive answers.

Inherent in the surgical candidates' informed consent for surgery is their motivation for surgery and expectations postsurgery, an understanding of the surgical procedure, potential complications and risks, any alternative treatments, and any postsurgical lifestyle adjustments that can be expected. It is important to identify the candidate's specific needs and any concerns the referring surgeon may have indicated. Obtaining information regarding the patient's expectations about both the surgery and any postsurgical changes is important to determine both the realistic nature of the patient's perceived surgical results and to address any unrealistic expectations that could lead to a poor or unsatisfied outcome. Another area to address is whether the patient is self-motivated to have the surgery or is being pressured by someone else to do so. For example, patients seeking elective cosmetic surgery may feel pressured to change their appearance with the belief that it will improve their interpersonal relationships or lead to greater acceptance or popularity (APS, 2018). In addition, when presurgical "assessment serves a gatekeeping function, ethical dilemmas may arise if the assessment itself is perceived by patients as a form of coercion" (Rouleau et al., 2014, p. 6). The patient should be informed that they can refuse to participate in a PPA as well as what the consequences of that decision will be.

The psychologist/mental health professional's role needs to be clearly delineated as well as who the client is (i.e., surgical candidate or referring surgeon). It is also important to address any confusion on the part of the candidate regarding the role of the assessment results in determining surgical decision making. The provider should inform the candidate that the assessment findings will be used to provide recommendations to the medical team regarding surgery. Of course, an informed consent process needs to occur for the PPA as well as for the surgery.

Information from the medical team needs to be provided in a clear and understandable manner. In addition, it is important to provide patients the ability to obtain additional information or ask questions specific to their situation. The mental health provider should inform the medical team if the patient has not received relevant information or if it appears that the patient does not have a good understanding of the surgical process.

A candidate may not have an adequate understanding of information covered in the informed consent process because of cognitive limitations or emotional factors, including poor attention when the information was provided, declining cognitive abilities, intellectual disability, high levels of anxiety or depression, or psychotic symptoms. Having the candidate repeat back in their own words the information that was provided can help assure their understanding of the information.

Assessment Process

The *assessment process*, from beginning to end, is designed to provide information that benefits the surgical candidate, even if the conclusions are contrary to the candidate's wishes, while not harming the candidate. These goals are reflected in the underlying ethical principles of beneficence and nonmaleficence. The psychometric testing component of the assessment is performed, adheres to, and is guided by, the same principles. In addition, specific ethical standards of the APA Ethics Code provide direction for clinicians. Professional competence for psychologists involves obtaining specialized educational and clinical training in selecting, administering, and interpreting intellectual, academic, and psychological measures. In addition, psychologists should have a good understanding of the psychometric properties of the measures they chose (see Chapter 2, this volume), and correlate their test findings to the patient populations with which they have been trained.

For presurgical assessments to be most effective, the provider should strive for consistency in the process and base any surgical decisions on scientifically reliable data (Block & Sarwer, 2013). Such consistency and reliance on objective evidence serve to reduce the likelihood of endorsing surgery that ultimately may not be successful or beneficial.

Assessment of a patient's social support can be an important part of the assessment process. Research indicates that patients with poor social support are more likely to have a poor postsurgical outcome (Block & Sarwer, 2013). Social support is most pertinent when one of the considerations to a successful surgical outcome is patient compliance, particularly with surgical procedures such as bariatric surgery or organ transplantation that require a postoperative regimen (Block & Sarwer, 2013). Social support is also helpful in assisting the patient—before surgery—in developing and maintaining lifestyle changes that may improve postsurgical outcome.

When assessment of social support is included as a part of the presurgical assessment process, the candidate's primary support system or caregiver should be identified, and informed consent for their involvement in the process should be obtained. The caregiver should be asked about their commitment to the process, their availability for the patient, and their personal health and mental status. Particularly for transplant patients, the medical team may ask that primary caregivers attend the transplant evaluation before a candidate's transplant listing. If a caregiver is not available, other forms of social support should be identified, such as extended family or friends, support groups, a mental health professional, or even a postsurgical patient who could serve as a caregiver and mentor. Patients may experience emotional changes during the recovery process and will likely need time postsurgery to return to activities of daily living. Both the patient and the caregiver may benefit from formal or informal emotional support.

Selection and Use of Measures

Ethical practice involves selecting assessment measures that are appropriate for the patient population with which they are to be used. APA Ethics Code Standard 9.01(a), Bases for Assessments, requires psychologists to base their opinions "on information and techniques sufficient to substantiate their findings." Toward that end, psychologists strive to select assessment instruments that assess mental health in general and instruments that are designed for surgical procedures. Standard 9.02(b), Use of Assessments, states: "Psychologists use assessment instruments whose validity and reliability have been established for use with members of the population tested. When such validity or reliability has not been established, psychologists describe the strengths and limitations of test results and interpretation."

The most commonly used broadband measure of psychological functioning and psychopathology across clinical contexts is the Minnesota Multiphasic Personality Inventory (MMPI) family of tests, such as the MMPI-2 (Butcher et al., 1989), MMPI-2–Restructured Form (MMPI-2-RF; Ben-Porath, 2012), and MMPI-3 (Ben-Porath & Tellegen, 2020a, 2020b). In addition, surgery-specific questionnaires, such as the Transplant Evaluation Rating Scale (Twillman et al., 1993), have been developed. This scale classifies 10 aspects of psychosocial functioning thought to help with adjusting to transplantation. The Cleveland Clinic Behavioral Rating System (Heinberg et al., 2010) is used to rate constructs found to be related to surgical outcome, including adherence, coping, expectations, social support, and substance abuse.

Although it is understood that appropriate normative data should be used whenever possible, it can sometimes be challenging for the psychologist/mental health professional to determine which norms are most appropriate for a given surgical candidate. For example, traditional psychological assessment norms are based on cisgender females and males (i.e., those whose sense of personal identity and gender are consistent with their birth sex vs. transgender). Thus, when scoring test protocols, it typically is necessary to identify the gender of the patient being assessed, with scores obtained dependent on the gender chosen. However, for transgender surgical candidates, determining which gender norms to use may be unclear. Consensus from APA Division 44 (Webb et al., 2016) suggests that mental health providers should "consider the stage of transition" (para. 14) a patient is in and the effect of that stage on the results of the assessment. In addition, the consensus indicates that providers could use both male and female norms, or they could ask the patient for their preference. Ultimately, the gender norms used should support the psychological characteristics of the candidate being assessed (see Standard 9.01[b] of the APA Ethics Code).

Once assessment measures have been selected, they must be used appropriately. APA Ethics Code Standard 9.02(a), Use of Assessments, states, "Psychologists administer, adapt, score, interpret, or use assessment techniques, interviews, tests, or instruments in a manner and for purposes that are appropriate in light of the research on or evidence of the usefulness and proper application of the techniques." In a practice context in which development of specific assessment measures is still in its infancy, it may be tempting, and even necessary in some instances, to depart from standardized procedures for a given test and a specific surgical candidate to obtain the best understanding of the constructs of interest and provide appropriate recommendations. However, clinicians should (a) do so only when necessary, (b) appreciate the risks of such departure (e.g., normative data may no longer apply), (c) explain the rationale for doing so, and (d) explain any anticipated effect of such deviation from standardized procedures on the results and recommendations.

Interpretation

Evidence-based interpretation should flow from the information obtained in the data-gathering components of the assessment process. Standard 9.06, Interpreting Assessment Results, of the APA Ethics Code instructs psychologists to

> take into account the purpose of the assessment as well as the various test factors, test-taking abilities, and other characteristics of the person being assessed, such as situational, personal, linguistic, and cultural differences that might affect psychologists' judgments or reduce the accuracy of their interpretations. [Psychologists] indicate any significant limitations of their interpretations.

In addition, Standard 9.09, Test Scoring and Interpretation Services, states, "Psychologists select scoring and interpretation services (including automated services) on the basis of evidence of the validity of the program and procedures as well as on other appropriate considerations" (Standard 9.09[b]) and "retain responsibility for the appropriate application, interpretation, and use of assessment instruments, whether they score and interpret such tests themselves or use automated or other services" (Standard 9.09[c]).

Report

The conclusions and recommendations of the psychological assessment of surgical candidates are typically reported to the referral source and other treatment team members and to the candidate or their representative (see APA Ethics Code Standard 9.10, Explaining Assessment Results). The report is commonly provided in writing and verbally. The information is typically best received when it is clear, is concise, uses nontechnical language, and is provided in a timely manner.

The process of report writing and patient feedback should be performed in a manner that continues to respect the patient and provides only necessary information. In the course of psychological assessment, surgical candidates share personal and often sensitive information, some of which may not be relevant to the surgical team or the candidate's postsurgical outcome.

APA Ethics Code Standard 4.04, Minimizing Intrusions on Privacy, holds that "only information germane to the purpose for which the communication is made" should be included in the assessment, whether provided verbally or in a written report, and only with the medical staff involved directly with the patient's care. Any cultural, situational, linguistic, or personal differences that may affect the provider's judgment or reduce the accuracy of interpretation should be explained. The clinician encourages and addresses questions or concerns that arise in the reporting process.

DIVERSITY ISSUES

This section focuses on ethnoracial, ethnocultural, and gender identity issues in the psychological assessment of presurgical candidates. APA Ethics Code General Principle E: Respect for People's Rights and Dignity is at the heart of the clinician's investment in these issues.

Ethnoracial and Ethnocultural Diversity

Although people of color or others from marginalized ethnic groups sometimes experience prejudice and discrimination purely because of their ethnic affiliation, the added stigma of select medical conditions (e.g., being overweight) can add a layer of bias that results in some persons foregoing medical assistance, which may include medically necessary or elective surgical procedures. In an effort to address the disparity in care provided to people of color, the APA established a task force to develop guidelines to mitigate unfair practices in psychology based on race and ethnicity. Guideline 9 is particularly relevant to psychological assessment, stating, "Psychologists strive to provide assessment, intervention, and consultation free from the negative effects of racial and ethnocultural bias" (APA Task Force on Race and Ethnicity Guidelines in Psychology, 2019, p. 9).

There has been recent debate about the use of race-based normative data sets. The American Academy of Clinical Neuropsychology (AACN, 2021) explained that "demographically-adjusted norms that include race along with other variables such as age, education, and gender were created to aid diagnostic precision and characterization of functional abilities, by ensuring comparison of individual test performance to appropriate normative reference groups" (p. 2). However, as AACN further noted,

> There can be a mix of positive and negative consequences of the use of race stratified norms. In some situations, it will be more important to avoid a false

> positive diagnosis, whereas in other situations the greater harm may arise from a false negative diagnosis, both of which can arise from applying race-stratified normative standards. . . . A false positive diagnosis in a clinical setting may result in needless medical intervention, but a false negative diagnosis may prevent timely access to potentially curative treatments. (p. 4)

To reduce the risk of diagnostic error for any given surgical candidate, clinical judgment is needed in the selection of a norm reference group.

Conversely, a patient may seek surgery to change a physical feature that connects them to a particular cultural or ethnic background, and once altered may result in a loss of personal identity or connection to others (APS, 2018). This may occur through the loss of the "shared physical familial or cultural characteristic" (APS, 2018, p. 7). In addition, for those with premorbid mental health issues, specifically body dysmorphic disorder, some may experience an increase in distressful symptoms, including potentially an increased risk for self-harm and suicide, Conversely, patients with the most positive post-surgical outcomes typically have the strongest correlation between presurgical self-concept and postsurgical appearance.

Sexual Orientation and Gender Identity

The classification of homosexuality as a medical or mental health condition was not eliminated until 1992, when the World Health Organization (1992) omitted the diagnosis from its 10th revision of the *International Classification of Mental and Behavioural Disorders*. Yet a stigma persists for many lesbians, gay men, bisexuals, and transgender individuals; transgender individuals experience gender dysphoria and wish to align or transition to their true gender. Not only do patients with gender dysphoria experience harassment and discrimination from outsiders, they may also experience it from those close to them, including family members.

Standards of care for transgender individuals seeking to change their gender have been outlined by the World Professional Association for Transgender Health (Dickey et al., 2016; see also Chapter 6, this volume, on gender embodiment surgery). These standards include assessment(s) by an informed and competent provider for the purpose of diagnosing the patient with gender dysphoria; for initiation of cross-sex hormones; and for presurgical assessments for procedures, such as breast augmentation, mastectomy, gonadectomy/hysterectomy, and vaginoplasty/phalloplasty (Odunze, 2020). Presurgical assessment gathers vital information for the surgical team regarding the patient's readiness to undergo surgery, including the patient's mental health and their expectations and surgical goals (Ettner, 2018). In addition to these standards, given the historical mistreatment and ostracization of such groups, ethical issues of privacy and confidentiality (including who will have access to their personal and medical information), respect for autonomy, and respect for people's rights and dignity are crucial considerations for clinicians.

TELEHEALTH

As with the rest of the health care community (American Hospital Association, n.d.), psychology is increasingly embracing technology-based services, including remote administration of psychological tests. Glueckauf et al. (2018) found that between 2013 and 2016, 43% of psychologists surveyed delivered psychological services to patients using telepsychology modalities for at least a few hours per week, of which 25% used videoconference platforms. It is almost certain that those percentages have increased dramatically since the onset of the novel coronavirus (COVID-19) and the move, internationally, to technology-based communication.

Remote assessments offer advantages, particularly ease of access for people who, primarily as a result of disability or distance, otherwise would have difficulty presenting to a clinic. However, disadvantages exist as well, including departure from conditions under which the measures were standardized and limited control over the security of select measures. Of course, the further one gets from standardized procedures, the more questionable the accuracy of the results as a reflection of the constructs of interest. In addition, for many tests, correspondence between traditional administration and technology-based administration has not been established. Given these advantages and disadvantages, the desire to benefit the patient (beneficence) must be balanced with the commitment to avoid outcomes that are harmful (nonmaleficence).

Telepsychology is the provision of psychological services using a telecommunication platform, which can range from videoconferencing to telephone conversations, texting or emailing, or online psychoeducational materials (Joint Task Force for the Development of Telepsychology Guidelines for Psychologists, 2013). To be considered telepsychology, the assessment need not be completely technology based; technology can serve as a supplement to traditional in-person services and assessment methodology.

There are two primary models for remote psychological assessment. The *assistant-proctored model* involves the psychologist/mental health professional's providing both clinical interview and testing using videoconference from one facility while assisted by an assistant, technician, or other staff member at a satellite or remote clinic. The psychologist/mental health professional either directly administers the measures or instructs the patient or staff member to open previously prepared folders containing test forms that require completion by the patient. With this model, the environment is relatively well controlled, and, depending on the site and the availability of hospital staff, it is possible for staff to guide patients if complications arise. Obstacles with assistant-proctored psychological assessment include modifications to the types of patients assessed (those who can go to a clinic and use technology), the need for continuous connectivity, and vulnerability to future clinic shutdowns.

The second model is the *direct-to-home model* through which psychologists and mental health professionals provide both clinical interview and testing using videoconference directly to a patient in their home. This is the quintessential videoconference model for other services (e.g., psychotherapy). Like the assistant-proctored model, this model involves the psychologist/mental health professional's directly administering measures to the patient; however, with this model, no additional assistance can be provided by staff, and the assessment must be modified to reduce or eliminate the need for test forms that require completion by the patient. Accessibility is the primary advantage of this model, allowing surgical candidates who otherwise would not be able to undergo an assessment to receive the needed service. In contrast, multiple challenges exist, including (a) problems with internet connectivity or other technology-based issues, (b) issues with information security (privacy and confidentiality), (c) emergency management, (d) alterations to service delivery, (e) potential threats to validity, and (f) the inability to assess a wide range of patient severity (International Test Commission, 2005; Joint Task Force for the Development of Telepsychology Guidelines for Psychologists, 2013).

The inability to control the assessment environment is a significant problem because of possible distractions and the potential for the patient's responses to be influenced by others or cues (e.g., phone). In addition, copyright laws frequently restrict the scanning or photocopying of test stimuli, which are needed for screen-sharing purposes, and mailing test materials to patients poses similar threats to test security (see APA Ethics Code Standard 9.11, Maintaining Test Security). As with selection of traditional assessment methods, having considered the various advantages and disadvantages, the clinician is responsible for choosing those procedures and measures that are most appropriate for a given patient (see APA Ethics Code Standard 9.01[b], Bases for Assessment). When indicated, involving the patient in the process of determining the manner of assessment is consistent with the principle of respect for patient autonomy.

PPA OF ONE'S OWN PATIENTS

Sometimes clinicians are asked to determine the psychological appropriateness of their own patients for a surgical procedure. Caution is warranted in such situations. The possibility of a dual or multiple relationship (see APA Ethics Code Standard 3.05, Multiple Relationships) emerges for a clinician who serves as both therapist and assessor and may create a conflict of interest that could be potentially harmful to the patient.

Standard 3.05(a), Multiple Relationships, states that a provider refrains from holding multiple relationships with a patient if doing so may impair the provider's "objectivity, competence, or effectiveness in performing his or her functions as a psychologist." For example, one concern would be that following a number of therapy sessions, the provider may develop a bias toward ensuring that the patient be approved for the surgical procedure.

ETHICAL DECISION-MAKING PROCESS

Ethical decision making is the process psychologists and mental health professionals use to establish ethical practices and address ethical challenges. Given the complexity of ethical dilemmas, a systematic process (i.e., a structured model) can facilitate sound decision making. Bush et al. (2017) presented such a model with a seven-letter mnemonic that may facilitate its retention and recall. The mnemonic CORE OPT can help psychologists and mental health professionals understand the ethical issues and possible solutions and select a correct option. The model consists of the following steps:

1. **C**larify the ethical issue, distinguishing it from clinical, legal, or other professional issues.
2. Identify the **o**bligations owed the relevant stakeholders.
3. Identify and review or consult ethical, legal, and professional **r**esources.
4. **E**xamine one's own personal beliefs and values as well as the potential effect of each on the decision-making process.
5. Consider the possible **o**ptions, including solutions and their consequences.
6. **P**ut the plan into practice.
7. **T**ake stock, evaluate the outcome, and revise as needed.

A key feature of the model is its reliance on multiple resources. Such resources include (a) general bioethical principles; (b) ethics codes of professional organizations; (c) practice guidelines and position statements of professional organizations; (d) scholarly publications, such as books, articles, and chapters; (e) jurisdictional laws; (f) professional liability insurance carriers; (g) institutional guidelines and resources; (h) ethics committees of professional organizations; and (i) experienced and knowledgeable colleagues. Although the recommendations or requirements detailed in the various publications do not always coincide, they illustrate the essential issues, and the decision-making model can help the clinician determine how to address the challenge.

LEGAL CONSIDERATIONS

Considerable moral consistency exists between professional ethical guidelines and the law because both were developed based on the shared values of a society to protect individuals within the society. Both support the concepts of confidentiality, privacy, and duty to inform (or informed consent) as well as require the patient to have the capacity to participate in a process, whether it be a psychological assessment or a legal proceeding. However, there are instances during which ethical standards and the law do not coincide. For example, if a clinician's employer requests that they send copyrighted materials to the patient for the purpose of a remote psychological assessment—an act that may violate copyright law and threaten the security of the materials—the clinician should clarify the nature of the conflict, make known their commitment to copyright law and professional ethics, and take reasonable steps to resolve the conflict in a manner that comports to APA Ethics Code Standards 1.02, Conflicts Between Ethics and Law, Regulations, or other Governing Legal Authority; and 1.03, Conflicts Between Ethics and Organizational Demands. There are instances, however, when, even after discussion, no reasonable solution is viable to satisfy the legal requirements. At that point, there could be legal consequences if the clinician did not follow the law.

CONCLUSION

Ethical issues serve as the foundation for effective psychological assessment of surgical candidates. Competence to provide services that benefit—without harming—candidates facilitates sound decision making about appropriateness for surgery. Respecting the candidates' autonomy includes providing them with the information needed to make informed decisions about both the surgical procedure and the psychological assessment.

A systematic ethical decision-making model can help clinicians arrive at good choices when making complex decisions. Psychologists and mental health professionals who attend to the ethical components of each step of the assessment process are well positioned to provide important contributions to the treatment team and the care of the patient.

REFERENCES

American Academy of Clinical Neuropsychology. (2021). *Position statement on use of race as a factor in neuropsychological test norming and performance prediction.* https://theaacn.org/wp-content/uploads/2021/11/AACN-Position-Statement-on-Race-Norms.pdf

American Hospital Association. (n.d.). *Telehealth.* https://www.AHA.org/telehealth

American Psychological Association. (2017). *Ethical principles of psychologists and code of conduct* (2002, amended effective June 1, 2010, and January 1, 2017). https://www.apa.org/ethics/code/

APA Task Force on Race and Ethnicity Guidelines in Psychology. (2019, August). *APA guidelines on race and ethnicity in psychology: Promoting responsiveness and equity.* American Psychological Association. https://www.apa.org/about/policy/guidelines-race-ethnicity.pdf

Australian Psychological Society. (2018). *Psychological evaluation of patients undergoing cosmetic procedures: Practice guide.* https://psychology.org.au/getmedia/5016efba-cb58-4cd5-a472-4313a1a70483/18aps-pp-cosmetic-surgery-p1a-web.pdf

Ben-Porath, Y. S. (2012). *Interpreting the MMPI-2-RF.* University of Minnesota Press.

Ben-Porath, Y. S., & Tellegen, A. (2020a). *The Minnesota Multiphasic Personality Inventory–3: Manual for administration, scoring, and interpretation.* University of Minnesota Press.

Ben-Porath, Y. S., & Tellegen, A. (2020b). *The Minnesota Multiphasic Personality Inventory–3: Technical manual.* University of Minnesota Press.

Block, A. R., & Marek, R. J. (2020). Presurgical psychological evaluation: Risk factor identification and mitigation. *Journal of Clinical Psychology in Medical Settings, 27*(2), 396–405. https://doi.org/10.1007/s10880-019-09660-0

Block, A. R., & Sarwer, D. B. (Eds.). (2013). *Presurgical psychological screening: Understanding patients, improving outcomes.* American Psychological Association. https://doi.org/10.1037/14035-000

Bush, S. S., Allen, R. S., & Molinari, V. A. (2017). *Ethical practice in geropsychology.* American Psychological Association. https://doi.org/10.1037/0000010-000

Butcher, J. N., Dahlstrom, W. G., Graham, J. R., Tellegen, A., & Kaemmer, B. (1989). *Manual for the restandardized Minnesota Multiphasic Personality Inventory: MMPI-2. An administrative and interpretive guide.* University of Minnesota Press.

Dickey, L. M., Karasic, D. H., & Sharon, N. G. (2016, May 28). *Mental health considerations with transgender and gender nonconforming clients.* University of California San Francisco Transgender Care & Treatment Guidelines. https://transcare.ucsf.edu/guidelines/mental-health

Ettner, R. (2018). Mental health evaluation for gender confirmation surgery. *Clinics in Plastic Surgery, 45*(3), 307–311. https://doi.org/10.1016/j.cps.2018.03.002

Farlex. (n.d.). Professional competence. In *The free dictionary: Medical dictionary.* Retrieved June 7, 2021, from https://medical-dictionary.thefreedictionary.com/professional+competence

Fouad, N. A., & Grus, C. G. (2014). Competency-based education and training in professional psychology. In W. B. Johnson & N. J. Kaslow (Eds.), *Oxford handbook of education and training in professional psychology* (pp. 105–119). Oxford University Press.

Glueckauf, R. L., Maheu, M. M., Drude, K. P., Wells, B. A., Wang, Y. X., Gustafson, D. J., & Nelson, E. L. (2018). Survey of psychologists' telebehavioral health practices: Technology use, ethical issues, and training needs. *Professional Psychology: Research and Practice*, *49*(3), 205–219. https://doi.org/10.1037/pro0000188

Health Service Psychology Education Collaborative. (2013). Professional psychology in health care services: A blueprint for education and training. *American Psychologist*, *68*(6), 411–426. https://doi.org/10.1037/a0033265

Heinberg, L. J., Ashton, K., & Windover, A. (2010). Moving beyond dichotomous psychological evaluation: The Cleveland Clinic Behavioral Rating System for weight loss surgery. *Surgery for Obesity and Related Diseases*, *6*(2), 185–190. https://doi.org/10.1016/j.soard.2009.10.004

International Test Commission. (2005). *International guidelines on computer-based and internet delivered testing*. https://www.intestcom.org/files/guideline_computer_based_testing.pdf

Joint Task Force for the Development of Telepsychology Guidelines for Psychologists. (2013). Guidelines for the practice of telepsychology. *American Psychologist*, *68*(9), 791–800. https://doi.org/10.1037/a0035001

Odunze, M. (2020). Preparation and procedures involved in gender affirmation surgeries. *Verywell Health*. https://www.verywellhealth.com/gender-affirmation-surgery-2710288

Rodolfa, E., Bent, R., Eisman, E., Nelson, P., Rehm, L., & Ritchie, P. (2005). A cube model for competency development: Implications for psychology educators and regulators. *Professional Psychology: Research and Practice*, *36*(4), 347–354. https://doi.org/10.1037/0735-7028.36.4.347

Rouleau, C. R., Rash, J. A., & Mothersill, K. J. (2014). Ethical issues in the psychosocial assessment of bariatric surgery candidates. *Journal of Health Psychology*. Advance online publication. https://doi.org/10.1177/1359105314556160

Twillman, R. K., Manetto, C., Wellisch, D. K., & Wolcott, D. L. (1993). The Transplant Evaluation Rating Scale. A revision of the psychosocial levels system for evaluating organ transplant candidates. *Psychosomatics*, *34*(2), 144–153. https://doi.org/10.1016/S0033-3182(93)71905-2

Webb, A., Heyne, G., Holmes, J. E., & Peta, J. L. (2016, April). Which box to check: Assessment norms for gender and implications for transgender, nonbinary populations. *Division 44 Newsletter*. https://www.apadivisions.org/division-44/publications/newsletters/division/2016/04/nonbinary-populations

World Health Organization. (1992). *The ICD-10 classification of mental and behavioural disorders: Clinical descriptions and diagnostic guidelines* (10th revision). https://apps.who.int/iris/bitstream/handle/10665/37958/9241544228_eng.pdf?sequence=8&isAllowed=y

4 METABOLIC AND BARIATRIC SURGERY

ALLYSON DIGGINS AND NINOSKA PETERSON

Almost 40% of U.S. adults meet the criteria for the disease of obesity (body mass index [BMI] ≥ 30 kg/m^2; Hales et al., 2018). Further, 5.6% of men and 9.7% of women have severe obesity (BMI ≥ 40 kg/m^2). In the last 20 years, the prevalence of severe obesity has increased more than 600% (Sturm & Hattori, 2013) and is associated with a rise in mortality and morbidity (e.g., Type 2 diabetes, certain cancers, obstructive sleep apnea, heart disease, stroke; Nguyen et al., 2014). Current criteria for metabolic and bariatric surgery (MBS) include Class II obesity (BMI = 30–39.9 kg/m^2) and two associated medical problems (e.g., hypertension and Type 2 diabetes) or Class III obesity (BMI ≥ 40 kg/m^2). The American Society for Metabolic and Bariatric Surgery (ASMBS) and the International Federation for the Surgery of Obesity and Metabolic Disorders (IFSO) are updating the "Statement of Indications for Metabolic and Bariatric Surgery" based on data from patients with lower BMI, Asian populations, adolescents, and long-term safety and efficacy outcomes over the past 30 years.

Metabolic and bariatric surgery is regarded as the most effective, efficient, and durable treatment for severe obesity. Recent estimates indicate that over

https://doi.org/10.1037/0000346-005
Psychological Assessment of Surgical Candidates: Evidence-Based Procedures and Practices, R. J. Marek and A. R. Block (Editors)

200,000 individuals undergo primary bariatric surgical procedures each year in the United States, with 61% undergoing sleeve gastrectomy (SG) and 17% undergoing Roux-en-Y gastric bypass (RYGB; Arterburn et al., 2020). Despite increases in acceptability, MBS continues to be underutilized, with only one in 100 Americans who meet the BMI criteria undergoing surgery (Gasoyan et al., 2019). Further, although Black and Hispanic Americans are disproportionately affected by severe obesity, they represent only 25% of individuals who undergo MBS annually (Gasoyan et al., 2019).

The mechanisms of action behind weight loss and metabolic changes from MBS are still being investigated. The surgeries described in this chapter are typically performed laparoscopically using five to six incisions. For the SG, 75% to 80% of the stomach is vertically cut, stapled, and removed, leaving behind a "sleeve" the shape and size of a banana; the portion of the stomach that is removed produces most of the hormone ghrelin, which has an effect of decreasing hunger cues. The smaller sleeve restricts the amount of food that can be eaten, thereby enhancing satiety. SG is nonreversible (ASMBS, 2021).

Although SG is currently the most common procedure, RYGB has been performed for more than 50 years (ASMBS, 2021). The typical surgical approach to RYGB involves two parts: (a) An egg-sized gastric pouch is created from the top of the stomach using a stapling device, which restricts the amount of food that can be eaten, and the larger part of the stomach is stapled shut and bypassed (i.e., it does not store or digest food); and (b) the small intestine is divided into two sections. The lower portion of the small intestine is attached to the new gastric pouch, allowing food to pass directly into the lower portion of the jejunum. The other end of the small intestine is reconnected further down to the lower end of the intestine (e.g., Roux limb), creating the "Y" shape described in the surgery's name. This "rerouting" of the intestines allows the stomach acids and digestive enzymes from the bypassed stomach to mix with food in the lower intestine, leading to malabsorption of calories and nutrients. The length of the upper and lower segments of the intestine can be increased to produce differing levels of malabsorption (ASMBS, 2021).

While RYGB and SG are increasing in procedural prevalence, rates of performing the laparoscopic adjustable gastric band (LAP band) have declined recently due to the likelihood of long-term complications and limited efficacy (Michalsky, 2021). Furthermore, there has been an increase in alternative procedures, including endoscopic procedures, such as intragastric balloon and endoscopic gastroplasty, that are considered safer and more cost-effective than traditional surgical therapies (Štimac & Majanović, 2012). More research is needed to determine the efficacy and durability of these procedures (Choi & Chun, 2017). Strong evidence from randomized controlled trials and observational studies shows that MBS results in greater long-term weight loss (20%–35% of total body weight) and improvements in comorbidities than nonsurgical interventions (Adams et al., 2017; Arterburn et al., 2020; Courcoulas et al., 2013, 2018). However, a significant subset of patients (~25%) do not achieve expected weight loss outcomes, and approximately 20% regain the majority of weight lost (Courcoulas et al., 2013). Postoperative weight regain has been attributed to physiological and behavioral factors (Sarwer et al., 2008, 2011) and often results in a lack of improvement or a recurrence of obesity-related comorbidities (Karmali et al., 2013).

Multidisciplinary assessment is standard, evidence-based practice for presurgical preparation to assess whether patients meet criteria for surgery, obtain informed consent, and address concerns that may interfere with optimal outcomes (Sarwer & Heinberg, 2020). Because psychosocial factors may influence long-term outcomes, mental health professionals (psychologists, psychiatrists, social workers, psychiatric nurses) were initially recommended to provide psychosocial assessments for MBS in the 1991 National Institutes of Health Consensus Development Conference statement and now have a central role in evaluating and caring for patients both before and after surgery (Peterson, 2018; Sogg et al., 2016). The clinical practice guidelines (CPG) are cosponsored by several professional societies and have been updated over the years; the most recent update is the 2019 CPG, and each update has provided revised management recommendations for perioperative nutritional, metabolic, and nonsurgical support of the patient seeking MBS (Mechanick et al., 2013, 2020).

PREVALENCE OF PSYCHOPATHOLOGY AMONG PATIENTS SEEKING METABOLIC AND BARIATRIC SURGERY

There is an overrepresentation of psychopathology among patients presenting for MBS, likely as a function of complicated biological and psychosocial factors (Kanji et al., 2019; Parikh et al., 2016). Lifetime rates of psychiatric diagnoses among patients presenting for MBS range from 36.8% to 72.6%, while current diagnoses are reported in 20.9% to 55.5% of candidates (Sarwer & Heinberg, 2020). Among the general population, 20.6% of adults report a current psychiatric diagnosis, thus highlighting the increased prevalence of psychopathology in bariatric populations (Substance Abuse and Mental Health Services Administration, 2020). Of these, the most diagnosed mental health concerns are depression and eating disorders. Other mental health conditions, such as anxiety, psychosis, posttraumatic stress disorder (PTSD), and personality disorders, are also prevalent (Dawes et al., 2016). Nearly 40%

of MBS candidates report current mental health treatment, and up to 50% report a history of mental health treatment, a rate higher than in the general population (Clark et al., 2003; Sarwer & Heinberg, 2020; Sarwer et al., 2004). Identifying mental health disorders has been noted to improve the quality of perioperative management and assists in predicting outcomes after MBS (Yen et al., 2014).

Mood Disorders

Mood disorders are common psychiatric comorbidities in MBS candidates, with up to 31.5% of individuals reporting a mood disorder (Sarwer & Heinberg, 2020). Antidepressants are the most frequently prescribed psychotropic medications in this population and are frequently continued postoperatively (Cunningham et al., 2012; McAlpine, 2006; Segal et al., 2009). Bariatric surgical patients often attribute depressive symptoms to concerns related to health-related quality of life, body image, weight bias, and discrimination (Sarwer & Heinberg, 2020). The presence of a mood disorder has been associated with less postoperative weight loss, albeit inconsistently (Dawes et al., 2016; de Zwaan et al., 2011; Marek et al., 2017; Müller et al., 2019). The literature has provided support for short-term improvements in mood symptoms following the first 24 months after MBS; however, depressive symptoms tend to rise after the first 2 years yet continue to be lower compared with baseline (Dawes et al., 2016; Gill et al., 2019). It is plausible that the increase in depressive symptoms long-term can be attributed in part to weight loss plateaus, weight regain, body dissatisfaction due to excess skin, and unrealistic expectations regarding the role of MBS in changing aspects of patients' lives (Alyahya & Alnujaidi, 2022).

Eating Disorders

A substantial percentage of bariatric surgical candidates report unhealthy and problematic eating behaviors, including binge eating disorder (BED), loss of control (LOC) eating, night eating syndrome (NES), and graze eating (Mitchell et al., 2015). NES is characterized by disproportionate consumption of calories at night and/or waking up from sleep to consciously eat, morning anorexia (i.e., lack of appetite in the morning), and insomnia (Allison et al., 2006). Graze eating is a construct without official recognition or criteria as a disorder in the fifth edition of the *Diagnostic and Statistical Manual of Mental Disorders* (*DSM-5*; American Psychiatric Association, 2013) and is defined as repetitive, unplanned eating of small amounts of food throughout the day (Conceição, Mitchell, Engel, et al., 2014).

Estimates suggest that up to 50% of individuals presenting for MBS evidence eating-disordered behaviors (Malik et al., 2014). BED is seen in 5% to 15% of patients and is the most common eating disorder diagnosis (Mitchell et al., 2012). LOC while eating, described as a subjective sense of loss of control while eating without reference to a specific amount of food, has been regarded as the most common form of disordered eating behavior (Sarwer & Heinberg, 2020). Approximately 33% of MBS candidates endorse graze eating, and 32% experience LOC (Goodpaster et al., 2016). Further, night eating is seen in 8% to 42% of patients seeking MBS (Allison et al., 2006; Goodpaster et al., 2016). All these maladaptive eating patterns likely contribute to and maintain severe obesity.

Anxiety Disorders

Up to 24% of bariatric surgical candidates are diagnosed with an anxiety disorder (Kalarchian et al., 2007). According to data from the Longitudinal Assessment of Bariatric Surgery (LABS) study and *DSM-IV* criteria, specific phobia, social anxiety, and PTSD are prevalent anxiety disorder diagnoses among bariatric surgical candidates (Kalarchian et al., 2016). A lifetime diagnosis of an anxiety disorder is negatively related to postoperative weight loss (de Zwaan et al., 2011). Interestingly, the point prevalence of anxiety disorders does not decrease after surgery. Moreover, untreated social anxiety may influence adherence to guidelines for physical activity, support group participation, and romantic and interpersonal relationships postoperatively (Sarwer et al., 2012).

Research on PTSD (classified in the *DSM-5* as a trauma- and stressor-related disorder; American Psychiatric Association, 2013) and bariatric surgery is relatively limited because it is often underrecognized or underreported during presurgical assessments. However, Walsh and colleagues (2017) found that among bariatric candidates with a history of abuse, individuals with a lifetime history of PTSD evidenced greater impairment. Further, there is a growing literature base evaluating trauma and adverse childhood experiences and bariatric surgery outcomes. For instance, research in this area has indicated that a high number of adverse childhood experiences negatively influences outcomes after bariatric surgery (e.g., postoperative BMI, total cholesterol, and LDL cholesterol; Lodhia et al., 2015).

Substance Use Disorders

Substance use (drugs and alcohol) occurs along a continuum, and not all persons who use substances abuse them. Before *DSM-5*, abuse and dependence were defined as two separate disorders; these are now combined into a single diagnosis of substance use disorder that includes use to fulfill a craving, compulsive, or difficult to control, despite harmful consequences (American Psychiatric Association, 2013). Preoperative substance use is common and reported by up to 60% of patients seeking MBS (Conason et al., 2013; Li & Wu, 2016). Specifically, up to 40% of patients report current tobacco use (Chow et al., 2021), while 6.2% to 8.3% report current marijuana use (Bauer et al., 2018; Shockcor et al., 2021). Approximately 8% of bariatric patients report chronic opioid use in the year before MBS (Raebel et al., 2013). Further, the majority of patients report alcohol consumption, with estimates from one study finding that 7.1% of patients meet criteria for alcohol abuse or dependence (Ertelt et al., 2008). Current substance misuse is seen in less than 2% of candidates for MBS and is less than population-based incidence rates (Kalarchian et al., 2007). Historical substance use disorders are seen in approximately 10% of presurgical candidates and are higher than population norms (King et al., 2012; Mitchell et al., 2012).

A history of substance abuse has been associated with greater postoperative weight loss (Clark et al., 2003; Heinberg et al., 2012); however, substance use and misuse before surgery may result in increased substance use postoperatively and an increased risk of new-onset substance use disorders (Heinberg et al., 2012; Kanji et al., 2019; Spadola et al., 2015). The prevalence of postoperative alcohol use among bariatric patients ranges from 7.6% to 11.8%, with up to 20% of patients reporting alcohol misuse after surgery (Ivezaj et al., 2019; King et al., 2017; Li & Wu, 2016). Moreover, Vidot and colleagues (2016) found that among those who endorsed cannabis use, 67.9% reported use within the past year, and 32.1% reported use within the last month. Furthermore, out of bariatric patients with no previous history of substance use problems, new-onset substance users range from 34.3% to 89.5% (Li & Wu, 2016). Overall, substance use is prevalent within this population, and active substance abuse is one of the most widely accepted contraindications for MBS and should be routinely assessed (Mechanick et al., 2020).

Cognitive Functioning

Cognitive dysfunction in areas such as memory and executive function is prevalent among MBS candidates (Alosco et al., 2014; Galioto et al., 2015; L. A. Miller et al., 2013; Spitznagel et al., 2015). Specifically, 25% of bariatric surgery candidates exhibit clinically meaningful levels of cognitive impairment preoperatively (> 1.5 SD below average), and up to 40%

evidence subtle impairments (> 1 SD below average) on neuropsychological testing (Gunstad et al., 2010). Taken together, it is evident that bariatric patients present with myriad psychosocial concerns that may impact outcomes; therefore, the presurgical assessment is essential.

THE PRESURGICAL ASSESSMENT

One of the main differences between a psychological assessment for MBS versus a general psychological assessment is that the former involves evaluating several domains specific to surgery and life after, including the patient's knowledge, motivation, and expectations as part of the informed consent (Bauchowitz et al., 2007; Heinberg, Ashton, & Windover, 2010; Sogg & Mori, 2004; Sogg et al., 2016). This collective information guides the clinician in assessing and increasing a patient's readiness for surgery during the preoperative process. The psychologist/mental health professional conducting the assessment should also have specialized and relevant knowledge, training, and experiences working with surgical and nonsurgical treatment of obesity (Sogg et al., 2016) and be available to provide postoperative care (Greenberg et al., 2009; Peterson, 2018).

Knowledge, Motivation, and Expectations

The patient should be able to demonstrate an understanding of the surgical procedures, risks, and benefits (Bauchowitz et al., 2007; Heinberg, Ashton, & Windover, 2010; Sogg et al., 2016). Brief education about the differences between surgical procedures can be provided during the initial assessment with pictures or videos, and the "teach-back method" of education can be used to reinforce understanding. Because long-term success is highly dependent on the patient's ability to adhere to postoperative lifestyle changes, the patient should also be able to discuss the basics of the diet, exercise recommendations, and vitamin regimen (Bauchowitz et al., 2007; Sogg et al., 2016). Gaps in a patient's nutritional knowledge can also be communicated to the dietitians and nurses so that the multidisciplinary team can collaborate in increasing the patient's readiness.

Expectations and motivation vary among patients, and these factors have not consistently been linked to postoperative outcomes (Bauchowitz et al., 2007; Sogg et al., 2016). As noted earlier, the average weight loss for SG and RYGB is 20% to 35% of total body weight (Arterburn et al., 2020); however, patients tend to expect weight losses that far exceed averages

(Heinberg, Keating, & Simonelli, 2010; Kaly et al., 2008). Patients primarily cite health concerns as their main motivation for MBS, but they may also share unrealistic expectations about the magnitude of weight loss and the impact this may have on their lives (e.g., being pain free or no longer experiencing depression; Peterson, 2018; Sogg & Mori, 2004). A discussion of expectations also provides a space for highlighting broad measures of success that include the reduction or resolution of obesity-related comorbidities, improvements in quality of life, and long-term maintenance of any resulting improved health status (Ames et al., 2009). Finally, exploring the impact of obesity on the patient's life offers greater insight into aspects of distress and disruption to functioning that a patient may be experiencing, in addition to building rapport and increasing empathic communication skills (Sogg & Mori, 2004). Patients with fair-to-poor knowledge and/or unrealistic expectations may benefit from additional individual or group intervention before proceeding to surgery.

Weight, Diet History, and Current Eating Patterns

A comprehensive assessment of the patient's weight trajectory and history of weight loss attempts is standard practice because it provides insight into the complexity of factors that contribute to the onset and maintenance of obesity (Sogg et al., 2016). Weight trajectory should include age of obesity onset, lowest and highest adult weight, and specific episodes and triggers for weight gain over the years (e.g., pregnancy, medication side effects, smoking cessation, injuries, sedentary jobs, night-shift work, or major life stressors). Kushner and Ryan (2014) recommended patients complete a "Lifestyle-Events-Body Weight Graph" before their medical appointments that show patterns of weight gain with associated life events; this information can be used in the psychological assessment to guide the conversation between patient and provider.

A history of weight loss attempts should include the method of weight loss attempted (e.g., commercial programs, diet pills, prescription medications), duration of adherence, and amount of weight lost and maintained. Patients may also provide reasons for the success or barriers related to each of these attempts, which may be useful for treatment planning. It is also important to assess for maladaptive weight loss attempts such as vomiting, use of laxatives or diuretics, starvation, and excessive exercise. Additional information should be gathered on when these maladaptive weight loss attempts occurred, how long these behaviors lasted, and if they ended due to professional treatment (Peterson, 2018).

The psychological assessment should also include a discussion of current eating patterns, exercise, and other health habits. Current eating patterns can provide insight into the timing of eating (e.g., skipped meals or excessive snacking), diet quality, portions, frequency of eating out (e.g., restaurants and/or fast food), consumption of sugar-sweetened and carbonated beverages, and caffeine intake (Peterson, 2018). Assessment of exercise patterns (i.e., frequency, intensity, time, type, and barriers) and other health habits (e.g., vitamin regimen, medication regimen, blood glucose monitoring, and sleep apnea treatments) is also common. Like weight loss attempts, this information provides a comprehensive understanding of the patient's successes and barriers to adherence and can be used as additional targets for behavior modification (Sogg et al., 2016).

Eating Disorder Assessment

Eating disorders and subclinical disordered eating should also be assessed using *DSM-5* criteria in a clinical interview, along with associated questionnaires; using diagnostic criteria will ensure objective assessment of symptoms, frequency, and distress. Individual or group treatment that facilitates learning and practicing behavioral, cognitive, and emotion-regulating skills may benefit patients before surgery. Patients should also be informed that MBS itself is not a treatment for eating disorders (Ames et al., 2009).

The most common eating disorders screened for in patients seeking MBS are BED, bulimia nervosa (BN), other specified feeding or eating disorders such as NES, and unspecified feeding or eating disorders such as graze eating, LOC while eating, or emotional eating. A diagnosis of anorexia nervosa (AN) is contradictory to a diagnosis of obesity, but a history of AN should be assessed nevertheless. Although rare, patients who currently meet criteria for BN should not move forward to surgery without treatment due to the increased risk for health complications (e.g., malnutrition, dehydration, electrolyte imbalances, esophageal or gastric erosion, gastroesophageal reflux disease, development of Barrett's esophagus, pancreatitis, dyspnea, cardiac issues, myopathy, and seizures; Sekuła et al., 2019).

Binge eating disorder, characterized by consumption of amounts of food that are larger than most people would eat in a similar time frame accompanied by LOC once a week for at least 3 months, is not a contraindication to having MBS; however, untreated symptoms (in particular, LOC) may lead to attenuated weight loss (Chao et al., 2016). While it may be difficult to eat large portions of food following MBS, patients may still report uncontrolled eating behaviors.

The association between NES and weight is inconsistent (Allison et al., 2006). Treatment of NES tends to address eating patterns, insomnia symptoms, depression, and beliefs about eating that are related to sleep.

Graze eating is also referred to as nibbling, picking, or unplanned snacking (Conceição, Mitchell, Engel, et al., 2014). This disordered eating pattern can occur with or without LOC and can be assessed during the clinical interview and/or with objective screening measures. Picking and nibbling behaviors appear to be the most frequently reported maladaptive eating behavior after MBS (Conceição, Mitchell, Vaz, et al., 2014). These maladaptive eating behaviors, in general, have been found to lead to suboptimal weight loss and ultimately can lead to weight regain (Ames et al., 2009; Conceição, Mitchell, Vaz, et al., 2014). Patients should be informed about the postoperative occurrence and consequences of graze eating, and LOC should be addressed as soon as possible.

Mental Health History

The assessment should also document a brief psychiatric history and mental status exam (Sogg & Mori, 2004). This section includes screening for past and present symptoms of depression, mania or bipolar disorder, psychosis, anxiety, panic disorder, obsessive-compulsive disorder, and trauma or other stress-related disorders. In addition to symptoms, distress and disruption to functioning should be documented. Untreated severe psychiatric illness is a potential contraindication according to consensus guidelines (Mechanick et al., 2013).

Past and current mental health treatment with counseling and psychotropic medications should be assessed with details of time frames (e.g., first and most recent treatment), intermittent versus continuous treatment, and response to treatment. For psychotropic medication management, it can be helpful to ask about what medications and doses were prescribed, who prescribed them, duration of use, response, and side effects. Patients should be educated about the risks of possible changes in medication effectiveness after RYGB due to altered absorption and should be encouraged to speak to their prescribers about postoperative medication management and the need for close follow-up. Collateral information should be requested from mental health treatment providers to confirm the patient's stability, response, and adherence to treatment (Peterson, 2018; Sogg et al., 2016).

Past and recent suicidal and homicidal ideation, plan, intent, and attempts, in addition to self-injurious behavior and psychiatric hospitalizations, should be assessed. Further details about dates of treatment, reasons for admission, duration, and discharge recommendations may also be documented (Peterson, 2018). Patients undergoing MBS are four times more likely to commit suicide compared with peers in the general population (Wagner et al., 2013). Patients with a diagnosis of self-harm in the 2 years preceding surgery are at an increased risk for self-harm or hospitalization for depression in the first 2 years after surgery (Lagerros et al., 2017). Concerns are higher for patients with a history of multiple or recent psychiatric hospitalizations (Sogg et al., 2016). While there is no current consensus regarding a period of stability, many programs require 1 year with no suicidal gestures, attempts, or treatment before proceeding with MBS (Sogg et al., 2016).

Substance Use History

Using a clinical interview and objective questionnaires, a thorough assessment of past and current alcohol, nicotine, and recreational drug use is warranted in patients seeking MBS. Assessment should include types of substances used, frequency, duration, and treatment history. Toxicology screening can be ordered to verify the cessation of substances. Alcohol dependence, illicit drug use, and prescription drug abuse are contraindications for surgery (Mechanick et al., 2013), and these patients should be referred to an alcohol or drug treatment program before returning for MBS consultations.

For alcohol, frequency of drinking, amounts and types of drinks consumed, and frequency of binge drinking (five plus alcoholic drinks per sitting) are important measures (Heinberg et al., 2012). Consistent evidence suggests an elevated risk of developing an alcohol use disorder (AUD) following MBS (Ivezaj et al., 2019). Data suggest that both RYGB and SG, but not LAP band, dramatically affect alcohol pharmacokinetics (Ivezaj et al., 2019; White et al., 2019). After metabolic and bariatric surgery, alcohol appears to peak at higher levels, reach the peak more quickly, and take longer to return to a sober state (Maluenda et al., 2010; Woodard et al., 2011). LABS data found that the prevalence of an AUD did not differ significantly from the year before surgery to the first year after bariatric surgery (7.6% vs. 7.3%) but was significantly higher in the second postoperative year (9.6%; King et al., 2012). Risk factors for postoperative AUD included male sex, younger age, smoking history, regular alcohol consumption (two plus drinks per week), history of AUD, recreational drug use, low support, and post-RYGB status (King et al., 2012, 2017; Svensson et al., 2013). Due to the overwhelming evidence of metabolic changes and effects of alcohol after MBS, all patients should be educated about the risks of alcohol use verbally and in writing, and patients should practice reducing alcohol use before surgery.

Nicotine use (frequency, duration, amounts, and quit attempts) with cigarettes, cigars, vapor, e-cigarettes, chew, snuff, and hookah should be assessed. Updated 2020 clinical guidelines (Mechanick et al., 2020) recommend avoiding tobacco by all patients before and after MBS. Before surgery, "patients who smoke should stop as soon as possible, preferably 1 year but at the very least 6 weeks before bariatric procedures" (Mechanick et al., 2020, pp. 186). Education about avoiding nicotine after surgery should be provided verbally and in writing because of the increased risk of anastomotic ulcer, poor wound healing, and overall impaired health. Further referral to a structured tobacco cessation program should be provided as needed.

Similarly, cannabis use should be assessed during the clinical interview, with attention to frequency, estimated dose, and route or type of administration (e.g., high-potency herbal cannabis, cannabis edibles, oils, concentrates, topical supplements, smoking; Diggins & Heinberg, 2021). As THC tends to impact parts of the brain in the limbic system associated with hunger and pleasure, cannabis use tends to lead to increased appetite and subsequent problematic eating behaviors (Vidot et al., 2016). Cannabis users may have increased pain and anxiety around the time of surgery compared with nonusers, with users having a greater postoperative pain and opioid demand; potential explanations include preoperative withdrawal, cross-tolerance to opioids, or lower pain threshold (Bauer et al., 2018).

Emerging data suggest that perhaps cannabis use should not be a contraindication for MBS because there are no differences in complication rates or weight loss at 2 weeks to 5 years after surgery between cannabis users and nonusers (Shockcor et al., 2021; Worrest et al., 2022). However, cannabis use may be illegal, may be consistent with a substance use disorder, may be recreational, or may be part of a physician-approved treatment regimen, thus complicating absolute recommendations. All patients should be informed about the perioperative risks associated with cannabis use and the potential for usage to impact their long-term health.

Background Information

As with a general psychological evaluation, an assessment of background information includes an overview of the patient's upbringing and family dynamics (Sogg et al., 2016). Psychologists and mental health professionals may want to obtain specific weight management details about a patient's family or cultural practices related to food, childhood eating patterns, food insecurity, weight stigma, bullying, or weight or body size shaming at home or school. Current marital status, number and ages of children, current occupants of the home, and the composition and quality of a patient's support network provide additional insight into potential factors that may encourage or hinder behavior modification efforts (Sogg & Mori, 2004). Patients seeking MBS tend to live with family members who also have obesity and engage in similar levels of sedentary behavior (Lent et al., 2016). Perceived support from family and friends was related to increased likelihood of successful postoperative outcomes (Livhits et al., 2011).

Other standard areas of assessment include highest level of education attained, difficulties in school, and current and past employment or disability status. Lower levels of education and health literacy were related to increased risk of postoperative emergency department visits and readmissions (Mahoney et al., 2018) because these factors appear to affect the patient's ability to adhere to postoperative instructions. Miller-Matero and colleagues (2021) found that higher health literacy was related to better weight maintenance (2–4 years postsurgery) when presumably physiological adaptation has occurred and the patient's adherence to lifestyle changes is driving success. Psychologists/mental health professionals may administer brief cognitive screening measures and refer to neuropsychology for additional testing to further evaluate for the presence, nature, and severity of potential cognitive deficits. The multidisciplinary team may also request that a patient's family attend appointments to increase understanding and support for the postoperative lifestyle.

Finally, the psychological assessment should evaluate the presence and impact of chronic and acute stress and coping strategies. Chronic stressors and maladaptive coping strategies may impact patient adherence to behavior modification and ultimate success (Sogg et al., 2016). Of note, patients who do not meet the criteria for an eating disorder diagnosis may still present with emotional eating or eating in response to emotional distress. Emotional eating is one example of a maladaptive coping strategy that may reoccur postsurgery even if patients cannot consume large portions (Chesler, 2012). Delaying surgery may be beneficial in cases where significant stressors may put a patient at risk for poor surgical outcomes (Sarwer et al., 2014). Additional individual or group treatment may be beneficial for patients to learn to increase adaptive coping skills in the meantime.

Psychological Testing

In addition to the clinical interview, psychologists and other mental health professionals use psychometric measures and/or personality inventories to further assess symptoms of mental health concerns and personality characteristics among candidates for MBS (Fabricatore et al., 2006; Sarwer & Heinberg, 2020). Psychological testing has several important functions, including assessing personality and related factors that have been linked with outcomes, identifying areas for further assessment during the clinical interview, detecting the extent to which patients may under- or overreport symptoms, and helping to determine differential diagnoses (Marek et al., 2016). Commonly, testing involves one broad measure of general psychopathology and several briefer and more specific assessments of depression, anxiety, substance use, and cognitive functioning (Goodpaster, 2017). For a thorough review of psychological testing, see Marek et al. (2016) and Goodpaster (2017).

Broadband psychological measures provide a comprehensive assessment of patients across the aforementioned psychological domains. There is wide support for the Minnesota Multiphasic Personality Inventory (MMPI) Restructured Form as a suitable broadband instrument due to its replicable normative data, good reliability and validity coefficients, and predictive utility (Marek et al., 2014, 2015). The updated version of the MMPI-3 contains a new scale aimed at assessing problematic eating; earlier versions do not directly assess eating behaviors (Marek et al., 2021). Other broadband instruments include the Personality Assessment Inventory (Morey, 1991), the Millon Behavioral Medicine Diagnostic (MBMD; Millon et al., 2006), and the Millon Clinical Multiaxial Inventory-III (MCMI-III; Millon et al., 2009). The MBMD and MCMI are considered secondary choices due to inadequate research supporting their psychometric properties within this population (Marek et al., 2016).

Narrowband or specific instruments include depression and anxiety, substance use, and eating behaviors measures. Commonly used measures to assess for depression and anxiety include Beck Depression Inventory-II (Beck et al., 1996), Patient Health Questionnaire-9 (PHQ-9; Kroenke & Spitzer, 2002), the Beck Anxiety Inventory (BAI; Beck & Steer, 1993), and the GAD-7 (Spitzer et al., 2006). According to psychometric properties, the PHQ-9 and BAI are top choices for measuring anxiety and depression (Marek et al., 2016).

Assessments for substance use may include the Alcohol Use Disorders Identification Test (AUDIT; Babor et al., 2001) and the Substance Abuse Subtle Screening Inventory–3 (F. Miller et al., 1997). The AUDIT and AUDIT-C are commonly used and have been studied and psychometrically established within MBS settings (Marek et al., 2016).

Last, eating pathology has been assessed with such measures including the Eating Disorders Examination Questionnaire (EDE-Q; Fairburn & Beglin, 2008), the Questionnaire of Eating and Weight Patterns–Revised (Spitzer et al., 1993), and the Binge Eating Scale (BES; Gormally et al., 1982). The EDE-Q and the BES are recommended as eating-related self-report instruments due to their strong reliability coefficients and good construct validity (Ashton et al., 2009; Hood et al., 2013; Marek et al., 2015).

RECOMMENDATIONS FOR MITIGATING RISK FACTORS AND OPTIMIZING READINESS

The majority of mental health professionals (85.6%) make recommendations to the multidisciplinary team about a patient's appropriateness for surgery based on psychological assessment (Fabricatore et al., 2006). A review of practices suggests that providers recommend 69% of patients for surgery without presurgical psychological intervention, recommend postponing surgery until specific concerns are addressed in 22.8% of patients, and recommend against surgery due to psychological contraindications in 4% of patients. The most widely accepted psychological contraindications to MBS include active substance abuse, psychosis, uncontrolled mood or eating disorders, current or recent suicidality, history of problematic adherence, and major life stressors (Sogg et al., 2016). For many patients, the evaluating psychologist/mental health professional will recommend additional management or intervention before and/or after surgery to reduce risks and optimize patient outcomes. Table 4.1 provides a review of recommendations for mitigating risk factors.

TABLE 4.1. Recommendations for Mitigating Risk Factors

Concern	Recommendations
Understanding of the surgical procedure	• Brief education about the surgical procedure, behavioral changes necessary, and realistic expectations using "teach-back" method • Collaborations with multidisciplinary team including dietitians and nurses • Individual or group intervention
Maladaptive eating patterns	• Individual or group intervention • Education about the postoperative occurrence and consequences of disordered eating behaviors
Psychiatric illness (e.g., depression, anxiety, bipolar disorder)	• Collateral information from mental health providers • Period of emotional stability • Referral to mental health treatment
Substance use	• Referral to drug and alcohol treatment • Verbal and written education on risk • Elimination of substances before surgery • Laboratory screening to confirm abstinence
Cognitive functioning	• Brief cognitive screens • Referral for neuropsychological evaluation • Enlist support person
Chronic stressors	• Individual or group intervention • Stress management and adaptive coping

CONCLUSION

Psychologists and other mental health providers are considered an important part of the multidisciplinary MBS team. Those who are conducting presurgical assessments should have a thorough understanding of the biopsychosocial contributors and consequences of obesity, as well as specialized knowledge and experience in MBS (Peterson, 2018; Sogg et al., 2016). Although there are no clear standards for psychological assessment and treatment of bariatric surgical candidates, generally accepted guidelines were reviewed in this chapter. The role of mental health in MBS will likely continue to evolve as additional research, especially longitudinal, becomes available to optimize medical, psychological, and behavioral outcomes.

REFERENCES

Adams, T. D., Davidson, L. E., Litwin, S. E., Kim, J., Kolotkin, R. L., Nanjee, M. N., Gutierrez, J. M., Frogley, S. J., Ibele, A. R., Brinton, E. A., Hopkins, P. N., McKinlay, R., Simper, S. C., & Hunt, S. C. (2017). Weight and metabolic outcomes 12 years after gastric bypass. *The New England Journal of Medicine*, *377*(12), 1143–1155. https://doi.org/10.1056/NEJMoa1700459

Allison, K. C., Wadden, T. A., Sarwer, D. B., Fabricatore, A. N., Crerand, C. E., Gibbons, L. M., Stack, R. M., Stunkard, A. J., & Williams, N. N. (2006). Night eating syndrome and binge eating disorder among persons seeking bariatric surgery: Prevalence and related features. *Obesity*, *14*(3S, Suppl. 2), 77S–82S. https://doi.org/10.1038/oby.2006.286

Alosco, M. L., Galioto, R., Spitznagel, M. B., Strain, G., Devlin, M., Cohen, R., Crosby, R. D., Mitchell, J. E., & Gunstad, J. (2014). Cognitive function after bariatric surgery: Evidence for improvement 3 years after surgery. *American Journal of Surgery*, *207*(6), 870–876. https://doi.org/10.1016/j.amjsurg.2013.05.018

Alyahya, R. A., & Alnujaidi, M. A. (2022). Prevalence and outcomes of depression after bariatric surgery: A systematic review and meta-analysis. *Cureus*, *14*(6), Article e25651. Advance online publication. https://doi.org/10.7759/cureus.25651

American Psychiatric Association. (2013). *Diagnostic and statistical manual of mental disorders* (5th ed.). https://doi.org/10.1176/appi.books.9780890425596

American Society for Metabolic and Bariatric Surgery. (2021). *Bariatric surgery procedures*. https://asmbs.org/patients/bariatric-surgery-procedures

Ames, G. E., Patel, R. H., Ames, S. C., & Lynch, S. A. (2009). Weight loss surgery: Patients who regain. *Obesity and Weight Management*, *5*(4), 154–161. https://doi.org/10.1089/obe.2009.0403

Arterburn, D. E., Telem, D. A., Kushner, R. F., & Courcoulas, A. P. (2020, September 1). Benefits and risks of bariatric surgery in adults: A review. *JAMA*, *324*(9), 879–887. https://doi.org/10.1001/jama.2020.12567

Ashton, K., Drerup, M., Windover, A., & Heinberg, L. (2009). Brief, four-session group CBT reduces binge eating behaviors among bariatric surgery candidates. *Surgery for Obesity and Related Diseases*, *5*(2), 257–262. https://doi.org/10.1016/j.soard.2009.01.005

Babor, T. F., Higgins-Biddle, J. C., Saunders, J. B., & Monteiro, M. G. (2001). *The Alcohol Use Disorders Identification Test: Guidelines for use in primary care* (2nd ed.). World Health Organization.

Bauchowitz, A., Azarbad, L., Day, K., & Gonder-Frederick, L. (2007). Evaluation of expectations and knowledge in bariatric surgery patients. *Surgery for Obesity and Related Diseases, 3*(5), 554–558. https://doi.org/10.1016/j.soard.2007.05.005

Bauer, F. L., Donahoo, W. T., Hollis, H. W., Jr., Tsai, A. G., Pottorf, B. J., Johnson, J. M., Silveira, L. J., & Husain, F. A. (2018). Marijuana's influence on pain scores, initial weight loss, and other bariatric surgical outcomes. *The Permanente Journal, 22*(3). https://doi.org/10.7812/TPP/18-002

Beck, A. T., & Steer, R. A. (1993). *Beck Anxiety Inventory*. Psychological Corporation.

Beck, A. T., Steer, R. A., & Brown, G. K. (1996). *Manual for the Beck Depression Inventory–II*. Psychological Corporation.

Chao, A. M., Wadden, T. A., Faulconbridge, L. F., Sarwer, D. B., Webb, V. L., Shaw, J. A., Thomas, J. G., Hopkins, C. M., Bakizada, Z. M., Alamuddin, N., & Williams, N. N. (2016). Binge-eating disorder and the outcome of bariatric surgery in a prospective, observational study: Two-year results. *Obesity, 24*(11), 2327–2333. https://doi.org/10.1002/oby.21648

Chesler, B. E. (2012). Emotional eating: A virtually untreated risk factor for outcome following bariatric surgery. *The Scientific World Journal, 2012*, Article 365961. https://doi.org/10.1100/2012/365961

Choi, H. S., & Chun, H. J. (2017). Recent trends in endoscopic bariatric therapies. *Clinical Endoscopy, 50*(1), 11–16. https://doi.org/10.5946/ce.2017.007

Chow, A., Neville, A., & Kolozsvari, N. (2021). Smoking in bariatric surgery: A systematic review. *Surgical Endoscopy, 35*(6), 3047–3066. https://doi.org/10.1007/s00464-020-07669-3

Clark, M. M., Balsiger, B. M., Sletten, C. D., Dahlman, K. L., Ames, G., Williams, D. E., Abu-Lebdeh, H. S., & Sarr, M. G. (2003). Psychosocial factors and 2-year outcome following bariatric surgery for weight loss. *Obesity Surgery, 13*(5), 739–745. https://doi.org/10.1381/096089203322509318

Conason, A., Teixeira, J., Hsu, C. H., Puma, L., Knafo, D., & Geliebter, A. (2013). Substance use following bariatric weight loss surgery. *JAMA Surgery, 148*(2), 145–150. https://doi.org/10.1001/2013.jamasurg.265

Conceição, E. M., Mitchell, J. E., Engel, S. G., Machado, P. P. P., Lancaster, K., & Wonderlich, S. A. (2014). What is "grazing"? Reviewing its definition, frequency, clinical characteristics, and impact on bariatric surgery outcomes, and proposing a standardized definition. *Surgery for Obesity and Related Diseases, 10*(5), 973–982. https://doi.org/10.1016/j.soard.2014.05.002

Conceição, E., Mitchell, J. E., Vaz, A. R., Bastos, A. P., Ramalho, S., Silva, C., Cao, L., Brandão, I., & Machado, P. P. P. (2014). The presence of maladaptive eating behaviors after bariatric surgery in a cross sectional study: Importance of picking or nibbling on weight regain. *Eating Behaviors, 15*(4), 558–562. https://doi.org/10.1016/j.eatbeh.2014.08.010

Courcoulas, A. P., Christian, N. J., Belle, S. H., Berk, P. D., Flum, D. R., Garcia, L., Horlick, M., Kalarchian, M. A., King, W. C., Mitchell, J. E., Patterson, E. J., Pender, J. R., Pomp, A., Pories, W. J., Thirlby, R. C., Yanovski, S. Z., & Wolfe, B. M. (2013). Weight change and health outcomes at 3 years after bariatric surgery among individuals with severe obesity. *JAMA*, *310*(22), 2416–2425. https://doi.org/10.1001/jama.2013.280928

Courcoulas, A. P., King, W. C., Belle, S. H., Berk, P., Flum, D. R., Garcia, L., Gourash, W., Horlick, M., Mitchell, J. E., Pomp, A., Pories, W. J., Purnell, J. Q., Singh, A., Spaniolas, K., Thirlby, R., Wolfe, B. M., & Yanovski, S. Z. (2018). Seven-year weight trajectories and health outcomes in the Longitudinal Assessment of Bariatric Surgery (LABS) study. *JAMA Surgery*, *153*(5), 427–434. https://doi.org/10.1001/jamasurg.2017.5025

Cunningham, J. L., Merrell, C. C., Sarr, M., Somers, K. J., McAlpine, D., Reese, M., Stevens, S. R., & Clark, M. M. (2012). Investigation of antidepressant medication usage after bariatric surgery. *Obesity Surgery*, *22*(4), 530–535. https://doi.org/10.1007/s11695-011-0517-8

Dawes, A. J., Maggard-Gibbons, M., Maher, A. R., Booth, M. J., Miake-Lye, I., Beroes, J. M., & Shekelle, P. G. (2016, January 12). Mental health conditions among patients seeking and undergoing bariatric surgery: A meta-analysis. *JAMA*, *315*(2), 150–163. https://doi.org/10.1001/jama.2015.18118

de Zwaan, M., Enderle, J., Wagner, S., Mühlhans, B., Ditzen, B., Gefeller, O., Mitchell, J. E., & Müller, A. (2011). Anxiety and depression in bariatric surgery patients: A prospective, follow-up study using structured clinical interviews. *Journal of Affective Disorders*, *133*(1-2), 61–68. https://doi.org/10.1016/j.jad.2011.03.025

Diggins, A., & Heinberg, L. (2021). Marijuana and bariatric surgery. *Current Psychiatry Reports*, *23*(2), 10. https://doi.org/10.1007/s11920-020-01218-4

Ertelt, T. W., Mitchell, J. E., Lancaster, K., Crosby, R. D., Steffen, K. J., & Marino, J. M. (2008). Alcohol abuse and dependence before and after bariatric surgery: A review of the literature and report of a new data set. *Surgery for Obesity and Related Diseases*, *4*(5), 647–650. https://doi.org/10.1016/j.soard.2008.01.004

Fabricatore, A. N., Crerand, C. E., Wadden, T. A., Sarwer, D. B., & Krasucki, J. L. (2006). How do mental health professionals evaluate candidates for bariatric surgery? Survey results. *Obesity Surgery*, *16*(5), 567–573. https://doi.org/10.1381/096089206776944986

Fairburn, C. G., & Beglin, S. J. (2008). Eating Disorder Examination Questionnaire. In C. G. Fairburn (Ed.), *Cognitive behavior therapy and eating disorders* (pp. 309–313). Guilford Press.

Galioto, R., Alosco, M. L., Spitznagel, M. B., Strain, G., Devlin, M., Cohen, R., Crosby, R. D., Mitchell, J. E., & Gunstad, J. (2015). Glucose regulation and cognitive function after bariatric surgery. *Journal of Clinical and Experimental Neuropsychology*, *37*(4), 402–413. https://doi.org/10.1080/13803395.2015.1023264

Gasoyan, H., Tajeu, G., Halpern, M. T., & Sarwer, D. B. (2019). Reasons for underutilization of bariatric surgery: The role of insurance benefit design. *Surgery for Obesity and Related Diseases*, *15*(1), 146–151. https://doi.org/10.1016/j.soard.2018.10.005

Gill, H., Kang, S., Lee, Y., Rosenblat, J. D., Brietzke, E., Zuckerman, H., & McIntyre, R. S. (2019). The long-term effect of bariatric surgery on depression and anxiety. *Journal of Affective Disorders*, *246*, 886–894. https://doi.org/10.1016/j.jad.2018.12.113

Goodpaster, K. P. (2017). The role of psychological testing in pre-surgical bariatric evaluations. *Journal of Health Service Psychology*, *43*(2), 67–73. https://doi.org/10.1007/BF03544652

Goodpaster, K. P. S., Marek, R. J., Lavery, M. E., Ashton, K., Merrell Rish, J., & Heinberg, L. J. (2016). Graze eating among bariatric surgery candidates: Prevalence and psychosocial correlates. *Surgery for Obesity and Related Diseases, 12*(5), 1091–1097. https://doi.org/10.1016/j.soard.2016.01.006

Gormally, J., Black, S., Daston, S., & Rardin, D. (1982). The assessment of binge eating severity among obese persons. *Addictive Behaviors, 7*(1), 47–55. https://doi.org/10.1016/0306-4603(82)90024-7

Greenberg, I., Sogg, S., & M Perna, F. (2009). Behavioral and psychological care in weight loss surgery: Best practice update. *Obesity, 17*(5), 880–884. https://doi.org/10.1038/oby.2008.571

Gunstad, J., Lhotsky, A., Wendell, C. R., Ferrucci, L., & Zonderman, A. B. (2010). Longitudinal examination of obesity and cognitive function: Results from the Baltimore Longitudinal Study of Aging. *Neuroepidemiology, 34*(4), 222–229. https://doi.org/10.1159/000297742

Hales, C. M., Fryar, C. D., Carroll, M. D., Freedman, D. S., Aoki, Y., & Ogden, C. L. (2018, June 19). Differences in obesity prevalence by demographic characteristics and urbanization level among adults in the United States, 2013–2016. *JAMA, 319*(23), 2419–2429. https://doi.org/10.1001/jama.2018.7270

Heinberg, L. J., Ashton, K., & Coughlin, J. (2012). Alcohol and bariatric surgery: Review and suggested recommendations for assessment and management. *Surgery for Obesity and Related Diseases, 8*(3), 357–363. https://doi.org/10.1016/j.soard.2012.01.016

Heinberg, L. J., Ashton, K., & Windover, A. (2010). Moving beyond dichotomous psychological evaluation: The Cleveland Clinic Behavioral Rating System for weight loss surgery. *Surgery for Obesity and Related Diseases, 6*(2), 185–190. https://doi.org/10.1016/j.soard.2009.10.004

Heinberg, L. J., Keating, K., & Simonelli, L. (2010). Discrepancy between ideal and realistic goal weights in three bariatric procedures: Who is likely to be unrealistic? *Obesity Surgery, 20*(2), 148–153. https://doi.org/10.1007/s11695-009-9982-8

Hood, M. M., Grupski, A. E., Hall, B. J., Ivan, I., & Corsica, J. (2013). Factor structure and predictive utility of the Binge Eating Scale in bariatric surgery candidates. *Surgery for Obesity and Related Diseases, 9*(6), 942–948. https://doi.org/10.1016/j.soard.2012.06.013

Ivezaj, V., Benoit, S. C., Davis, J., Engel, S., Lloret-Linares, C., Mitchell, J. E., Pepino, M. Y., Rogers, A. M., Steffen, K., & Sogg, S. (2019). Changes in alcohol use after metabolic and bariatric surgery: Predictors and mechanisms. *Current Psychiatry Reports, 21*(9), 85. Advance online publication. https://doi.org/10.1007/s11920-019-1070-8

Kalarchian, M. A., King, W. C., Devlin, M. J., Marcus, M. D., Garcia, L., Chen, J. Y., Yanovski, S. Z., & Mitchell, J. E. (2016). Psychiatric disorders and weight change in a prospective study of bariatric surgery patients: A 3-year follow-up. *Psychosomatic Medicine, 78*(3), 373–381. https://doi.org/10.1097/PSY.0000000000000277

Kalarchian, M. A., Marcus, M. D., Levine, M. D., Courcoulas, A. P., Pilkonis, P. A., Ringham, R. M., Soulakova, J. N., Weissfeld, L. A., & Rofey, D. L. (2007). Psychiatric disorders among bariatric surgery candidates: Relationship to obesity and functional health status. *The American Journal of Psychiatry, 164*(2), 328–334. https://doi.org/10.1176/ajp.2007.164.2.328

Kaly, P., Orellana, S., Torrella, T., Takagishi, C., Saff-Koche, L., & Murr, M. M. (2008). Unrealistic weight loss expectations in candidates for bariatric surgery. *Surgery for Obesity and Related Diseases*, *4*(1), 6–10. https://doi.org/10.1016/j.soard.2007.10.012

Kanji, S., Wong, E., Akioyamen, L., Melamed, O., & Taylor, V. H. (2019). Exploring pre-surgery and post-surgery substance use disorder and alcohol use disorder in bariatric surgery: A qualitative scoping review. *International Journal of Obesity*, *43*(9), 1659–1674. https://doi.org/10.1038/s41366-019-0397-x

Karmali, S., Brar, B., Shi, X., Sharma, A. M., de Gara, C., & Birch, D. W. (2013). Weight recidivism post-bariatric surgery: A systematic review. *Obesity Surgery*, *23*(11), 1922–1933. https://doi.org/10.1007/s11695-013-1070-4

King, W. C., Chen, J.-Y., Courcoulas, A. P., Dakin, G. F., Engel, S. G., Flum, D. R., Hinojosa, M. W., Kalarchian, M. A., Mattar, S. G., Mitchell, J. E., Pomp, A., Pories, W. J., Steffen, K. J., White, G. E., Wolfe, B. M., & Yanovski, S. Z. (2017). Alcohol and other substance use after bariatric surgery: Prospective evidence from a U.S. multicenter cohort study. *Surgery for Obesity and Related Diseases*, *13*(8), 1392–1402. https://doi.org/10.1016/j.soard.2017.03.021

King, W. C., Chen, J. Y., Mitchell, J. E., Kalarchian, M. A., Steffen, K. J., Engel, S. G., Courcoulas, A. P., Pories, W. J., & Yanovski, S. Z. (2012, June 20). Prevalence of alcohol use disorders before and after bariatric surgery. *JAMA*, *307*(23), 2516–2525. https://doi.org/10.1001/jama.2012.6147

Kroenke, K., & Spitzer, R. L. (2002). The PHQ-9: A new depression diagnostic and severity measure. *Psychiatric Annals*, *32*(9), 509–515. https://doi.org/10.3928/0048-5713-20020901-06

Kushner, R. F., & Ryan, D. H. (2014, September 3). Assessment and lifestyle management of patients with obesity: Clinical recommendations from systematic reviews. *JAMA*, *312*(9), 943–952. https://doi.org/10.1001/jama.2014.10432

Lagerros, Y. T., Brandt, L., Hedberg, J., Sundbom, M., & Bodén, R. (2017). Suicide, self-harm, and depression after gastric bypass surgery: A nationwide cohort study. *Annals of Surgery*, *265*(2), 235–243. https://doi.org/10.1097/SLA.0000000000001884

Lent, M. R., Bailey-Davis, L., Irving, B. A., Wood, G. C., Cook, A. M., Hirsch, A. G., Still, C. D., Benotti, P. N., & Franceschelli-Hosterman, J. (2016). Bariatric surgery patients and their families: Health, physical activity, and social support. *Obesity Surgery*, *26*(12), 2981–2988. https://doi.org/10.1007/s11695-016-2228-7

Li, L., & Wu, L. T. (2016). Substance use after bariatric surgery: A review. *Journal of Psychiatric Research*, *76*, 16–29. https://doi.org/10.1016/j.jpsychires.2016.01.009

Livhits, M., Mercado, C., Yermilov, I., Parikh, J. A., Dutson, E., Mehran, A., Ko, C. Y., Shekelle, P. G., & Gibbons, M. M. (2011). Is social support associated with greater weight loss after bariatric surgery?: A systematic review. *Obesity Reviews*, *12*(2), 142–148. https://doi.org/10.1111/j.1467-789X.2010.00720.x

Lodhia, N. A., Rosas, U. S., Moore, M., Glaseroff, A., Azagury, D., Rivas, H., & Morton, J. M. (2015). Do adverse childhood experiences affect surgical weight loss outcomes? *Journal of Gastrointestinal Surgery*, *19*(6), 993–998. https://doi.org/10.1007/s11605-015-2810-7

Mahoney, S. T., Tawfik-Sexton, D., Strassle, P. D., Farrell, T. M., & Duke, M. C. (2018). Effects of education and health literacy on postoperative hospital visits in bariatric surgery. *Journal of Laparoendoscopic & Advanced Surgical Techniques*, *28*(9), 1100–1104. https://doi.org/10.1089/lap.2018.0093

Malik, S., Mitchell, J. E., Engel, S., Crosby, R., & Wonderlich, S. (2014). Psychopathology in bariatric surgery candidates: A review of studies using structured diagnostic interviews. *Comprehensive Psychiatry*, *55*(2), 248–259. https://doi.org/10.1016/j.comppsych.2013.08.021

Maluenda, F., Csendes, A., De Aretxabala, X., Poniachik, J., Salvo, K., Delgado, I., & Rodriguez, P. (2010). Alcohol absorption modification after a laparoscopic sleeve gastrectomy due to obesity. *Obesity Surgery*, *20*(6), 744–748. https://doi.org/10.1007/s11695-010-0136-9

Marek, R. J., Ben-Porath, Y. S., Ashton, K., & Heinberg, L. J. (2014). Minnesota Multiphasic Personality Inventory–2 Restructured Form (MMPI-2-RF) scale score differences in bariatric surgery candidates diagnosed with binge eating disorder versus BMI-matched controls. *International Journal of Eating Disorders*, *47*(3), 315–319. https://doi.org/10.1002/eat.22194

Marek, R. J., Ben-Porath, Y. S., Dulmen, M. H. M. V., Ashton, K., & Heinberg, L. J. (2017). Using the presurgical psychological evaluation to predict 5-year weight loss outcomes in bariatric surgery patients. *Surgery for Obesity and Related Diseases*, *13*(3), 514–521. https://doi.org/10.1016/j.soard.2016.11.008

Marek, R. J., Ben-Porath, Y. S., Sellbom, M., McNulty, J. L., & Heinberg, L. J. (2015). Validity of Minnesota Multiphasic Personality Inventory–2–Restructured Form (MMPI-2-RF) scores as a function of gender, ethnicity, and age of bariatric surgery candidates. *Surgery for Obesity and Related Diseases*, *11*(3), 627–634. https://doi.org/10.1016/j.soard.2014.10.005

Marek, R. J., Heinberg, L. J., Lavery, M., Merrell Rish, J., & Ashton, K. (2016). A review of psychological assessment instruments for use in bariatric surgery evaluations. *Psychological Assessment*, *28*(9), 1142–1157. https://doi.org/10.1037/pas0000286

Marek, R. J., Martin-Fernandez, K., Heinberg, L. J., & Ben-Porath, Y. S. (2021). An investigation of the Eating Concerns Scale of the Minnesota Multiphasic Personality Inventory–3 (MMPI-3) in a postoperative bariatric surgery sample. *Obesity Surgery*, *31*(5), 2335–2338. https://doi.org/10.1007/s11695-020-05113-y

McAlpine, D. E. (2006). How to adjust drug dosing after bariatric surgery. *Current Psychiatry*, *5*(1), 27.

Mechanick, J. I., Apovian, C., Brethauer, S., Garvey, W. T., Joffe, A. M., Kim, J., Kushner, R. F., Lindquist, R., Pessah-Pollack, R., Seger, J., Urman, R. D., Adams, S., Cleek, J. B., Correa, R., Figaro, M. K., Flanders, K., Grams, J., Hurley, D. L., Kothari, S., . . . Still, C. D. (2020). Clinical practice guidelines for the perioperative nutrition, metabolic, and nonsurgical support of patients undergoing bariatric procedures—2019 update: Cosponsored by American Association of Clinical Endocrinologists/American College of Endocrinology, The Obesity Society, American Society for Metabolic & Bariatric Surgery, Obesity Medicine Association, and American Society of Anesthesiologists. *Surgery for Obesity and Related Diseases*, *16*(2), 175–247. https://doi.org/10.1016/j.soard.2019.10.025

Mechanick, J. I., Youdim, A., Jones, D. B., Timothy Garvey, W., Hurley, D. L., Molly McMahon, M., Heinberg, L. J., Kushner, R., Adams, T. D., Shikora, S., Dixon, J. B., & Brethauer, S. (2013). Clinical practice guidelines for the perioperative nutritional, metabolic, and nonsurgical support of the bariatric surgery patient—2013 update: Cosponsored by American Association of Clinical Endocrinologists, the Obesity Society, and American Society for Metabolic & Bariatric Surgery. *Surgery for Obesity and Related Diseases*, *9*(2), 159–191. https://doi.org/10.1016/j.soard.2012.12.010

Michalsky, M. P. (2021). Perhaps it's time to move on from the LAP-band entirely? *Obesity Surgery*, *31*(12), 5475. https://doi.org/10.1007/s11695-021-05557-w

Miller, F., Roberts, J., Brooks, M., & Lazowski, L. (1997). *SASSI-3 user's guide*. Baugh Enterprises.

Miller, L. A., Crosby, R. D., Galioto, R., Strain, G., Devlin, M. J., Wing, R., Cohen, R. A., Paul, R. H., Mitchell, J. E., & Gunstad, J. (2013). Bariatric surgery patients exhibit improved memory function 12 months postoperatively. *Obesity Surgery*, *23*(10), 1527–1535. https://doi.org/10.1007/s11695-013-0970-7

Miller-Matero, L. R., Hecht, L., Patel, S., Martens, K. M., Hamann, A., & Carlin, A. M. (2021). The influence of health literacy and health numeracy on weight loss outcomes following bariatric surgery. *Surgery for Obesity and Related Diseases*, *17*(2), 384–389. https://doi.org/10.1016/j.soard.2020.09.021

Millon, T., Antoni, M. H., Millon, C., Minor, S., & Grossman, S. (2006). *Millon Behavioral Medicine Diagnostic (MBMD) manual* (2nd ed.). Pearson Assessments.

Millon, T., Millon, C., Davis, R. D., & Grossman, S. (2009). *Millon Clinical Multiaxial Inventory-III (MCMI-III): Manual*. Pearson/PsychCorp.

Mitchell, J. E., King, W. C., Courcoulas, A., Dakin, G., Elder, K., Engel, S., Flum, D., Kalarchian, M., Khandelwal, S., Pender, J., Pories, W., & Wolfe, B. (2015). Eating behavior and eating disorders in adults before bariatric surgery. *International Journal of Eating Disorders*, *48*(2), 215–222. https://doi.org/10.1002/eat.22275

Mitchell, J. E., Selzer, F., Kalarchian, M. A., Devlin, M. J., Strain, G. W., Elder, K. A., Marcus, M. D., Wonderlich, S., Christian, N. J., & Yanovski, S. Z. (2012). Psychopathology before surgery in the Longitudinal Assessment of Bariatric Surgery–3 (LABS-3) psychosocial study. *Surgery for Obesity and Related Diseases*, *8*(5), 533–541. https://doi.org/10.1016/j.soard.2012.07.001

Morey, L. C. (1991). *Personality Assessment Inventory*. Psychological Assessment Resources.

Müller, A., Hase, C., Pommnitz, M., & de Zwaan, M. (2019). Depression and suicide after bariatric surgery. *Current Psychiatry Reports*, *21*(9), 84. https://doi.org/10.1007/s11920-019-1069-1

Nguyen, J. C., Killcross, A. S., & Jenkins, T. A. (2014). Obesity and cognitive decline: Role of inflammation and vascular changes. *Frontiers in Neuroscience*, *8*, 375. https://doi.org/10.3389/fnins.2014.00375

Parikh, M., Johnson, J. M., Ballem, N., & the American Society for Metabolic and Bariatric Surgery Clinical Issues Committee. (2016). ASMBS position statement on alcohol use before and after bariatric surgery. *Surgery for Obesity and Related Diseases*, *12*(2), 225–230. https://doi.org/10.1016/j.soard.2015.10.085

Peterson, N. D. (2018). The role of the psychologist in the management of the bariatric patient. In K. Reavis, A. Barrett A., & M. Kroh (Eds.), *The SAGES manual of bariatric surgery* (pp. 137–159). Springer International. https://doi.org/10.1007/978-3-319-71282-6_14

Raebel, M. A., Newcomer, S. R., Reifler, L. M., Boudreau, D., Elliott, T. E., DeBar, L., Ahmed, A., Pawloski, P. A., Fisher, D., Donahoo, W. T., & Bayliss, E. A. (2013, October 2). Chronic use of opioid medications before and after bariatric surgery. *Journal of the American Medical Association*, *310*(13), 1369–1376. https://doi.org/10.1001/jama.2013.278344

Sarwer, D. B., Allison, K. C., Bailer, B. A., & Faulconbridge, L. F. (2014). Psychosocial characteristics of bariatric surgery candidates. In C. Still, D. B. Sarwer, & J. Blankenship (Eds.), *The ASMBS textbook of bariatric surgery: Vol. 2. Integrated health* (pp. 3–9). Springer. https://doi.org/10.1007/978-1-4939-1197-4_1

Sarwer, D. B., Cohn, N. I., Gibbons, L. M., Magee, L., Crerand, C. E., Raper, S. E., Rosato, E. F., Williams, N. N., & Wadden, T. A. (2004). Psychiatric diagnoses and psychiatric treatment among bariatric surgery candidates. *Obesity Surgery*, *14*(9), 1148–1156. https://doi.org/10.1381/0960892042386922

Sarwer, D. B., Dilks, R. J., & West-Smith, L. (2011). Dietary intake and eating behavior after bariatric surgery: Threats to weight loss maintenance and strategies for success. *Surgery for Obesity and Related Diseases*, *7*(5), 644–651. https://doi.org/10.1016/j.soard.2011.06.016

Sarwer, D. B., & Heinberg, L. J. (2020). A review of the psychosocial aspects of clinically severe obesity and bariatric surgery. *American Psychologist*, *75*(2), 252–264. https://doi.org/10.1037/amp0000550

Sarwer, D. B., Lavery, M., & Spitzer, J. C. (2012). A review of the relationships between extreme obesity, quality of life, and sexual function. *Obesity Surgery*, *22*(4), 668–676. https://doi.org/10.1007/s11695-012-0588-1

Sarwer, D. B., Wadden, T. A., Moore, R. H., Baker, A. W., Gibbons, L. M., Raper, S. E., & Williams, N. N. (2008). Preoperative eating behavior, postoperative dietary adherence, and weight loss after gastric bypass surgery. *Surgery for Obesity and Related Diseases*, *4*(5), 640–646. https://doi.org/10.1016/j.soard.2008.04.013

Segal, J. B., Clark, J. M., Shore, A. D., Dominici, F., Magnuson, T., Richards, T. M., Weiner, J. P., Bass, E. B., Wu, A. W., & Makary, M. A. (2009). Prompt reduction in use of medications for comorbid conditions after bariatric surgery. *Obesity Surgery*, *19*(12), 1646–1656. https://doi.org/10.1007/s11695-009-9960-1

Sekuła, M., Boniecka, I., & Paśnik, K. (2019). Bulimia nervosa in obese patients qualified for bariatric surgery—clinical picture, background and treatment. *Wideochirurgia i Inne Techniki Malo Inwazyjne*, *14*(3), 408–414. https://doi.org/10.5114/wiitm.2019.81312

Shockcor, N., Adnan, S. M., Siegel, A., Wise, E., Zafar, S. N., & Kligman, M. (2021). Marijuana use does not affect the outcomes of bariatric surgery. *Surgical Endoscopy*, *35*(3), 1264–1268. https://doi.org/10.1007/s00464-020-07497-5

Sogg, S., Lauretti, J., & West-Smith, L. (2016). Recommendations for the presurgical psychosocial evaluation of bariatric surgery patients. *Surgery for Obesity and Related Diseases*, *12*(4), 731–749. https://doi.org/10.1016/j.soard.2016.02.008

Sogg, S., & Mori, D. L. (2004). The Boston interview for gastric bypass: Determining the psychological suitability of surgical candidates. *Obesity Surgery*, *14*(3), 370–380. https://doi.org/10.1381/096089204322917909

Spadola, C. E., Wagner, E. F., Dillon, F. R., Trepka, M. J., De La Cruz-Munoz, N., & Messiah, S. E. (2015). Alcohol and drug use among postoperative bariatric patients: A systematic review of the emerging research and its implications. *Alcoholism, Clinical and Experimental Research*, *39*(9), 1582–1601. https://doi.org/10.1111/acer.12805

Spitzer, R. L., Kroenke, K., Williams, J. B., & Löwe, B. (2006). A brief measure for assessing generalized anxiety disorder: The GAD-7. *Archives of Internal Medicine*, *166*(10), 1092–1097. https://doi.org/10.1001/archinte.166.10.1092

Spitzer, R. L., Yanovski, S., & Marcus, M. (1993). *The questionnaire on eating and weight patterns-revised (QEWP-R)*. New York State Psychiatric Institute.

Spitznagel, M. B., Hawkins, M., Alosco, M., Galioto, R., Garcia, S., Miller, L., & Gunstad, J. (2015). Neurocognitive effects of obesity and bariatric surgery. *European Eating Disorders Review, 23*(6), 488–495. https://doi.org/10.1002/erv.2393

Štimac, D., & Majanović, S. K. (2012). Endoscopic approaches to obesity. *Digestive Diseases, 30*(2), 187–195. https://doi.org/10.1159/000336683

Sturm, R., & Hattori, A. (2013). Morbid obesity rates continue to rise rapidly in the United States. *International Journal of Obesity, 37*(6), 889–891. https://doi.org/10.1038/ijo.2012.159

Substance Abuse and Mental Health Services Administration. (2020). *Key substance use and mental health indicators in the United States: Results from the 2019 National Survey on Drug Use and health*. https://www.samhsa.gov/data/sites/default/files/reports/rpt29393/2019NSDUHFFRPDFWHTML/2019NSDUHFFR090120.htm

Svensson, P.-A., Anveden, Å., Romeo, S., Peltonen, M., Ahlin, S., Burza, M. A., Carlsson, B., Jacobson, P., Lindroos, A.-K., Lönroth, H., Maglio, C., Näslund, I., Sjöholm, K., Wedel, H., Söderpalm, B., Sjöström, L., & Carlsson, L. M. S. (2013). Alcohol consumption and alcohol problems after bariatric surgery in the Swedish Obese Subjects study. *Obesity, 21*(12), 2444–2451. https://doi.org/10.1002/oby.20397

Vidot, D. C., Prado, G., De La Cruz-Munoz, N., Spadola, C., Cuesta, M., & Messiah, S. E. (2016). Postoperative marijuana use and disordered eating among bariatric surgery patients. *Surgery for Obesity and Related Diseases, 12*(1), 171–178. https://doi.org/10.1016/j.soard.2015.06.007

Wagner, B., Klinitzke, G., Brähler, E., & Kersting, A. (2013). Extreme obesity is associated with suicidal behavior and suicide attempts in adults: Results of a population-based representative sample. *Depression and Anxiety, 30*(10), 975–981. https://doi.org/10.1002/da.22105

Walsh, E., Rosenstein, L., Dalrymple, K., Chelminski, I., & Zimmerman, M. (2017). The importance of assessing for childhood abuse and lifetime PTSD in bariatric surgery candidates. *Journal of Clinical Psychology in Medical Settings, 24*(3–4), 341–354. https://doi.org/10.1007/s10880-017-9518-7

White, G. E., Courcoulas, A. P., & King, W. C. (2019). Drug- and alcohol-related mortality risk after bariatric surgery: Evidence from a 7-year prospective multicenter cohort study. *Surgery for Obesity and Related Diseases, 15*(7), 1160–1169. https://doi.org/10.1016/j.soard.2019.04.007

Woodard, G. A., Downey, J., Hernandez-Boussard, T., & Morton, J. M. (2011). Impaired alcohol metabolism after gastric bypass surgery: A case-crossover trial. *Journal of the American College of Surgeons, 212*(2), 209–214. https://doi.org/10.1016/j.jamcollsurg.2010.09.020

Worrest, T., Malibiran, C. C., Welshans, J., Dewey, E., & Husain, F. (2022). Marijuana use does not affect weight loss or complication rate after bariatric surgery. *Surgical Endoscopy*. Advance online publication. https://doi.org/10.1007/s00464-022-09038-8

Yen, Y. C., Huang, C. K., & Tai, C. M. (2014). Psychiatric aspects of bariatric surgery. *Current Opinion in Psychiatry, 27*(5), 374–379. https://doi.org/10.1097/YCO.0000000000000085

5 SPINE SURGERY

JULIE MURRAY, JAYME S. WARNER, AND M. SCOTT DeBERARD

An estimated 75% of adults in the United States have experienced back pain (Murphy et al., 2017). For the majority of patients, back pain is acute and resolves within days or weeks, whereas for others, back pain persists or worsens. An estimated 12% of adults in the United States have chronic low back pain that lasts for more than 6 months (Von Korff et al., 2016). First-line treatments for acute back pain are typically conservative and may include the use of nonsteroidal anti-inflammatory drugs, heating pads, chiropractic care, injections, or physical therapy (Oliveira et al., 2018). It is estimated that approximately 10% of patients with persistent spine pain receive a surgical intervention (Trivedi, 2021). Despite these surgical efforts, an estimated 20% or more of such patients will experience *failed back surgery syndrome*, which is patient dissatisfaction with outcomes and residual symptoms that continue, worsen, or manifest after one or more spine surgeries (e.g., pain, ongoing neurological symptoms; Inoue et al., 2017).

https://doi.org/10.1037/0000346-006
Psychological Assessment of Surgical Candidates: Evidence-Based Procedures and Practices, R. J. Marek and A. R. Block (Editors)

COMMON SURGICAL PROCEDURES

Common surgical procedures include lumbar discectomy, lumbar fusion, artificial disc replacement, lumbar laminectomy, spinal cord stimulation, and rhizotomy. The goals of these procedures are to correct or minimize the effect of diseased or damaged structures, reduce pain, and improve the patient's function. The success of these procedures in achieving these goals, however, is variable.

Lumbar Discectomy

A *lumbar discectomy* is typically an outpatient spinal surgery in which the damaged part of an intervertebral disc is removed by either an orthopedic surgeon or a neurosurgeon. Discectomies are largely performed to repair weakened, degenerative, bulging, or herniated discs. When intervertebral discs bulge or herniate, the damaged, protruding portion of the disc can press on the spinal cord, creating pain, tingling, numbness or weakness (Johns Hopkins Medicine, n.d.-b).

The goal of this procedure is to surgically remove the protruding portion to relieve the symptoms caused by the pressure from the disc on the spinal cord. Thus, lumbar discectomy is intended to reduce the symptoms of bulging, herniated, or degenerative intervertebral discs. Approximately 285,000 discectomies are performed each year in the United States (McDermott & Liang, 2021), with an estimated 79% of patients experiencing good or excellent outcomes (Dohrmann & Mansour, 2015).

Lumbar Fusion

Lumbar fusion, or "spinal fusion," is a more invasive procedure that involves the use of a bone graft to permanently connect or fuse two vertebrae together to create a single bone and ultimately prevent motion in that segment of the spine entirely. The bone graft may be created with bone from a bone bank, from the patient's own body (typically from the pelvis), or occasionally from synthetic material (Mayo Clinic, 2020). The surgeon may use metal plates, rods, and screws to hold the graft in place while it heals.

The main goal of this surgery is to eliminate motion between vertebrae, creating more stability in the spine. The technique used for this surgery depends on the location of the affected vertebral joint. For the lumbar fusion, incision may be made either directly over the spine or on either side of the spine if a posterior approach is preferred, or it may be made in the abdomen if an anterior approach is preferred. Using retraction devices, the muscles are moved aside, and the bone graft and any necessary supportive hardware are placed. If the patient has pain in their arms or legs as well as their spine, the surgeon may also perform a decompressive laminectomy (see the discussion in the Lumbar Laminectomy section of this chapter) during the fusion procedure.

Lumbar fusion may be used to address symptoms and complications from herniated disks; spinal injuries; diseases, such as arthritis; infections; tumors; deformities; and congenital defects, such as scoliosis (American Academy of Orthopaedic Surgeons, n.d.). This surgery is best for patients whose source of pain is motion of the joint (Carreon et al., 2009). Approximately 500,000 fusions are performed each year in the United States (McDermott & Liang, 2021), with success rates varying widely, depending on type of procedure and presurgical pathology.

Artificial Disc Replacement

Artificial disc replacement is a procedure that is generally used as an alternative to lumbar fusion in the treatment of degenerative disc disease. This procedure involves replacing worn or degenerative discs in the cervical or lumbar spine with an artificial disc (Othman et al., 2019). Artificial discs, made of metal or a combination of metals and plastics, are designed to emulate the qualities of natural discs to allow them to perform similarly in function.

Although fusion of vertebrae can reduce range of motion in the spine, artificial disc replacement aims to maintain movement and flexibility. In addition, lumbar fusion can result in load transfer to unfused adjacent vertebra, resulting in the development or acceleration of degeneration of adjacent spinal segments. Artificial disc replacement aims to overcome this complication by maintaining a balanced spinal load (Othman et al., 2019).

A recent meta-analysis suggested that artificial disc replacement may have some benefits over lumbar fusion in the treatment of degenerative disc disease, including greater patient satisfaction, shorter hospital stay, less postoperative pain, and lower complication rates (Li et al., 2020). However, no significant differences were found between lumbar fusion and artificial disc replacement in the context of blood loss, return to work status, or reoperation rate (Li et al., 2020).

Lumbar Laminectomy

Each vertebra in the spine has a bony spinous process that protrudes from the rear of the spine. These spinous processes are connected to posterior facets of the vertebrae by the lamina on either side. During a *lumbar laminectomy*, the surgeon creates an incision directly above the affected area of the spine and moves the muscles aside to access the spinal column. Special surgical instruments are used to remove the spinous processes, followed by the removal of the lamina on either side (Johns Hopkins Medicine, n.d.-a). The surgeon may remove the lamina from one or more vertebrae, and this surgery may be done in combination with a discectomy or fusion, depending on the size of the affected area, the extent of damage, and the causes of pain. The surgeon can use several methods to perform a lumbar laminectomy, and research shows no difference in the long-term outcomes of each (Bouknaitir et al., 2020).

Lumbar laminectomy may be used to address pain, numbness, and weakness caused by pressure on the spinal cord that results from *stenosis*, a narrowing of the spinal canal. This narrowing is often caused by bony growths, most commonly resulting from arthritis or the normal aging process (Mayo Clinic, 2022) as well as displaced intervertebral discs. Removing the lamina from the spine in the affected area relieves that pressure by creating more space in the spinal canal. For that reason, this surgery is often called a "decompressive laminectomy." As is the case with other spinal surgeries, this surgery is typically only recommended if nonsurgical treatments, such as physical therapy, medication, and injections, have failed (Mayo Clinic, 2022). Laminectomy is a procedure that is often performed in conjunction with both discectomy and fusion surgeries.

Spinal Cord Stimulation

Spinal cord stimulation, the use of an implanted device to send electrical pulses to select areas of the spinal cord, has been used to treat chronic back pain; postoperative pain; arachnoiditis; spinal cord injury–related pain; other nerve-related pain (e.g., diabetic neuropathy); complex regional pain syndrome; in some cases, even angina untreatable by other means; visceral abdominal or perineal pain; peripheral vascular disease; and pain after amputation (Johns Hopkins Medicine, n.d.-d). Chronic back pain can develop for a variety of reasons and can have a significant negative effect on the ability of an individual to function and on their overall quality of life. When conservative treatments have failed to relieve chronic back pain, spinal cord stimulation may be an option.

Spinal cord stimulation surgery begins with a trial period (typically lasting about a week) to ensure that the treatment is the correct option for the patient and to identify the best location for the electrodes that will be implanted if it is. If the trial period is successful, the surgeon makes an incision and places one or more electrodes in the form of thin wires into the spinal column using the guidance of X-ray or ultrasound. After the electrodes have been implanted, the patient can send electrical impulses using a remote control to stimulate their spinal cord and relieve pain. The mechanism is not fully understood, and the technology is still developing.

Spinal cord stimulation is considered successful if half of the patient's pain can be reduced (Anderson & Cockroft, n.d.). Outcomes are widely varied in terms of success, with some longitudinal studies showing that the operation is unsuccessful for more than half of patients (Nissen et al., 2019). Manchikanti et al. (2021) reported significantly increased utilization rates of spinal cord stimulation among Medicare enrollees from 2009 to 2018, with more than 59,000 units implanted in 2018.

Rhizotomy

Sometimes referred to as an "ablation" or "neurotomy," a *rhizotomy* is a surgical procedure performed to intentionally destroy nerves or nerve fibers that carry pain signals and are causing chronic pain (Johns Hopkins Medicine, n.d.-c). This is a minimally invasive procedure, and the destruction of the nerves can be done either by severing them or burning them with chemicals or electricity. The surgeon uses three main methods to destroy the problematic nerves or nerve fibers. The first is by injecting either glycerol or glycerin into the nerve root. The second method uses a radiofrequency current to coagulate the fibers. It is more effective than the chemical destruction of glycerol/glycerin and takes less time to complete. The third method, called an *endoscopic rhizotomy*, involves the insertion of an endoscope through a small incision and a tubular retractor system that allows the surgeon access to the affected nerve, where they can then sever the fibers. The destruction of the nerves through the rhizotomy procedure may result in immediate pain relief that lasts until the nerves recover, which typically takes a few months (as is the case with radiofrequency neurotomy) to years if the nerve is completely severed.

Rhizotomies are performed to treat chronic pain that results specifically from abnormal nerve activity. This includes trigeminal neuralgia (most commonly) and spasticity among more traditional causes of back pain, such as herniated discs, arthritis, stenosis, and degenerative diseases (Johns Hopkins Medicine, n.d.-c).

OUTCOMES AND RATIONALE FOR PRESURGICAL ASSESSMENT

The health outcomes of spinal surgeries need to be considered in both the short and long term. The goals of spinal surgeries are generally to reduce pain, reduce pain medication intake, improve spine stability, increase mobility, and improve overall quality of life. The success of these surgeries, however, is variable. For example, Atlas et al. (2005) surveyed nonsurgical patients with chronic back pain and spinal surgery patients annually for 8 to 10 years and determined that pain improvement was about the same among the two groups. Fifty-three percent of nonsurgical patients reported an improvement in their pain, whereas 54% of surgical patients reported improvement. Further, a study of discectomy patients found that 28% had less than favorable outcomes (Sherman et al., 2010).

In addition to health outcomes, spine surgeries are often accompanied by significant financial burden. Financial considerations include time off work before and after surgery, the cost of the surgery itself, postoperative physical therapy, any subsequent operations, and complications that may arise. These considerations are important because only 29% of workers' compensation patients who undergo lumbar discectomy have good outcomes after a 40-week follow-up (Klekamp et al., 1998). However, some research has determined that with advancing technology, patients who undergo a spinal discectomy surgery have significantly increased quality of life, with an average savings of $971 to $1,655 per patient (Sherman et al., 2010).

CONSIDERATIONS FOR ASSESSMENT

A variety of psychosocial, medical, and occupational factors have been found to be associated with the various spine surgery outcomes. Assessment and consideration of these factors before surgery is essential for identifying and managing risk for spine surgery candidates.

Psychosocial Risk Factors

A well-established body of literature links psychosocial factors with adverse spine surgery outcomes, such as increased postsurgical disability status and poor health-related quality of life. Indeed, one study found that although presurgical medical variables were better able to predict pain and symptom-specific well-being at 6 months postsurgery, psychosocial predictors were able to explain a higher proportion of the variance in postsurgical back function, general well-being, and disability (Mannion et al., 2007). Other studies have found that a combination of presurgical medical and psychosocial variables were most predictive of a variety of surgical outcomes related to pain, disability, satisfaction, and general well-being (Costelloe et al., 2020; DeBerard et al., 2009; Macki et al., 2019). As such, it is important to screen for such factors before surgery to identify patients who may be at high risk for adverse outcomes or whose outcomes may be improved by presurgical intervention.

Depression

Spine injuries and chronic pain—two conditions that often precede spine surgery—are frequently accompanied by difficulty sleeping, loss of income, and diminished functional ability. As such, it is not surprising that symptoms of depression are found in an as many as 85% of patients with a significant spine injury (Sørensen & Mors, 1988). Across studies, a variety of methods have been used to identify depression in spine patients, including the Minnesota Multiphasic Personality Inventory–2–Restructured Form (MMPI-2-RF; Ben-Porath & Tellegen, 2008/2011), Hospital Anxiety and Depression Scale (HADS; Zigmond & Snaith, 1983), Patient Health Questionnaire–9 (Kroenke & Spitzer, 2002), and Beck Depression Inventory (Beck et al., 1961), and less formal measures, such as medical chart review and observation (Bendinger et al., 2015; Block et al., 2017; Järvimäki et al., 2016; Menendez et al., 2014).

A growing body of literature has found presurgical depression to be related to adverse outcomes of spinal surgeries, including increased postoperative pain, lower functional improvement, and higher health care expenditure costs (Adogwa et al., 2014; Costelloe et al., 2020; Walid & Robinson, 2011). Of note, depression is often undiagnosed after back injuries because of the overlap in the symptoms of injury and depression, thus resulting in difficulty determining whether symptoms are normal and expected responses to stress and disability or are indicative of a comorbid depressive disorder (Zepinic & Kuzmanovski, 2019). For instance, both depression and functional limitations from injury can lead to the inability of a person to engage in pleasurable activities, lead to excessive fatigue, and lead to difficulty sleeping. Presurgical identification of depression is important because some research suggests that presurgical treatment of depression with antidepressants may improve postsurgical perception of pain and functional disability (Elsamadicy et al., 2016).

Anxiety and Fear

Anxiety is characterized by fear, worry, and avoidance. Symptoms of anxiety occur in nearly one third of patients with chronic back pain undergoing surgery (Arts et al., 2012). Spine patients may have fears related to undergoing surgery. They may worry about when they will be able to return to normal activities or about the financial burden that can come with spine surgeries. In addition, spine patients may avoid certain activities for fear of aggravating their injury or further damaging the spine.

A systematic review of the literature found anxiety to be a positive predictor for short-term (up to 3 months postsurgery), medium-term (3 to 12 months postsurgery), and long-term (12 or more months postsurgery) pain following lumbar surgery (Dorow et al., 2017). In a recent study, spine patients with presurgical anxiety that persisted postoperation demonstrated less improvement in physical function and in sleep disturbance (Rahman et al., 2020). Presurgical identification and treatment of anxiety may be meaningful—for example, one study suggested that presurgical treatment of anxiety with joint pharmacological treatment and psychotherapy may improve postsurgical outcomes in patients undergoing anterior cervical discectomy and fusion (Adogwa et al., 2016). However, more research in this area is needed, particularly larger scale trials. Across studies, a variety of methods have been used to measure anxiety in spine patients, including the MMPI-2-RF (Ben-Porath & Tellegen, 2008/2011), HADS (Zigmond & Snaith, 1983), Fear-Avoidance Beliefs Questionnaire (Waddell et al., 1993), and medical chart review (Bendinger et al., 2015; Block et al., 2017; Mannion et al., 2007; Menendez et al., 2014).

Substance Use

Over the past 2 decades, the increased prescription and subsequent misuse of opioid medications in the United States has led to the development of a national crisis, ultimately leading the U.S. Department of Health and Human Services (2017) to declare the opioid epidemic a public health emergency. Widespread concern related to the opioid epidemic has led to a decrease in opioid prescriptions in recent years, yet the number of prescriptions still remains high in the United States, with more than 191 million opioid prescriptions dispensed in 2017 (Centers for Disease Control and Prevention, 2018). It is estimated that up to 30% of patients presenting with low back pain in primary care and up to 60% of patients presenting with low back pain in emergency departments are prescribed opioids (Kamper et al., 2020). In addition to concerns about misuse and dependence, opioid use has been negatively linked to postsurgical outcomes. More specifically, presurgical opioid use was found to be a negative predictor of return-to-work status within 3 years postsurgery and was positively associated with reoperation and permanent disability after cervical fusion (Faour et al., 2018).

Similar to opioid misuse, alcohol abuse has been found to be associated with negative clinical outcomes following spine surgery. More specifically, alcohol abuse is an independent risk factor for readmission after anterior lumbar fusion and is associated with greater risk of surgical site infection (Dobran et al., 2017; Phan et al., 2018). Further, alcohol abuse is associated with respiratory, cardiac, gastrointestinal, urinary, renal, venous thromboembolism, and wound-related complications in patients undergoing elective spinal fusion (Han et al., 2021). Some research suggests that these associations may, in part, be explained by the presence of alcohol withdrawal (Han et al., 2021).

In addition to opioid and alcohol abuse, patients with any presurgical substance use disorders have been found to be at higher risk for adverse outcomes. Those with substance use disorders have been found to have higher rates of leaving the hospital against medical advice, poorer follow-up compliance, and higher readmission rates when they did attend follow-up appointments (Ferari et al., 2020). Further, drug abuse has been associated with postsurgery surgical site infection (Dobran et al., 2017). As such, it is important that providers assess for all types of substance abuse in spine surgery candidates.

Social Support

Spine injuries can lead to physical limitations and emotional burdens that necessitate help from others. Some research suggests that social support, as measured by the Duke–UNC Functional Social Support Questionnaire (Broadhead et al., 1988), is positively associated with both postsurgical health-related and non–health-related quality of life (Laxton & Perrin, 2003). Further, some evidence points to an association between social support and length of hospital stay after spine surgery, such that patients who reported adequate social support had shorter length of stay (Adogwa et al., 2017; Mancuso et al., 2018).

Patient Expectations and Activation

Spine surgery patients whose presurgical expectations are fulfilled experience higher postsurgical satisfaction, regardless of functional outcomes (Soroceanu et al., 2012; Waljee et al., 2014). Further, positive presurgical expectations have been found to be associated with greater postsurgical quality of life (Saban & Penckofer, 2007). As such, it is important for patients to have positive, yet realistic expectations for surgery. *Patient activation* refers to a patient's beliefs in the importance in taking an active role in their care, and the knowledge, skills, and confidence to manage their condition (Hibbard et al., 2004). High presurgical patient activation, as measured by the Patient

Activation Measure (PAM; Hibbard et al., 2004), is associated with higher postsurgical satisfaction (Harris et al., 2020). In addition to postsurgical satisfaction, PAM scores have been associated with greater improvements in functional ability, potentially because of increased postsurgical adherence to physical therapy in highly activated patients (Skolasky et al., 2011). Remarkably, PAM scores have been found to mediate the relationship between presurgical psychosocial risk factors and poor outcomes (Block et al., 2019). As such, patient activation may be a protective factor that can help mitigate psychosocial risks.

Medical Risk Factors

Medical factors, including obesity, smoking, and comorbid health problems, can affect surgical outcomes for spine patients. As such, consideration of these factors is important for identifying and managing risk for spine surgery candidates.

Obesity

Obesity is defined by the World Health Organization (2021) as having a body mass index greater than or equal to 30 kg/m^2. In spine patients, obesity is associated with high risk of complications and reoperation. More specifically, a systematic review of the literature found that spine patients with obesity have significantly longer operative times, higher estimated blood loss, and more perioperative complications than spine patients without obesity (Goyal et al., 2019). Further, patients with obesity who underwent open spine surgeries were found to have significantly higher incidence of reoperation. Notably, the reoperation rate between patients with and without obesity undergoing minimally invasive spine surgeries was found to be similar (Goyal et al., 2019). Although patients with obesity may be at greater risk for complications and reoperation, postoperative functional status, back pain, and disability status have been found to be similar in patients with and without obesity after lumbar surgery (Brennan et al., 2017; Goyal et al., 2019) This suggests that both patients with and without obesity may benefit from surgery.

Smoking

The negative effects of smoking and tobacco use have been well established. For spine patients, smoking has been associated with higher risk of postoperative infection, a lower rate of return to work, and higher rates of overall dissatisfaction with surgical outcomes (Berman et al., 2017; Jackson & Devine, 2016). Further, smoking places fusion patients at increased risk for nonunion (Berman et al., 2017). Smoking has also been found to be strongly associated with spine pain (Smuck et al., 2020). Although smoking increases risks of negative outcomes and complications for spine patients, research has demonstrated that smoking cessation can help mitigate some risk (Jackson & Devine, 2016). More specifically, refraining from smoking after surgery has been found to be associated with improvements in fusion rates, return-to-work rates, and patient satisfaction (Glassman et al., 2000). These improvements tended to be better in individuals who quit for more than 6 months after surgery (Glassman et al., 2000).

Comorbid Health Problems

Spine surgery candidates often deal with other medical ailments and conditions. Research has demonstrated that having more comorbid health conditions is predictive of poorer outcomes for lumbar discectomy patients (DeBerard et al., 2009).

Occupational Risk Factors

Several occupational factors, such as workers' compensation status, litigation history, and unemployment, before surgery are associated with negative surgical outcomes. For instance, receiving workers' compensation has been found to predict decreased physical function, postsurgical pain, and disability after lumbar fusion surgery (Trief et al., 2006). Further, among workers' compensation cases, involvement of a patient's private lawyer in the compensation case has been associated with worse physical function, pain severity, social function, and overall health (DeBerard et al., 2009). In addition to workers' compensation and litigation, patients not working for more than 2 months before surgery tend to have poorer outcomes (Marek et al., 2021).

CONDUCTING A PRESURGICAL ASSESSMENT

At this time, no standard approach exists to conducting presurgical psychological assessments (PPAs) for spine surgeries. However, a risk identification and mitigation (RIM) model based in the literature has been proposed that provides a flexible framework for conducting presurgical assessments (Block & Marek, 2020). The RIM model consists of five steps and draws on three main sources of information—(a) psychometric testing, (b) medical record review, and (c) a semistructured interview—to inform treatment recommendations.

Step 1 is to use psychometric testing to identify objective psychosocial risk factors that have been empirically linked to a full range of surgical outcomes. In this step, careful selection of psychometric testing is imperative so as to choose appropriate, reliable, and valid tests that have norms within the specific surgical population of interest. Step 2 is to substantiate the risk factors identified in psychometric testing and to capture a more complete picture of the patient's experience through a clinical interview and medical chart review. Step 3 in the RIM model involves consideration of risk factor mitigation. Although some psychosocial factors may increase risk for adverse outcomes, other factors, such as positive realistic expectations, patient activation, and social support, have been found to mitigate some risk for surgical candidates (Adogwa et al., 2017; Block et al., 2019; Harris et al., 2020; Mancuso et al., 2018; Saban & Penckofer, 2007; Soroceanu et al., 2012; Waljee et al., 2014). It is important, then, for the psychologist/mental health professional to consider these factors that may offset some of the overall level of risk for adverse outcomes.

Step 4 involves integrating the collected data and making determinations about risk. This step requires the psychologist/mental health professional to integrate the information collected with clinical judgment and experience to obtain an overall picture of surgical risk. Several researchers have created algorithms or scorecards to aid in this process. For example, Block et al. (2001) created an algorithm that synthesizes psychological, medical, and social factors and stratifies patients into risk categories. More recently, this algorithm has been revised for use with the MMPI-2-RF (Ben-Porath & Tellegen, 2008/2011; Block & Sarwer, 2013). Using this algorithm, 97% of the 435 patients predicted to have an excellent prognosis were classified in longitudinal analyses to have excellent ($n = 320$) or good ($n = 102$) surgical outcomes at 1 year postsurgery (Marek et al., 2021). Further, 52% of the 43 patients predicted to have poor or very poor prognosis obtained poor surgical outcomes at 1 year postsurgery, and only 16% of predicted poor prognosis patients achieved excellent outcomes (Marek et al., 2021).

Step 5 of the RIM model is to make informed treatment recommendations. In some cases, it may be determined that risk of adverse outcome is low to moderate. In these cases, the use of psychological or behavioral interventions may serve to supplement surgery and increase the patient activation and ability to manage symptoms (Block & Marek, 2020). In patients with moderate psychosocial risk, treatment recommendations may include participation in presurgical interventions to reduce risk, such as smoking cessation, treatment for depression, weight loss, or reduction of opioid medication (Block & Marek, 2020). In patients determined to be at high risk for adverse outcomes, it may be prudent to recommend alternatives to surgical interventions, at least temporarily (Block & Marek, 2020).

CONCLUSION

Despite widespread use and technological advances, the outcomes of spine surgeries are variable. One reason may be the wide variety of outcomes to consider, from physical and emotional health-related outcomes to financial burden and functional outcomes. In addition, the studies reviewed in this chapter demonstrate the strong influence of psychosocial factors on the different outcomes. These psychosocial influences may also play an important role in the variable results.

Although, at this time, there is no standard approach to PPAs for spine surgeries, the RIM model reviewed in this chapter provides a flexible framework for gathering and integrating information from psychometric testing, medical record review, and semistructured interview to inform treatment recommendations (Block & Marek, 2020). For patients with low psychosocial risk, psychological or behavioral interventions may supplement surgery to increase patient activation and ability to manage symptoms (Block & Marek, 2020). For example, cognitive behavior therapy has demonstrated efficacy as a supplemental or preoperative intervention for patients undergoing bariatric surgery, cardiac surgery, and lumbar surgery (Hwang et al., 2015; Parrish et al., 2021; Paul et al., 2015). Specifically, a meta-analysis of cognitive behavior therapy interventions for patients undergoing spine surgeries found improvements in quality of life, psychological outcomes, and postoperative disability and pain scores (Parrish et al., 2021).

For patients who are determined to be at moderate psychosocial risk for poor surgical outcomes, treatment recommendations may include delaying surgery while patients participate in presurgical interventions to reduce risk, such as smoking cessation, treatment for depression, weight loss, or reduction of opioid medication (Block & Marek, 2020). For patients who are determined to be at high psychosocial risk, treatment recommendations may include less invasive alternatives to surgical interventions, including multidisciplinary chronic pain management programs (Block & Marek, 2020)—which have demonstrated effectiveness in reducing pain intensity and functional disability in patients with chronic back pain (Salathé et al., 2018). In addition, these programs are often more cost effective than surgery (Rivero-Arias et al., 2005).

PPAs can be a useful tool for helping to identify and manage risk for spine surgery candidates. However, ultimately it is the responsibility of the surgeon to weigh the mental health professional's recommendations with other considerations and make the final determination about whether to proceed with surgery.

REFERENCES

Adogwa, O., Elsamadicy, A. A., Cheng, J., & Bagley, C. (2016). Pretreatment of anxiety before cervical spine surgery improves clinical outcomes: A prospective, single-institution experience. *World Neurosurgery*, *88*, 625–630. https://doi.org/10.1016/j.wneu.2015.11.014

Adogwa, O., Elsamadicy, A. A., Vuong, V. D., Mehta, A. I., Vasquez, R. A., Cheng, J., Bagley, C. A., & Karikari, I. O. (2017). Effect of social support and marital status on perceived surgical effectiveness and 30-day hospital readmission. *Global Spine Journal*, *7*(8), 774–779. https://doi.org/10.1177/2192568217696696

Adogwa, O., Verla, T., Thompson, P., Penumaka, A., Kudyba, K., Johnson, K., Fulchiero, E., Miller, T., Jr., Hoang, K. B., Cheng, J., & Bagley, C. A. (2014). Affective disorders influence clinical outcomes after revision lumbar surgery in elderly patients with symptomatic adjacent-segment disease, recurrent stenosis, or pseudarthrosis: Clinical article. *Journal of Neurosurgery: Spine*, *21*(2), 153–159. https://doi.org/10.3171/2014.4.SPINE12668

American Academy of Orthopaedic Surgeons. (n.d.). *Spinal fusion*. Retrieved August 14, 2022, from https://orthoinfo.aaos.org/en/treatment/spinal-fusion

Anderson, B., & Cockroft, K. M. (n.d.). *Spinal cord stimulation*. https://www.aans.org/en/Patients/Neurosurgical-Conditions-and-Treatments/Spinal-Cord-Stimulation

Arts, M. P., Kols, N. I., Onderwater, S. M., & Peul, W. C. (2012). Clinical outcome of instrumented fusion for the treatment of failed back surgery syndrome: A case series of 100 patients. *Acta Neurochirurgica*, *154*(7), 1213–1217. https://doi.org/10.1007/s00701-012-1380-7

Atlas, S. J., Keller, R. B., Wu, Y. A., Deyo, R. A., & Singer, D. E. (2005). Long-term outcomes of surgical and nonsurgical management of lumbar spinal stenosis: 8 to 10 year results from the Maine lumbar spine study. *Spine*, *30*(8), 936–943. https://doi.org/10.1097/01.brs.0000158953.57966.c0

Beck, A. T., Ward, C. H., Mendelson, M., Mock, J., & Erbaugh, J. (1961). An inventory for measuring depression. *Archives of General Psychiatry*, *4*, 561–571.

Bendinger, T., Plunkett, N., Poole, D., & Turnbull, D. (2015). Psychological factors as outcome predictors for spinal cord stimulation. *Neuromodulation*, *18*(6), 465–471. https://doi.org/10.1111/ner.12321

Ben-Porath, Y. S., & Tellegen, A. (2008/2011). *Minnesota Multiphasic Personality Inventory–2–Restructured Form (MMPI-2-RF): Manual for administration, scoring, and interpretation*. University of Minnesota Press.

Berman, D., Oren, J. H., Bendo, J., & Spivak, J. (2017). The effect of smoking on spinal fusion. *The International Journal of Spine Surgery*. Advance online publication. https://doi.org/10.14444/4029

Block, A. R., & Marek, R. J. (2020). Presurgical psychological evaluation: Risk factor identification and mitigation. *Journal of Clinical Psychology in Medical Settings*, *27*(2), 396–405. https://doi.org/10.1007/s10880-019-09660-0

Block, A. R., Marek, R. J., & Ben-Porath, Y. S. (2019). Patient activation mediates the association between psychosocial risk factors and spine surgery results. *Journal of*

Clinical Psychology in Medical Settings, 26(2), 123–130. https://doi.org/10.1007/s10880-018-9571-x

Block, A. R., Marek, R. J., Ben-Porath, Y. S., & Kukal, D. (2017). Associations between pre-implant psychosocial factors and spinal cord stimulation outcome: Evaluation using the MMPI-2-RF. *Assessment, 24*(1), 60–70. https://doi.org/10.1177/1073191115601518

Block, A. R., Ohnmeiss, D. D., Guyer, R. D., Rashbaum, R. F., & Hochschuler, S. H. (2001). The use of presurgical psychological screening to predict the outcome of spine surgery. *The Spine Journal, 1*(4), 274–282. https://doi.org/10.1016/S1529-9430(01)00054-7

Block, A. R., & Sarwer, D. B. (Eds.). (2013). *Presurgical psychological screening: Understanding patients, improving outcomes*. American Psychological Association. https://doi.org/10.1037/14035-000

Bouknaitir, J. B., Carreon, L. Y., Brorson, S., Pederson, C. F., & Andersen, M. (2020). Comparison of five-year outcomes between wide laminectomy, segmental bilateral laminotomies and unilateral hemi-laminectomy for lumbar spinal stenosis. *The Spine Journal, 20*(9), S203. https://doi.org/10.1016/j.spinee.2020.05.517

Brennan, P. M., Loan, J. J. M., Watson, N., Bhatt, P. M., & Bodkin, P. A. (2017). Preoperative obesity does not predict poorer symptom control and quality of life after lumbar disc surgery. *British Journal of Neurosurgery, 31*(6), 682–687. https://doi.org/10.1080/02688697.2017.1354122

Broadhead, W. E., Gehlbach, S. H., DeGruy, F. V., & Kaplan, B. H. (1988). The Duke-UNC Functional Social Support Questionnaire: Measurement of social support in family medicine patients. *Medical Care, 26*(7), 709–723.

Carreon, L. Y., Glassman, S. D., Djurasovic, M., Dimar, J. R., Johnson, J. R., Puno, R. M., & Campbell, M. J. (2009). Are preoperative health-related quality of life scores predictive of clinical outcomes after lumbar fusion? *Spine, 34*(7), 725–730. https://doi.org/10.1097/BRS.0b013e318198cae4

Centers for Disease Control and Prevention. (2018, August 31). *2018 annual surveillance report of drug-related risks and outcomes: United States.* U.S. Department of Health and Human Services. https://www.cdc.gov/drugoverdose/pdf/pubs/2018-cdc-drug-surveillance-report.pdf

Costelloe, C., Burns, S., Yong, R. J., Kaye, A. D., & Urman, R. D. (2020). An analysis of predictors of persistent postoperative pain in spine surgery. *Current Pain and Headache Reports, 24*(4), Article 11. https://doi.org/10.1007/s11916-020-0842-5

DeBerard, M. S., LaCaille, R. A., Spielmans, G., Colledge, A., & Parlin, M. A. (2009). Outcomes and presurgery correlates of lumbar discectomy in Utah Workers' Compensation patients. *The Spine Journal, 9*(3), 193–203. https://doi.org/10.1016/j.spinee.2008.02.001

Dobran, M., Marini, A., Nasi, D., Gladi, M., Liverotti, V., Costanza, M. D., Mancini, F., & Scerrati, M. (2017). Risk factors of surgical site infections in instrumented spine surgery. *Surgical Neurology International, 8*(1), Article 212. https://doi.org/10.4103/sni.sni_222_17

Dohrmann, G. J., & Mansour, N. (2015). Long-term results of various operations for lumbar disc herniation: Analysis of over 39,000 patients. *Medical Principles and Practice, 24*(3), 285–290. https://doi.org/10.1159/000375499

Dorow, M., Löbner, M., Stein, J., Konnopka, A., Meisel, H. J., Günther, L., Meixensberger, J., Stengler, K., König, H.-H., & Riedel-Heller, S. G. (2017). Risk factors for postoperative pain intensity in patients undergoing lumbar disc surgery: A systematic review. *PLOS ONE*, *12*(1), Article e0170303. https://doi.org/10.1136/bmj.g6380

Elsamadicy, A. A., Adogwa, O., Cheng, J., & Bagley, C. (2016). Pretreatment of depression before cervical spine surgery improves patients' perception of postoperative health status: A retrospective, single institutional experience. *World Neurosurgery*, *87*, 214–219. https://doi.org/10.1016/j.wneu.2015.11.067

Faour, M., Anderson, J. T., Haas, A. R., Percy, R., Woods, S. T., Ahn, U. M., & Ahn, N. U. (2018). Preoperative opioid use: A risk factor for poor return to work status after single-level cervical fusion for radiculopathy in a workers' compensation setting. *Clinical Spine Surgery*, *31*(1), E19–E24. https://doi.org/10.1097/BSD.0000000000000545

Ferari, C. S., Katsevman, G. A., Dekeseredy, P., & Sedney, C. L. (2020). Implications of drug use disorders on spine surgery. *World Neurosurgery*, *136*, e334–e341. https://doi.org/10.1016/j.wneu.2019.12.177

Glassman, S. D., Anagnost, S. C., Parker, A., Burke, D., Johnson, J. R., & Dimar, J. R. (2000). The effect of cigarette smoking and smoking cessation on spinal fusion. *Spine*, *25*(20), 2608–2615. https://doi.org/10.1097/00007632-200010150-00011

Goyal, A., Elminawy, M., Kerezoudis, P., Lu, V. M., Yolcu, Y., Alvi, M. A., & Bydon, M. (2019). Impact of obesity on outcomes following lumbar spine surgery: A systematic review and meta-analysis. *Clinical Neurology and Neurosurgery*, *177*, 27–36. https://doi.org/10.1016/j.clineuro.2018.12.012

Han, L., Han, H., Liu, H., Wang, C., Wei, X., He, J., & Lu, X. (2021). Alcohol abuse and alcohol withdrawal are associated with adverse perioperative outcomes following elective spine fusion surgery. *Spine*, *46*(9), 588–595. https://doi.org/10.1097/BRS.0000000000003868

Harris, A. B., Kebaish, F., Riley, L. H., Kebaish, K. M., & Skolasky, R. L. (2020). The engaged patient: Patient activation can predict satisfaction with surgical treatment of lumbar and cervical spine disorders. *Journal of Neurosurgery: Spine*, *32*(6), 914–920. https://doi.org/10.3171/2019.11.SPINE191159

Hibbard, J. H., Stockard, J., Mahoney, E. R., & Tusler, M. (2004). Development of the Patient Activation Measure (PAM): Conceptualizing and measuring activation in patients and consumers. *Health Services Research*, *39*(4p1), 1005–1026. https://doi.org/10.1111/j.1475-6773.2004.00269.x

Hwang, B., Eastwood, J. A., McGuire, A., Chen, B., Cross-Bodán, R., & Doering, L. V. (2015). Cognitive behavioral therapy in depressed cardiac surgery patients: Role of ejection fraction. *The Journal of Cardiovascular Nursing*, *30*(4), 319–324. https://doi.org/10.1097/JCN.0000000000000155

Inoue, S., Kamiya, M., Nishihara, M., Arai, Y. P., Ikemoto, T., & Ushida, T. (2017). Prevalence, characteristics, and burden of failed back surgery syndrome: The influence of various residual symptoms on patient satisfaction and quality of life as assessed by a nationwide Internet survey in Japan. *Journal of Pain Research*, *10*, 811–823. https://doi.org/10.2147/JPR.S129295

Jackson, K. L., II, & Devine, J. G. (2016). The effects of smoking and smoking cessation on spine surgery: A systematic review of the literature. *Global Spine Journal*, *6*(7), 695–701. https://doi.org/10.1055/s-0036-1571285

Järvimäki, V., Kautiainen, H., Haanpää, M., Koponen, H., Spalding, M., Alahuhta, S., & Vakkala, M. (2016). Depressive symptoms are associated with poor outcome for lumbar spine surgery. *Scandinavian Journal of Pain*, *12*(1), 13–17. https://doi.org/10.1016/j.sjpain.2016.01.008

Johns Hopkins Medicine. (n.d.-a). *Laminectomy*. https://www.hopkinsmedicine.org/health/treatment-tests-and-therapies/laminectomy

Johns Hopkins Medicine. (n.d.-b). *Minimally invasive lumbar discectomy*. https://www.hopkinsmedicine.org/health/treatment-tests-and-therapies/minimally-invasive-lumbar-discectomy

Johns Hopkins Medicine. (n.d.-c). *Rhizotomy*. https://www.hopkinsmedicine.org/health/treatment-tests-and-therapies/rhizotomy

Johns Hopkins Medicine. (n.d.-d). *Spinal cord stimulator.* https://www.hopkinsmedicine.org/health/treatment-tests-and-therapies/treating-pain-with-spinal-cord-stimulators

Kamper, S. J., Logan, G., Copsey, B., Thompson, J., Machado, G. C., Abdel-Shaheed, C., Williams, C. M., Maher, C. G., & Hall, A. M. (2020). What is usual care for low back pain? A systematic review of health care provided to patients with low back pain in family practice and emergency departments. *Pain*, *161*(4), 694–702. https://doi.org/10.1097/j.pain.0000000000001751

Klekamp, J., McCarty, E., & Spengler, D. M. (1998). Results of elective lumbar discectomy for patients involved in the workers' compensation system. *Journal of Spinal Disorders*, *11*(4), 277–282.

Kroenke, K., & Spitzer, R. L. (2002). The PHQ-9: A new depression diagnostic and severity measure. *Psychiatric Annals*, *32*(9), 509–515. https://doi.org/10.3928/0048-5713-20020901-06

Laxton, A. W., & Perrin, R. G. (2003). The relations between social support, life stress, and quality of life following spinal decompression surgery. *Spinal Cord*, *41*(10), 553–558. https://doi.org/10.1038/sj.sc.3101432

Li, Y.-Z., Sun, P., Chen, D., Tang, L., Chen, C.-H., & Wu, A.-M. (2020). Artificial total disc replacement versus fusion for lumbar degenerative disc disease: An update systematic review and meta-analysis. *Turkish Neurosurgery*, *30*(1), 1–10.

Macki, M., Alvi, M. A., Kerezoudis, P., Xiao, S., Schultz, L., Bazydlo, M., Bydon, M., Park, P., Chang, V., & the MSSIC Investigators. (2019). Predictors of patient dissatisfaction at 1 and 2 years after lumbar surgery. *Journal of Neurosurgery: Spine*, *32*(3), 1–10. https://doi.org/10.5137/1019-5149.JTN.24799-18.2

Manchikanti, L., Pampati, V., Vangala, B. P., Soin, A., Sanapati, M. R., Thota, S., & Hirsch, J. A. (2021). Spinal cord stimulation trends of utilization and expenditures in fee-for-service (FFS) Medicare population from 2009 to 2018. *Pain Physician*, *24*(5), 293–308.

Mancuso, C. A., Duculan, R., Craig, C. M., & Girardi, F. P. (2018). Psychosocial variables contribute to length of stay and discharge destination after lumbar surgery independent of demographic and clinical variables. *Spine*, *43*(4), 281–286. https://doi.org/10.1097/BRS.0000000000002312

Mannion, A. F., Elfering, A., Staerkle, R., Junge, A., Grob, D., Dvorak, J., Jacobshagen, N., Semmer, N. K., & Boos, N. (2007). Predictors of multidimensional outcome after spinal surgery. *European Spine Journal*, *16*(6), 777–786. https://doi.org/10.1007/s00586-006-0255-0

Marek, R. J., Lieberman, I., Derman, P., Nghiem, D. M., & Block, A. R. (2021). Validity of a pre-surgical algorithm to predict pain, functional disability, and emotional functioning 1 year after spine surgery. *Psychological Assessment*. Advance online publication. https://doi.org/10.1037/pas0001008

Mayo Clinic. (2020, November 14). *Spinal fusion*. https://www.mayoclinic.org/tests-procedures/spinal-fusion/about/pac-20384523

Mayo Clinic. (2022, June 30). *Laminectomy*. https://www.mayoclinic.org/tests-procedures/laminectomy/about/pac-20394533

McDermott, K. W., & Liang, L. (2021). Overview of operating room procedures during Inpatient stays in U.S. hospitals, 2018 (Statistical Brief No. 281). In *Healthcare Cost and Utilization Project (HCUP) statistical briefs*. Agency for Healthcare Research and Quality. https://www.hcup-us.ahrq.gov/reports/statbriefs/sb281-Operating-Room-Procedures-During-Hospitalization-2018.pdf

Menendez, M. E., Neuhaus, V., Bot, A. G., Ring, D., & Cha, T. D. (2014). Psychiatric disorders and major spine surgery: Epidemiology and perioperative outcomes. *Spine*, *39*(2), E111–E122. https://doi.org/10.1097/BRS.0000000000000064

Murphy, K. R., Han, J. L., Yang, S., Hussaini, S. M., Elsamadicy, A. A., Parente, B., Xie, J., Pagadala, P., & Lad, S. P. (2017). Prevalence of specific types of pain diagnoses in a sample of United States adults. *Pain Physician*, *20*(2), E257–E268.

Nissen, M., Ikäheimo, T. M., Huttunen, J., Leinonen, V., & von und zu Fraunberg, M. (2019). Long-term outcome of spinal cord stimulation in failed back surgery syndrome: 20 years of experience with 224 consecutive patients. *Neurosurgery*, *84*(5), 1011–1018. https://doi.org/10.1093/neuros/nyy194

Oliveira, C. B., Maher, C. G., Pinto, R. Z., Traeger, A. C., Lin, C. C., Chenot, J. F., van Tulder, M., & Koes, B. W. (2018). Clinical practice guidelines for the management of non-specific low back pain in primary care: An updated overview. *European Spine Journal*, *27*(11), 2791–2803. https://doi.org/10.1007/s00586-018-5673-2

Othman, Y. A., Verma, R., & Qureshi, S. A. (2019). Artificial disc replacement in spine surgery. *Annals of Translational Medicine*, *7*(Suppl. 5), Article S170. https://doi.org/10.21037/atm.2019.08.26

Parrish, J. M., Jenkins, N. W., Parrish, M. S., Cha, E. D. K., Lynch, C. P., Massel, D. H., Hrynewycz, N. M., Mohan, S., Geoghegan, C. E., Jadczak, C. N., Westrick, J., Van Horn, R., & Singh, K. (2021). The influence of cognitive behavioral therapy on lumbar spine surgery outcomes: A systematic review and meta-analysis. *European Spine Journal*, *30*(5), 1365–1379. https://doi.org/10.1007/s00586-021-06747-x

Paul, L., van Rongen, S., Van Hoeken, D., Deen, M., Klaassen, R., Biter, L. U., Hoek, H. W., & van der Heiden, C. (2015). Does cognitive behavioral therapy strengthen the effect of bariatric surgery for obesity? Design and methods of a randomized and controlled study. *Contemporary Clinical Trials*, *42*, 252–256. https://doi.org/10.1016/j.cct.2015.04.001

Phan, K., Lee, N. J., Kothari, P., Kim, J. S., & Cho, S. K. (2018). Risk factors for readmissions following anterior lumbar interbody fusion. *Spine*, *43*(5), 364–369. https://doi.org/10.1097/BRS.0000000000001677

Rahman, R., Ibaseta, A., Reidler, J. S., Andrade, N. S., Skolasky, R. L., Riley, L. H., Cohen, D. B., Sciubba, D. M., Kebaish, K. M., & Neuman, B. J. (2020). Changes in patients' depression and anxiety associated with changes in patient-reported outcomes after spine surgery. *Journal of Neurosurgery: Spine*, *32*(6), 871–890. https://doi.org/10.3171/2019.11.SPINE19586

Rivero-Arias, O., Campbell, H., Gray, A., Fairbank, J., Frost, H., & Wilson-MacDonald, J. (2005). Surgical stabilisation of the spine compared with a programme of intensive rehabilitation for the management of patients with chronic low back pain: Cost utility analysis based on a randomised controlled trial. *BMJ*, *330*(7502), Article 1239. https://doi.org/10.1136/bmj.38441.429618.8F

Saban, K. L., & Penckofer, S. M. (2007). Patient expectations of quality of life following lumbar spinal surgery. *The Journal of Neuroscience Nursing*, *39*(3), 180–189. https://doi.org/10.1097/01376517-200706000-00009

Salathé, C. R., Melloh, M., Crawford, R., Scherrer, S., Boos, N., & Elfering, A. (2018). Treatment efficacy, clinical utility, and cost-effectiveness of multidisciplinary biopsychosocial rehabilitation treatments for persistent low back pain: A systematic review. *Global Spine Journal*, *8*(8), 872–886. https://doi.org/10.1177/2192568218765483

Sherman, J., Cauthen, J., Schoenberg, D., Burns, M., Reaven, N. L., & Griffith, S. L. (2010). Economic impact of improving outcomes of lumbar discectomy. *The Spine Journal*, *10*(2), 108–116. https://doi.org/10.1016/j.spinee.2009.08.453

Skolasky, R. L., Mackenzie, E. J., Wegener, S. T., & Riley, L. H., III. (2011). Patient activation and functional recovery in persons undergoing spine surgery. *The Journal of Bone & Joint Surgery*, *93*(18), 1665–1671. https://doi.org/10.2106/JBJS.J.00855

Smuck, M., Schneider, B. J., Ehsanian, R., Martin, E., & Kao, M. J. (2020). Smoking is associated with pain in all body regions, with greatest influence on spinal pain. *Pain Medicine*, *21*(9), 1759–1768. https://doi.org/10.1093/pm/pnz224

Sørensen, L. V., & Mors, O. (1988). Presentation of a new MMPI scale to predict outcome after first lumbar diskectomy. *Pain*, *34*(2), 191–194. https://doi.org/10.1016/0304-3959(88)90165-0

Soroceanu, A., Ching, A., Abdu, W., & McGuire, K. (2012). Relationship between preoperative expectations, satisfaction, and functional outcomes in patients undergoing lumbar and cervical spine surgery: A multicenter study. *Spine*, *37*(2), E103–E108. https://doi.org/10.1097/BRS.0b013e3182245c1f

Trief, P. M., Ploutz-Snyder, R., & Fredrickson, B. E. (2006). Emotional health predicts pain and function after fusion: A prospective multicenter study. *Spine*, *31*(7), 823–830. https://doi.org/10.1097/01.brs.0000206362.03950.5b

Trivedi, K. (2021, July 21). *Just 10% of back pain requires surgery—and minimally invasive procedures work for many*. UT Southwestern Medical Center. https://utswmed.org/medblog/back-pain-surgery-alternatives/#:~:text=Not%20all%20of%20these%20sensitive,with%20spine%20disorders%20without%20surgery

U.S. Department of Health and Human Services. (2017, October 26). *Determination that a public health emergency exists*. https://www.hhs.gov/sites/default/files/opioid%20PHE%20Declaration-no-sig.pdf

Von Korff, M., Scher, A. I., Helmick, C., Carter-Pokras, O., Dodick, D. W., Goulet, J., Hamill-Ruth, R., LeResche, L., Porter, L., Tait, R., Terman, G., Veasley, C., & Mackey, S. (2016). United States national pain strategy for population research: Concepts, definitions, and pilot data. *The Journal of Pain*, *17*(10), 1068–1080. https://doi.org/10.1016/j.jpain.2016.06.009

Waddell, G., Newton, M., Henderson, I., Somerville, D., & Main, C. J. (1993). A Fear-Avoidance Beliefs Questionnaire (FABQ) and the role of fear-avoidance beliefs in chronic low back pain and disability. *Pain*, *52*(2), 157–168. https://doi.org/10.1016/0304-3959(93)90127-B

Walid, M. S., & Robinson, J. S., Jr. (2011). Economic impact of comorbidities in spine surgery. *Journal of Neurosurgery: Spine*, *14*(3), 318–321. https://doi.org/10.3171/2010.11.SPINE10139

Waljee, J., McGlinn, E. P., Sears, E. D., & Chung, K. C. (2014). Patient expectations and patient-reported outcomes in surgery: A systematic review. *Surgery*, *155*(5), 799–808. https://doi.org/10.1016/j.surg.2013.12.015

World Health Organization. (2021, June 9). *Obesity and overweight.* https://www.who.int/news-room/fact-sheets/detail/obesity-and-overweight

Zepinic, V., & Kuzmanovski, B. (2019). Chronic pain and depression in low back (spinal) injured patients. *American Journal of Applied Psychology*, *8*(5), 89–97. https://doi.org/10.11648/j.ajap.20190805.11

Zigmond, A. S., & Snaith, R. P. (1983). The Hospital Anxiety and Depression Scale. *Acta Psychiatrica Scandinavica*, *67*(6), 361–370. https://doi.org/10.1111/j.1600-0447.1983.tb09716.x

6 GENDER EMBODIMENT SURGERY

ZO AMARO JIMENEZ AND COLT ST. AMAND

The first accounts of transgender people having surgery to meet their embodiment goals date back to the 1930s (Blumberg, 2021). *Embodiment goals* refer to the specific primary and secondary sex characteristics desired (Hastings et al., 2021). As an example, a person's gender embodiment goals may include a beard, breasts, and lower pitched voice. Over the past few decades, access to these procedures has increased at incredible rates as more surgeons are offering affirming care and more trans people are seeking such procedures.[1]

GENDER EMBODIMENT SURGERIES

Terms like "sex change surgery" (considered offensive), "sex reassignment surgery" (considered outdated and offensive), "gender confirming surgery," and "gender affirming surgery" have all been used to describe the set of more than 10 different surgeries one might desire to undergo to achieve their gender embodiment goals. Because these terms have commonly been

[1]Reading this chapter is not sufficient training for providing presurgical psychological assessments for gender embodiment surgery.

https://doi.org/10.1037/0000346-007
Psychological Assessment of Surgical Candidates: Evidence-Based Procedures and Practices, R. J. Marek and A. R. Block (Editors)

interpreted to refer only to surgery on the external genitalia, it is more appropriate to name the particular surgery to which one is referring when discussing surgical procedures for transgender people. For simplicity, surgical options for gender embodiment can be thought of in the following categories: face, voice, chest, gonadal, genital, and body contouring. Many surgical procedures end in "-plasty" or "-ectomy." As a rule, *-plasty* indicates the addition of something, whereas *-ectomy* specifies the removal of something. In this chapter, we refer to the range of surgeries as "gender embodiment surgery."

Facial Surgery

Facial surgery includes procedures that alter any part of the face and neck based on individual embodiment goals. Historically, these have been referred to as "facial feminization surgery" or "facial masculinization surgery." This categorical convention limits options and is not inclusive of intersex people and those with gender embodiment goals that do not fit into a gender binary. In addition, it does not use a person-centered, trauma informed, individualized approach; therefore, we refer to individual procedures without categorizing them into a binary.

Through facial surgery procedures, the surgeon can, for example, change the length and predominance of the forehead through *contouring*; perform a *lift* to change the appearance of the brow; alter the skin around the eyes via a *blepharoplasty*; perform a *rhinoplasty* to change the nose; alter the cheeks, lips, chin, or jaw; perform a *thyroid chondroplasty/tracheal shave* or *thyroid cartilage enhancement* to reshape the Adam's apple; reposition the skin through a *face lift* or *neck lift*; or perform a *hairline advancement* to lower the hairline. Some surgeons offer technology that shows a patient what their face will look like after surgery. Many dermatologists offer temporary treatments, such as fillers and botox, that may assist patients in visualizing changes to their face so they can determine if a more permanent procedure is right for them.

Voice Surgery

Voice surgery options are much newer than other gender embodiment surgeries. Vocal cord shortening, known as a *glottoplasty* or *anterior glottal web formation*, aims to eliminate the production of lower pitches yet also narrows the airway, but long-term results have been variable. Elongation of the vocal cords—*cricothyroid approximation surgery*—aims to provide a higher pitch but has not been found to have a lasting effect. *Relaxation thyroplasty*—that is, vocal fold tension reduction—is thought to reduce pitch yet can result in a rougher voice with less volume production.

Experts in this field agree that working with specialized speech language pathologists and gender voice specialists is the appropriate route, and surgery is thought to be a second- or third-line intervention (Davies et al., 2015). Because voice surgery targets the pitch, and many aspects to the voice are thought to be as important if not more important than pitch range—including resonance and intonation—behavioral approaches and testosterone therapy are thought to be first-line options for changing the voice.

Breast/Chest Surgery

Breast/chest surgery includes procedures that modify breast tissue. Breast augmentation surgery, or *mammoplasty*, involves choosing both the size and material for the postoperative breast appearance. Silicone and saline are the most commonly selected materials for breast implants. Breast reduction surgery can reduce the size of the breast based on the individual's goals without completely removing all breast tissue.

For those with size A or smaller breasts, a *periareolar breast reduction mastectomy* may be an option to achieve a flat chest and maintain nipple sensation. A *double mastectomy* with or without nipple grafts removes the breast tissue and mammary folds. It typically uses one or two large incisions across the chest and often results in the loss of nipple sensation postoperatively. The incisions and nipple grafts require postoperative care. Patients who undergo breast/chest surgery often require surgical drains postoperatively.

Gonadal Surgery

Gonadal surgery involves removal of *gonads*, which include testicles, ovaries, and intersex variations of gonadal tissue. *Orchiectomy* is the removal of the testicles and generally leaves scrotal tissue behind. *Oophorectomy*, the removal of one or two ovaries, can be performed at the same time as *hysterectomy*, which is the removal of the uterus. *Hysterectomy with bilateral salpingo-oophorectomy* is the removal of the uterus, fallopian tubes, and ovaries.

Some may choose to retain one or two ovaries to use them for reproductive or sex hormone production purposes. If all gonads are removed, a person is no longer thought to have eggs or sperm and is considered infertile.

Genital Surgery

Genital surgery alters the appearance and function of the external genitalia. Of the three major surgeries in this category, all can be customized to meet the goals of the individual. Surgeons may recommend that patients undergo hair removal from the pubic region or sites where grafts will be created, such as the forearm. *Vaginoplasty* has been used as an umbrella term for the creation of a vulva—through a *vulvoplasty*—and a vagina. This can be accomplished with creation of a clitoris using the glans of a penis, called a *clitoroplasty*; creation of the labia using scrotal skin and excess urethral tissue through a procedure called a *labiaplasty*; removal of testicles from the scrotal sac—an *orchiectomy*; and creation of a vagina using penile skin (most common) or portions of the colon or omentum (i.e., vaginoplasty). If individuals would like to prevent their vagina from prolapsing (essentially falling outside of the body), they will need to dilate the vagina on a schedule provided by their surgeon for their lifetime. Surgeons should be able to accommodate individualized gender embodiment goals—for example, prominent protrusion of labia minora or vulvoplasty without vaginoplasty (i.e., clitoris and labia without a vagina).

Phalloplasty is the most complex of the gender embodiment surgeries and is typically performed in multiple stages—that is, via multiple separate surgeries that require long periods of recovery. *Phalloplasty* has been used as an umbrella term for creation of a penis most commonly by using grafts of the forearm, called a *radial forearm flap phalloplasty*, or thigh, called an *anterolateral thigh phalloplasty*; urethral lengthening most commonly by using labia minora or buccal tissue;, creation of a scrotal sac using the labia majora, a procedure called a *scrotoplasty*; removal of the vagina via a *vaginectomy*; insertion of testicular prostheses; and insertion of an erectile device. Individuals seeking this procedure decide which aspects are most important to them—for example, urinating out of the end of their penis, engaging in sexual penetration using their penis, experiencing penile erogenous sensation, or having a certain penile aesthetic appearance.

Metoidioplasty uses growth of the glans resulting from testosterone treatment to create a penis. Metoidioplasty can include procedures such as scrotoplasty with testicular implants, urethral lengthening, vaginectomy, use of labia minora tissue around the glans to increase penile girth, and mons lift/resection. For both phalloplasty and metoidioplasty, individualized gender embodiment goals—for instance, creation of a penis without removal of the vagina or without creation of a scrotal sac or without urethral lengthening (i.e., patients urinate from their original urethral opening)—can be accommodated by the surgeon. Patient priorities should guide the surgical treatment plan.

Additional Surgeries

Several other surgical procedures make up gender embodiment surgeries. Surgical procedures designed to change body contours have been desired or accessed by both cisgender (people who are not transgender) and transgender people alike. Historically, these procedures have been considered cosmetic, yet the World Professional Association for Transgender Health (WPATH) has referred to these procedures as medically necessary (Knudson et al., 2016). Examples include lipofilling of hips, thighs, and buttocks and liposuction of abdomen, flanks, hips, and thighs. Several implants can be done, including buttocks, pectoral, and calf implants. A lift and reduction of the mons pubis can serve to reduce the size of the fat pad of the mons.

Additional procedures related to accessing surgical procedures include electrolysis, laser hair removal, and hair grafts. Skin grafts and care are necessary for sites (e.g., leg, forearm) used in phalloplasty surgeries that require skin, vessels, and tissue. Although the aforementioned additional procedures are less commonly covered by insurance, Starbucks made history by being the first company in the United States to provide comprehensive insurance benefits to transgender employees that cover all of these procedures (Anapol, 2018).

HISTORY OF PSYCHOLOGICAL ASSESSMENTS FOR GENDER EMBODIMENT SURGERIES

WPATH is a professional multidisciplinary association with a stated mission of promoting awareness and advancement in the care and research of transgender and gender nonconforming individuals. Since 1979, WPATH has set forth its international *Standards of Care for the Health of Transsexual, Transgender, and Gender Nonconforming People* (*SOC*) that include criteria that transgender people need to meet to access surgical procedures. As of this writing, seven versions of the WPATH *SOC* have been published. A huge shift from version 6 to 7 (*SOC7*; Coleman et al., 2012) was that a duration of psychotherapy was no longer a requirement for accessing surgical care. The *SOC7* requires one or more mental health assessments, depending on which surgery is being accessed.

Criteria for accessing breast/chest surgery in adults are (a) persistent, well-documented gender dysphoria (GD); (b) capacity to make a fully informed decision and to consent for treatment; (c) age of majority in a given country; and (d) if significant medical or mental health concerns are present, they must be reasonably well controlled (Coleman et al., 2012). Hormone therapy is not a prerequisite for mastectomy but is commonly required by surgeons for breast augmentation to maximize breast development from estrogen treatment.

Criteria for gonadectomy/internal genital surgery (hysterectomy with salpingo-oophorectomy and orchiectomy) to address GD—not for other medical reasons—include the aforementioned four criteria. They also include 12 months of hormone therapy as appropriate for a patient's treatment goals—unless hormone therapy is not indicated in their case.

Criteria for external genital surgery (i.e., vaginoplasty, phalloplasty, and metoidioplasty) include all previous criteria plus 12 continuous months of living as their true gender self. This has historically been called the "real-life test" and has been fiercely criticized by transgender community advocates and health professionals, who maintain that this requirement can be dangerous for many people, especially trans people of color who are at higher risk of being murdered than their White counterparts.

Two mental health assessments that result in letters approving a person for surgery are required for gonadectomy and genital surgeries; in many cases, one letter is required to come from a psychologist/mental health professional who holds a doctoral degree. One letter is required for breast/chest surgeries. No criteria are provided for facial surgery or body-contouring surgery. Psychotherapy is not a requirement for accessing gender embodiment surgery.

Several criticisms of requiring mental health assessments for access to surgery hold merit. The majority of psychologists and mental health professionals have neither received adequate nor comprehensive training in providing this type of assessment. Further, they are neither familiar with the multiple surgical options available nor the process of recovering from a major surgery. No research supports the guidelines and criteria listed in the WPATH *SOC7* (Coleman et al., 2012; see also Deutsch, 2016). It has been argued that *gatekeeping*—the positioning of psychologists and mental health professionals between transgender people seeking to access surgery and surgeons for the purpose of conducting mental health assessments—provides more anxiety reduction for psychologists and mental health professionals, including surgeons, as well as legal protection for surgeons rather than a care service for the patients themselves (Puckett et al., 2018).

Historically, the purpose of gatekeeping was to determine if patients were *really* transgender or not. Clinicians typically came from an *endocisheteronormative framework* (Hastings et al., 2021), which favored transgender people who wanted their postoperative bodies to closely approximate those of *endosex*—individuals born with physical characteristics that can be clearly categorized as male or female (Carpenter et al., 2022)—and not *intersex*—an umbrella term for differences in sex traits, genitalia, hormones, internal anatomy, or chromosomes (InterACT Advocates for Intersex Youth, n.d.)—cisgender people and function in heteronormative sexual activity. This led to denials of access to care if a person acknowledged that they would not be using their new genitals for "heterosexual" (i.e., penovaginal penetration) sexual practices. Thus, lesbian, bisexual, gay, and queer people were denied access to surgery. Many clinicians would comment on how "passable" they thought the patient would be postoperatively, with those who were more "convincing" (i.e., gender conforming, heteronormative, with specific body shapes) being more likely to be allowed access to care (Meyerowitz, 2004). Patients who were allowed access to surgery also had to be gender conforming—meaning stereotypically feminine women or masculine men. Many patients would spend hours dressing up for their assessments.

Many clinicians who routinely provided presurgical psychological assessments (PPAs) for transgender individuals came from a psychosexual perspective. In 2007, one of us (C. St. Amand) was asked details about his masturbatory practices and sexual fantasies when being assessed for double mastectomy surgery. Today, we argue this line of questioning is highly inappropriate and unnecessary because it was not related to the process of undergoing or recovering from surgery. He would have much preferred information about how undergoing this surgery would affect resulting chest and nipple sensation.

Endonormativity—that is, privileging endosex phenotypes over intersex phenotypes—has been and still is inherent in access to gender embodiment surgery. Historically, surgeons have proceeded with complex procedures, such as phalloplasty with vaginectomy, without asking patients about their embodiment goals. The endonormative assumption was that the patient would not desire to keep their vagina/G spot because "he is a man" (a WPATH surgeon in Belgium,[2] June 18, 2009). Although that reasoning appears to be gender affirming, the assumption that having both a penis and a vagina is less desirable than one or the other is an example of endonormativity.

The transgender population is vibrant and full of strongly resilient people. Black and Brown transgender people have faced unimaginable barriers to accessing care. They have used their creativity and resilience to create what is known as the *trans-script* from which they learn what answers given to the psychologists and mental health professionals conducting assessments will result in access to care (shuster, 2021). Thus, the community has shared this knowledge and provided these answers to access care that was needed. This, of course, has resulted in further distrust and mistrust on the part of trans people in most—if not all—cisgender psychologists and mental health professionals.

Psychologists and mental health professionals in trans health have taken different approaches to their positioning as gatekeepers. Some who reject

[2]The communicator requested anonymity.

the position as gatekeepers write letters without a providing a comprehensive mental health assessment out of an ethical stance that a person has the autonomy to access surgery and are able to provide their own consent without need for a comprehensive psychological assessment. They point to examples of cisgender patients' accessing major life-altering surgeries without the need for psychological assessments (shuster, 2021). Thus, requiring transgender people to undergo comprehensive mental health assessments to access surgery is a form of discrimination in which many psychologists and mental health professionals do not want to take part.

HISTORY OF PATHOLOGIZING OF TRANSGENDER IDENTITY THROUGH DIAGNOSES

Beginning with the first and second editions of the *Diagnostic and Statistical Manual of Mental Disorders* (*DSM-I*; American Psychiatric Association, 1952; *DSM-II*; American Psychiatric Association, 1968), the diagnoses of transvestism and homosexuality were present, pathologizing cross-dressing and attraction to members of the same sex as "sexual deviations." The third edition of the *Diagnostic and Statistical Manual of Mental Disorders* (*DSM-III*; American Psychiatric Association, 1980) introduced gender identity disorders (GIDs) that describe the incongruence between anatomic sex and gender identity as a mental health disorder and include transvestism. The classification of the transgender identity as a mental health disorder is pathologizing; however, it allowed an avenue for insurance to cover gender embodiment surgeries and hormone therapy (American Psychiatric Association, 1980). The classification caused an uproar in the transgender community: Some stated their contentment with an avenue for insurance coverage for affirming procedures, whereas others lamented the classification of the transgender identity as a mental health disorder. This second group argued that the classification also opened the door for practitioners of conversion therapy to harm transgender people through shaming the individuals for having a mental disorder (Langer & Martin, 2004).

The fourth edition of the *Diagnostic and Statistical Manual of Mental Disorders* (*DSM-IV*; American Psychiatric Association, 1994), released in 1994, replaced GIDs with a singular version, GID, and eliminated the use of "transsexualism" as a descriptor of those with GID. It also was reclassified as a sexual disorder rather than a psychological one. The criteria described stereotypical cross-gender behaviors and implied abnormal sexuality. The criteria did not include many mentions of the different psychosocial difficulties that come from being transgender in a society that punishes gender-variant behavior and identity. Notably, the GID diagnosis for children noted the cross-gender behaviors often exhibited as symptoms of a sexual disorder and imply abnormal gender identity development (American Psychiatric Association, 1994).

With the publication in 2013 of the fifth edition of the *Diagnostic and Statistical Manual of Mental Disorders* (*DSM-5*; American Psychiatric Association, 2013), GID was replaced with the diagnosis of GD, a label that can be removed from the medical record if the need for gender embodiment surgery or hormone treatment is no longer present. Although GID focused on adult cross-gender behavior and its pathologization, GD focuses on the desires of the individual to transition and identify as transgender. Notably, the language in the GD diagnosis is broader to include nonbinary and gender nonconforming individuals who require the diagnosis to access treatment (American Psychiatric Association, 2013).

In a press release in June 2018, the World Health Organization (2018), the body that publishes the *International Statistical Classification of Diseases and Related Health Problems*, announced that the new 11th edition (WHO, 2019) would reclassify "gender incongruence" as a sexual health condition, rather than the previous classification as a mental health disorder.

THE PPA FOR GENDER EMBODIMENT SURGERY

With the tarnished history of the gatekeeping and discriminatory nature of mental health assessments, many may wonder: How do we move forward? Although reading this chapter is an important step in the process, it will not fully prepare one to effectively or ethically complete a PPA. This is a developing field involving a variety of personal considerations (e.g., examination of personal biases, lack of education in this area) to address before being competent to assess for these procedures. No consensus on best practice for assessments for gender embodiment surgery exists. No personality, intelligence, or neuropsychological testing batteries have been validated for assessment and psychological testing on transgender adults for the purpose of PPAs (Keo-Meier & Fitzgerald, 2017) and are not recommended for use as part of this process.

In considering all of this, we, the chapter authors, have found a middle ground: focusing on facilitating a person's access to desired treatments and ensuring that they are psychologically and practically prepared to undergo and recover from surgery. Although at least one PPA by a psychologist/mental health professional is required to access surgery, neither the American Psychological Association (APA) nor WPATH has presented a comprehensive example of such an assessment. They do suggest domains to cover, including emotional functioning, social history, family history, and relationship history (APA, 2015; Coleman et al., 2012). The purpose of covering these domains is to collaboratively identify sources of support and resources as well as potential factors that would affect individuals' ability to recover safely. Examples of such factors include unstable housing, active opioid misuse, and lack of an identified caregiver. To our knowledge, the only comprehensive assessment is the Gender Affirmative Supportive Surgery Evaluation Tool (Gender ASSET; St. Amand & Keo, 2016); a 6-hour APA continuing education webinar is available that offers training for the provision of this PPA (see https://thegenderu.com/). At this time, more than 200 providers have been trained to use this evaluation tool, the major components of which we summarize later in the chapter.

The *SOC7* (Coleman et al., 2012) states that the purpose of a PPA is to provide information on a person's psychological and practical preparation to undergo and recover from a surgical procedure. This assessment is not to determine whether a person is transgender or not, nor is it a universal evaluation to assess capacity; a capacity evaluation is unnecessary unless there is a question about a person's capacity. In a 2016 article, Maddie Deutsch argued that patients benefit from education during the PPA to develop realistic expectations about surgery and the recovery process as well as resources to undergo and recover well from surgery.

Criteria for Access to Surgery

Surgeons and insurance companies commonly require "the letter" from psychologists and mental health professionals for clients to access gender embodiment surgery per the *SOC7* (Coleman et al., 2012). Although the APA (2015) *Guidelines for Psychological Practice With Transgender and Gender Nonconforming People* directly address the importance of offering care that affirms the patient's gender identity (see Guideline 11), the guidelines do not provide any specific recommendations for how to conduct the assessment or discuss the role of psychologists and mental health professionals in granting access to gender embodiment surgery through letters of support (APA, 2015).

Because that letter is what clients are seeking and ultimately provides them with access to surgery, it is critical that evaluators understand the required letter content that includes at least three sources of criteria: (a) the surgeon, (b) the insurance company, and (c) the *SOC7* (Coleman et al., 2012). The first two vary by individual client, and the third one does not. The *SOC7* recommends that the letter includes the patient's general identifying characteristics; results of the patient's psychosocial assessment, including any diagnoses; the duration of the psychologist/mental health professional's relationship with the patient, including the type of evaluation and therapy or counseling to date; an explanation that the criteria for surgery have been met as well as a brief description of the clinical rationale for supporting the patient's request for surgery; a statement about the fact that informed consent has been obtained from the patient; and a statement that the psychologist/mental health professional is available for coordination of care and welcomes a phone call to establish such (Coleman et al., 2012). It is important for the psychologist/mental health professional to speak with their client and ask that the client attempt to provide their surgeon's and insurance's list of letter criteria. Having this information from the outset can make a big difference in the amount of time it takes for the client to access care because, if the letter is missing one of their insurance policy's criteria, the psychologist/mental health professional may have to appeal the decision and include another letter with the additional criteria.

The Gender ASSET (St. Amand & Keo, 2016) is a comprehensive, collaborative, clinical interview that comprises three sections: (a) gender history, (b) psychosocial history, and (c) practical preparation. The purpose of the Gender ASSET is to facilitate access to treatment, provide clients with accurate information, ensure that they make a fully informed decision, prepare them for the recovery process, and reduce the likelihood of dissatisfaction or regret. Client's chosen name, pronouns (e.g., they, she, he), and honorifics (e.g., Ms., Mx., Mr., Mrs., Dr.) should be used throughout the evaluation and letter-writing process. If the client's legal name is different from their chosen name, for insurance coverage, the legal name only needs to appear one time on the letter (see Appendix 6.1 for sample text). When providing informed consent for the PPA, it is important to inform clients of possible outcomes from the assessment. Outcomes include a letter for surgery or further preparation with the evaluator or another clinician to support their preparation for surgery. In both cases, the evaluator should still be willing to provide a letter as the client becomes prepared to undergo and recover from surgery, and should clearly communicate what the client needs to obtain the letter as well as ensure that the client is connected with the resources to meet these needs.

Section 1: Gender History

Clinicians should use the gender history questions to learn information relevant to the client's specific gender embodiment goals (e.g., size C breasts with silicone implants penis with glans, radial forearm flap, testicular implants, retention of the vagina, ability to urinate) and the status of their planning process. Possible questions to explore in gender history include these:

- What surgery are they seeking?
- What are their embodiment goals? Say the client presents for evaluation for double mastectomy. Ask, for example, "Do you want nipples? If so, what size? Do you want nipple grafts or nipples tattooed on postoperatively?"
- Have they chosen a surgeon?
- Do they have a timeline in mind?
- Where will they stay to recover?
- Will they be able to get off of work or school?
- Who will take them to appointments, provide postoperative care and meals, and organize and administer medications?
- Do they have a primary doctor to complete their preoperative medical evaluation?
- What is their understanding of what their desired procedure and recovery entail?
- What is their experience since coming out as transgender?

The APA (2015) *Guidelines for Psychological Practice With Transgender and Gender Nonconforming People* recommend gathering, during a psychosocial assessment of life domains, information about the person's experience with externalized and internalized prejudice and discrimination as well as their means of coping and resilience.

When assessing a client who is seeking to access external genital surgery, many psychologists and mental health professionals will benefit from a review of genital anatomy with the client to facilitate communication of embodiment goals and encourage the client to choose what feels right for them, regardless if it is thought to be "normal." Evaluators should also realize that some client's goals and priorities may change over time; therefore, completing evaluations for external genital surgery in two to three sessions can be helpful because the client has time to process information and solidify plans for undergoing and recovering from surgery. This is in contrast to assessments for face, chest, and body-contouring surgeries, which providers are more likely to complete in one to two sessions.

Section 2: Psychosocial History

A psychosocial history should be similar to what the clinician typically uses for a general psychological assessment and include information about the client's living situation, education, work, mental health history (e.g., previous diagnoses, medications, therapy, hospitalizations, access to care, abuse history, substance use), medical history, fertility goals, and sexual history as relevant to the specific surgery. Although a mental health assessment is neither necessary nor recommended for assessment of suitability of a client for surgery, the client can consent to additional mental health support from the clinician. If the client has a significant mental health history and consents to further exploration of mental health history, evaluators may consider using nongendered symptom inventories—for example, the Beck Depression Inventory (Beck et al., 1996), Beck Anxiety Inventory (Beck & Steer, 1993), Life Events Checklist for the *DSM-5* (American Psychiatric Association, 2013), or Mood Disorder Questionnaire (Hirschfield et al., 2000)—to confirm diagnoses and inform individual recommendations. Those with severe depression may take longer to recover from surgery than those without depression and therefore would benefit from knowing this information. Those with a history of trauma may benefit from additional time with nursing to review the process of surgery and who will see or touch their body. Those with specific fears, such as going under anesthesia, may benefit from having nurses be aware of this fear before intravenous placement. Providing these recommendations can aid in normalizing the client's individual experience of their recovery and provide information to aid in successful recovery.

To inform more accurate case conceptualizations, evaluators should be well versed in the gender affirmative model (Keo-Meier & Ehrensaft, 2018), gender minority stress theory (Hendricks & Testa, 2012), and the effects of GD on mental health. Mental health conditions are not in and of themselves contraindications for gender embodiment surgery unless they affect a person's ability to recover from surgery, such as a current active psychotic episode (Coleman et al., 2012). It is sometimes the case that mental health conditions that may concern the evaluator are alleviated by the treatment in and of itself (Pflum et al., 2015). One criterion for surgery is that mental health conditions should be reasonably well controlled (Coleman et al., 2012). We, the chapter authors, interpret this as whether the mental health condition significantly affects the client's ability to undergo and recover from surgery (e.g., housing instability). In this case, it is the responsibility of the evaluator and care team to connect the client with resources to address the factors that affect the client's ability to undergo and recover from surgery.

Section 3: Practical Preparation

This third section of the Gender ASSET (St. Amand & Keo, 2016) tends to be the most useful for the client and their caregiver(s) who, if at all possible, accompany the client to this portion of the assessment. This portion of the assessment addresses considerations for practical preparation. The evaluator, client, and caregiver review information relevant to the surgeon's pre- and postoperative care instructions; time line for operation(s) and hospital stay; plans for transportation; and possible risks and complications, including plans to respond to them. They also review the expectations for postoperative appearance and functioning, plans to take off of school or work, accommodations for recovery, preparation for undergoing anesthesia, common medications during recovery (e.g., antibiotics, stool softeners, pain medication), comfort levels with changing wound dressings postsurgery and emptying drains/catheter bags, help with bathing, how to handle surgical drains, how to organize and administer medications, assurance that the client has adequate hydration and nutrition, a discussion of bowel habits, dressing of the client, opioid pain medication use, and activity limitations during recovery.

A psychologist/mental health professional may not be best suited to complete this section of the Gender ASSET. Indeed, a nurse, social worker, transgender peer navigator, or another care team members may be better prepared to conduct this part of the assessment with the client and caregiver (see Table 6.1 for an example of a recovery diary for a caregiver to keep).

TABLE 6.1. Sample Recovery Diary for Caregiver

Medications (dosage, time given)	**Day 0**	**Day 1**	**Day 2**
Pain			
Antibiotics			
Stool softeners			
Vitamin C			
Zinc			
Intake (amount, time)	**Day 0**	**Day 1**	**Day 2**
Water			
Food			
Output (amount, description, time)	**Day 0**	**Day 1**	**Day 2**
Bowel movement			
Catheter			
Drains (if applicable)			
Dilation (if applicable)			
Complications			

Evaluator Preparedness

Providers should conduct their own self-assessment of psychological and practical preparedness to provide PPAs for gender embodiment surgery. This is especially relevant if the evaluator is endosex and cisgender and therefore will never have to be the client who is being assessed by someone else in this context. First, the evaluator needs to make sure to have the proper training, supervision, and consultation to provide this service. It is not ethical to provide a PPA for someone seeking a surgery that the evaluator is not familiar with. Attending a conference presentation is not sufficient to provide best care, and psychologists and mental health professionals are encouraged to complete their first PPA under supervision and seek ongoing consultation as they provide more of these assessments in the future. Providers should operate with a gender affirmative lens, thus endorsing the ethical mindset that each individual is the expert in their own experience and gender embodiment goals. This is a patient-centered, collaborative, trauma-informed approach that moves to empower the client to know what they know and make decisions about their own life. The evaluator's goal should be to facilitate access to and healthy recovery from the desired intervention.

Using a trauma-informed approach, evaluators should be transparent and up-front with their PPA process, including anticipated costs. This is especially true in light of the history of gatekeeping and positioning of a psychologist/mental health professional as another "hoop to jump through" to access surgery. It is important to delineate the difference between psychotherapy and evaluation/assessment services because a client may not be aware of the difference, and this is an important part of the informed consent process. Unlike many other circumstances outside of transgender care, if a therapist has been working with a client for support with their gender journey, it is absolutely appropriate for them to provide PPA services to their client—assuming the therapist has appropriate training. In these cases, the therapist should already have a gender history and psychosocial history on the client and will really only need to complete the practical preparation section.

If an evaluator and client complete an evaluation together and *collaboratively* determine that the client is not ready to access surgery, the work of the evaluator is not done. Hundreds of anecdotal reports within the community have indicated that trans people attempted to get a letter for surgery and were either told that they needed to attend therapy longer—and then never actually received a letter—or the therapist decided, after hundreds of dollars were spent on therapy, that they were unable to provide the letter. These experiences have further traumatized the population and increased the already present distrust of the field of mental health held by many trans people. Again, the role of the evaluator is to help facilitate access. Specific recommendations should be provided for what would help prepare the client to access surgery. Perhaps the person does not have stable housing, a place to recover safely, or someone to provide postoperative care. Another client may be actively using substances that may interfere with a healthy recovery. Evaluators should work to connect the client to relevant resources and work collaboratively with the surgeon's office staff to make sure the client has what they need for a safe and healthy recovery. Recognizing systemic barriers to accessing and recovering from surgery as well as supporting clients to overcome these barriers can facilitate an improved perioperative course (Deutsch, 2016).

MOVING FORWARD

It is our hope that all transgender people will be able to access the care they need to obtain their desired gender embodiment—and the requirement of a universal mental health assessment before accessing surgery will no longer exist. Although a mental health assessment may be helpful if questions exist about a client's ability to make an informed consent or to undergo and recover from surgery, requiring mental health assessments for all people who are accessing gender embodiment surgery is a form of continued psychopathologization of the transgender community.

Instead of focusing on mental health assessments, we hope gender care providers will focus more on interdisciplinary care in which clients are provided with the information and resources they need about the processes of undergoing and recovering from gender embodiment surgeries in a way that prioritizes autonomy, collaboration, and wellness. We believe that although psychologists and mental health professionals can be an important part of a gender care team, they should not be positioned as gatekeepers, and their evaluation of clients should not be a universal requirement to access gender embodiment surgeries in the future.

APPENDIX 6.1: EXAMPLE LETTER

Date: [DATE]
TO: [NAME OF SURGEON]
Client Name: [NAME] **Pronouns:** [PRONOUNS] **Age:** [AGE] **DOB:** [DATE OF BIRTH]
Legal Name: [LEGAL NAME OF CLIENT]

Referring Provider: [NAME OF PSYCHOLOGIST/MENTAL HEALTH PROFESSIONAL AND CREDENTIALS]
Dates of Assessment: [DATES]
Surgery: [MEDICAL TERM FOR SURGICAL PROCEDURE(S) WITH SPECIFIC GOALS]

Examples:

- Double mastectomy with nipple grafts
- Penile inversion vaginoplasty with adequate depth for receptive penetration, orchiectomy, clitoroplasty, and labiaplasty with protruding labia minora
- Radial forearm flap phalloplasty with urethral lengthening and nerve hookup, glansplasty, endogenous glans (clitoris) burial, scrotoplasty with testicular implants, and erectile device implantation
- Anterolateral thigh phalloplasty with phallus (7 inches), with nerve hookup, glansplasty, urethral lengthening, and vaginectomy; at this time, [PRONOUN] is considering whether [PRONOUN] desires scrotoplasty with testicular implants and erectile device implantation. [PRONOUN] postoperative goals, in order of prioritization, are: appearance, sensate penis, penetrative sex, and stand to pee

Reason for Referral

[NAME OF CLIENT] is a [NUMBER]-year-old transgender person who presented for an independent assessment before undergoing [MEDICAL TERM FOR PROCEDURE(S)] with [NAME OF SURGEON] as part of [PRONOUN] gender transition. [PRONOUN] was self-referred for a comprehensive presurgical assessment for [MEDICAL TERM FOR PROCEDURE(S)]. Following version 7 of the World Professional Association for Transgender Health (WPATH) *Standards of Care for the Health of Transsexual, Transgender, and Gender Nonconforming People* (*SOC7*), this report is derived from my independent evaluation in addition to the additional independent evaluation from a licensed therapist, [NAME OF THERAPIST], who supports [PRONOUN] plan for [MEDICAL TERM FOR SURGICAL PROCEDURE(S)].

I assessed [NAME OF CLIENT]'s psychological and practical preparedness for surgery according to *SOC7* set forth by WPATH. We completed a comprehensive psychosocial assessment and surgery recovery preparation education using the Gender Affirmative Supportive Surgery Evaluation Tool (Gender ASSET; St. Amand & Keo, 2016). Their close friend and family member, [NAME OF CAREGIVER], has agreed to be their caretaker throughout the surgery and recovery process. I met with [NAME OF CAREGIVER] to review the expected postoperative course and plan for emergencies, and I also answered their questions.

Psychologist/Mental Health Professional's Background

Sample text:

I am a licensed psychologist specializing in work with transgender and gender expansive individuals. My experience with transgender individuals includes 10 years serving more than 200 individual, couples, and group therapy clients. I am a certified member of the World Professional Association for Transgender Health (WPATH) *Standards of Care for the Health of Transsexual, Transgender, and Gender Nonconforming People*, version 7 (*SOC7*), and a WPATH Global Education Institute mentor who trains providers for certification. I have been a member of WPATH for 10 years and follow the *SOC* set forth by this organization.

My practice has included psychotherapy and assessment of transgender and gender expansive individuals—both those who do and do not wish to make a physical transition via hormone therapy and/or surgery. I have published research in peer-reviewed journals on the effects of hormone therapy and surgery on the mental health and sexuality of transgender people.

Expectations and Qualifications for Care

Circle one: Y = Yes, N = No.

- Client has been diagnosed with persistent, well documented gender dysphoria. Y N
- Client's gender dysphoria is not a symptom of another mental health disorder. Y N
- Client's gender dysphoria causes clinically significant distress or impairment in social, occupational, or other important areas of functioning. Y N
- Client has completed over 2 years of living as [PRONOUN] true gender self across all environments. Y N

- Client has been treated with and prescribed hormone therapy. Y N
- Client has completed a minimum of 12 continuous months of living in a gender role that is congruent with [PRONOUN] gender identity across a wide range of life experience and events that may occur throughout the year. Y N
- Client has been informed of the expectations for care and risks and benefits, and client has shown the ability give informed consent and understand this information. Y N

WPATH Criteria for Surgery

1. [NAME OF CLIENT] has a history of persistent, well-documented gender dysphoria.
2. Psychologically, there are no indicators that [PRONOUN] is not making a fully informed and reasonable decision.
3. [PRONOUN] is of majority age.
4. There are no significant mental health issues present that would prevent [PRONOUN] from making a fully informed consent for or undergoing and recovering from surgery.
5. [NAME OF CLIENT] has undergone more than 12 months of hormone therapy.

Treatment Recommendation and Plan for Support

Sample text:

We have discussed the expectations for surgery, including surgical outcomes, the next steps in the process, the risks associated with this procedure, and the components of recovering from multiple surgeries. [NAME OF CLIENT] understands how smoking and alcohol use affect outcomes. Denies the use of cigarettes and other drugs. Smokes 5 cigarettes/day, has a plan to quit smoking by [DATE]. Currently drinks alcohol socially. Drinks alcohol excessively on weekends; does have a plan to decrease alcohol use and abstain from alcohol before surgery and during recovery. Plans for postoperative recovery were discussed with [NAME OF CLIENT] and [NAME OF CAREGIVER]. [PRONOUN] is able to comply with long-term follow-up requirements.

Support/Care Plan

[Sample plan]

Plan	Yes	No	In process	Notes
Client has made plans for pre- and postcare, including transportation, support network, how to meet basic needs, ongoing maintenance	X			Plans to stay at home and have [NAME OF CAREGIVER] provide support throughout the process
Client has been made aware of possible complications, including the effects of medications used in procedure	X			

Summary

The current assessment results indicate that [NAME OF CLIENT] meets WPATH criteria for [TYPE OF SURGERY], is capable of making informed decisions regarding medical treatment, and has given informed consent for surgery. [NAME OF CLIENT] has realistic expectations of the effects and risks of surgery.

I fully support [NAME OF CLIENT]'s decision to undergo [MEDICAL TERM FOR PROCEDURE(S)] as part of [PRONOUN] gender transition and believe it to be clinically indicated and medically necessary in this case. It is my professional opinion that [PRONOUN] [is/are] approaching this decision rationally and exercising good judgment. I anticipate that [PRONOUN] will find the effects of surgery satisfying and rewarding. Please feel free to contact me should you have any questions or need any further information. Thank you in advance for the care that you will provide to [NAME OF CLIENT].

____

[NAME OF PSYCHOLOGIST/MENTAL HEALTH PROFESSIONAL],
[CREDENTIALS], [EMAIL ADDRESS]
[LICENSE AND NUMBER] [PHONE NUMBER]
Signed Electronically [DATE]

Note. For this letter, use the clinician's letterhead.

REFERENCES

American Psychiatric Association. (1952). *Diagnostic and statistical manual of mental disorders*.

American Psychiatric Association. (1968). *Diagnostic and statistical manual of mental disorders* (2nd ed.).

American Psychiatric Association. (1980). *Diagnostic and statistical manual of mental disorders* (3rd ed.).

American Psychiatric Association. (1994). *Diagnostic and statistical manual of mental disorders* (4th ed.).

American Psychiatric Association. (2013). *Diagnostic and statistical manual of mental disorders* (5th ed.).

American Psychological Association. (2015). Guidelines for psychological practice with transgender and gender nonconforming people. *American Psychologist, 70*(9), 832–864. https://doi.org/10.1037/a0039906

Anapol, A. (2018, June 26). Starbucks expands health benefits for transgender employees. *The Hill*. https://thehill.com/blogs/blog-briefing-room/394221-starbucks-expands-health-benefits-for-transgender-employees Accessed September 23, 2018.

Beck, A. T., & Steer, R. A. (1993). *Beck Anxiety Inventory*. Psychological Corporation.

Beck, A. T., Steer, R. A., & Brown, G. K. (1996). *Manual for the Beck Depression Inventory-II*. Psychological Corporation.

Blumberg, N. (2021, September 9). Lili Elbe. *Britannica*. https://www.britannica.com/biography/Lili-Elbe

Carpenter, M., Dalke, K. B., & Earp, B. D. (2022). Endosex. *Journal of Medical Ethics*. Advance online publication. https://doi.org/10.1136/medethics-2022-108317

Coleman, E., Bockting, W., Botzer, M., Cohen-Kettenis, P., DeCuypere, G., Feldman, J., Fraser, L., Green, J., Knudson, G., Meyer, W. J., Monstrey, S., Adler, R. K., Brown, G. R., Devor, A. H., Ehrbar, R., Ettner, R., Eyler, E., Garofalo, R., Karasic, D. H., . . . Zucker, K. (2012). Standards of Care for the Health of Transsexual, Transgender, and Gender-Nonconforming People, version 7. *International Journal of Transgenderism, 13*(4), 165–232. https://doi.org/10.1080/15532739.2011.700873

Davies, S., Papp, V. G., & Antoni, C. (2015). Voice and communication change for gender nonconforming individuals: Giving voice to the person inside. *International Journal of Transgenderism, 16*(3), 117–159. https://doi.org/10.1080/15532739.2015.1075931

Deutsch, M. B. (2016). Gender-affirming surgeries in the era of insurance coverage: Developing a framework for psychosocial support and care navigation in the perioperative period. *Journal of Health Care for the Poor and Underserved, 27*(2), 386–391. https://doi.org/10.1353/hpu.2016.0092

Hastings, J., Bobb, C., Wolfe, M., Amaro Jimenez, Z., & St. Amand, C. (2021). Medical care for nonbinary youth: Individualized gender care beyond a binary framework. *Pediatric Annals, 50*(9), e384–e390. https://doi.org/10.3928/19382359-20210818-03

Hendricks, M. L., & Testa, R. J. (2012). A conceptual framework for clinical work with transgender and gender nonconforming clients: An adaptation of the minority stress model. *Professional Psychology: Research and Practice, 43*(5), 460467. https://doi.org/10.1037/a0029597

Hirschfield, R. M. A., Williams, J. B. W., Spitzer, R. L., Calabrese, J. R., Flynn, L., Keck, P E., Jr., Lewis, L., McElroy, S. L., Post, R. M., Rapport, D. J., Russell, J. M., Sachs, G. S., & Zajecka, J. (2000). Development and validation of a screening instrument for bipolar spectrum disorder: The Mood Disorder Questionnaire. *The American Journal of Psychiatry, 157*(11), 1873–1875. https://doi.org/10.1176/appi.ajp.157.11.1873

InterACT Advocates for Intersex Youth. (n.d.). *Intersex definitions.* https://interactadvocates.org/intersex-definitions/

Keo-Meier, C., & Ehrensaft, D. (2018). *The gender affirmative model: An interdisciplinary approach to supporting transgender and gender expansive children.* American Psychological Association.

Keo-Meier, C. L., & Fitzgerald, K. M. (2017). Affirmative psychological testing and neurocognitive assessment with transgender adults. *Psychiatric Clinics, 40*(1), 51–64. https://doi.org/10.1016/j.psc.2016.10.011

Knudson, G., Tangpricha, V., Green, J., Bouman, W. P., Ettner, R., Adrian, T., & Winter, S. (2016). *Position Statement on Medical Necessity of Treatment, Sex Reassignment, and Insurance Coverage in the USA.* World Professional Association for Transgender Health.

Langer, S. J, & Martin, J. I (2004). How dresses can make you mentally ill: Examining gender identity disorder in children. *Child and Adolescent Social Work Journal, 21*, 5–23. https://doi.org/10.1023/B:CASW.0000012346.80025.f7

Meyerowitz, J. (2004). *How sex changed: A history of transsexuality in the United States.* Harvard University Press. https://doi.org/10.2307/j.ctv1c7zfrv

Pflum, S. R., Testa, R. J., Balsam, K. F., Goldblum, P. B., & Bongar, B. (2015). Social support, trans community connectedness, and mental health symptoms among transgender and gender nonconforming adults. *Psychology of Sexual Orientation and Gender Diversity, 2*(3), 281–286. https://doi.org/10.1037/sgd0000122

Puckett, J. A., Cleary, P., Rossman, K., Mustanski, B., & Newcomb, M. E. (2018). Barriers to gender-affirming care for transgender and gender nonconforming individuals. *Sexuality Research and Social Policy, 15*(1), 48–59. https://doi.org/10.1007/s13178-017-0295-8

shuster, s. m. (2021). *Trans medicine: The emergence and practice of treating gender.* New York University Press. https://doi.org/10.18574/nyu/9781479836291.001.0001

St. Amand, C. M., & Keo, B. (2016). *The Gender ASSET: Gender Affirmative Supportive Surgery Evaluation Tool* [Online course]. The Gender U. https://thegenderu.com/courses/thegenderasset

World Health Organization. (2018, June 22). *ICD-11: Classifying disease to map the way we live and die* [Press release]. https://www.afro.who.int/news/icd-11-classifying-disease-map-way-we-live-and-die

World Health Organization. (2019). *International statistical classification of diseases and related health problems* (11th ed.). https://icd.who.int/

7 SURGERY FOR TREATMENT AND PREVENTION OF BREAST CANCER

ANDREA BRADFORD

Breast cancer is the most common type of cancer in women worldwide (Sung et al., 2021). In the United States, approximately 13% of women are diagnosed with breast cancer at some point in their lifetimes. Because of advances in treatment, mortality from the disease has gradually declined over the past 3 decades. Most breast cancers are diagnosed at an early stage before cancer cells have spread to distant areas of the body (metastasis). According to the National Cancer Institute (n.d.), approximately 90% of women with breast cancer survive at least 5 years after diagnosis. Breast cancer now accounts for 30% of cancer diagnoses but only about 15% of cancer-related deaths in U.S. women (American Cancer Society, 2021). Breast cancer occurs in men relatively rarely (just under 1% of breast cancers) but is associated with somewhat greater mortality. This is likely because of disparities in breast cancer detection and treatment in men compared with women (Wang et al., 2019).

Risk factors for breast cancer include female sex, increasing age, and a strong family history of breast cancer. Other risk factors include certain types of hormonal exposures (e.g., longer than average menstrual history;

https://doi.org/10.1037/0000346-008
Psychological Assessment of Surgical Candidates: Evidence-Based Procedures and Practices, R. J. Marek and A. R. Block (Editors)

use of hormone replacement therapy with estrogen and progestin after menopause); a history of benign atypical cell growth in the breast; and lifestyle factors, including low physical activity level, excess weight (only in postmenopausal women), and higher alcohol use. About 5% to 10% of breast cancers are linked to a strong family history of breast cancer or hereditary risk factors, including inherited mutations in the *BRCA1* and *BRCA2* genes as well as less common mutations (e.g., *PALB2, CHEK2,* Lynch syndrome). More than two thirds of women with high-risk *BRCA1* or *BRCA2* mutations will develop breast cancer in their lifetimes without preventive intervention (Kuchenbaecker et al., 2017).

The vast majority of patients with breast cancer are treated with surgery to partially or completely remove the affected breast(s). Increasingly, breast surgery is also used for cancer prevention in women who have a strong family history of breast cancer or a high-risk genetic mutation. Although surgery is not a routine component of treatment in patients who have distant metastases (i.e., cancer that has spread beyond the primary site of the tumor), surgery may be used for palliative purposes on a case-by-case basis.

There are a number of compelling reasons to implement psychological screening and assessment in people with breast cancer. First, people with breast cancer and hereditary cancer syndromes have a high burden of adjustment difficulties, anxiety, mood disturbance, sleep disturbance, and body image concerns after treatment. Psychological problems in this population are treatable and can be comanaged effectively alongside cancer therapy and other medical management (Ye et al., 2018). Second, although most breast cancer survivors adapt well over time, a significant minority experience long-term psychological difficulty after treatment. Several risk factors for poorer long-term adjustment are identifiable early in the course of cancer treatment and may be able to be addressed before problems escalate. Third, psychological difficulties may complicate recovery from cancer treatment. For example, depression is a risk factor for increased surgical complications and increased length of stay in patients who undergo breast reconstruction (Drinane et al., 2019). Although early identification of psychological difficulties is a desirable goal, some patients with persistent or worsening distress may not be referred for psychological assessment until well after surgery.

In the United States, assessment of psychological distress before or after breast cancer surgery is implemented variably, if at all, across clinicians and health care organizations. However, professional societies and accrediting bodies are increasingly recognizing the importance of addressing patients' psychosocial needs in cancer care. In 2012, the American College of Surgeons Commission on Cancer (2012) adopted new standards for accrediting cancer care programs, requiring that programs implement distress screening by 2015 as a condition of accreditation (see also Lazenby et al., 2015). Clinical practice guidelines adopted by the American Society of Clinical Oncology (Andersen et al., 2015) and the National Comprehensive Cancer Network (NCCN, 2021) provide specific recommendations for screening, assessment, and management of distress.

The remainder of this chapter presents an overview of breast surgery for women with breast cancer or elevated risk for developing breast cancer. I provide an orientation to screening and referral practices that are commonly applied in cancer care settings, and I offer recommendations to guide assessment of common manifestations of psychological distress and maladjustment in this population.

OVERVIEW OF SURGERY FOR BREAST CANCER

Surgery for breast cancer involves excision of the tumor(s) and some or all of the surrounding breast tissue. A pathologist tests the tumor to determine the subtype of breast cancer and also examines the tissue surrounding the tumor (the "margin") for cancerous cells. Often, the surgeon and pathologist test for evidence that cancer cells have spread (metastasized) to the lymph nodes in the axilla (armpit) and possibly other lymph nodes near the breast. The surgeon may remove one or more of these lymph nodes for further evaluation by the pathologist. The findings of the surgeon and pathologist help determine the stage of the cancer, a classification that informs prognosis and treatment recommendations.

Surgery is commonly the first step in a multicomponent approach that includes other treatments, called *adjuvant therapies*, to prevent disease spread and recurrence. Adjuvant therapies include radiation, chemotherapy, and medications that are used for certain subtypes of breast cancer, such as targeted therapy, immunotherapy, and hormone therapy. Patients with more advanced tumors may receive treatment before surgery, termed *neoadjuvant therapy*, to shrink the tumor and reduce the need for more extensive surgery.

Types of Breast Cancer Surgery

The choice of surgery depends on the type of breast cancer, tumor size and location(s), existing conditions that could affect further treatment, and patient preference. Over time, development of more effective and targeted adjuvant therapies has made it possible to offer less aggressive surgery without compromising survival.

Following is a summary of common approaches to surgery:

- *Breast-conserving surgery* (BCS; also referred to as "lumpectomy" or "partial mastectomy") entails removal of the tumor, the immediately surrounding tissue, and sometimes the skin overlying the area of the tumor. This approach is often feasible in patients with early stage disease, and survival outcomes are comparable between BCS and total mastectomy. If cancer cells are found very close to the margin, further surgery (re-excision or conversion to total mastectomy) may be recommended. BCS is usually followed by adjuvant radiation therapy to treat residual disease.
- With a *total mastectomy* (also referred to as "simple mastectomy"), the entire breast is removed, including the nipple, areola, and the skin on the breast surface. The surgeon also removes the fascia overlying the chest muscle.
- A *modified radical mastectomy* entails complete removal of the breast as well as removal of axillary lymph nodes. This procedure is limited to patients with locally advanced breast cancer, which is characterized by larger tumors or spread of cancer cells to the surrounding lymph nodes. A more aggressive procedure known as a *radical mastectomy* (or "Halsted mastectomy") includes removal of the underlying chest muscles but is rarely used in modern practice.
- A *skin- and nipple-sparing mastectomy* entails the following: If the tumor is relatively small and not near the surface of the breast, most of the overlying skin, and possibly the nipple and areola, can be preserved by removing only the internal breast tissue. If clinically appropriate, these procedures can be performed as an alternative to total or modified radical mastectomy. In the case of a nipple-sparing procedure, the preserved nipple and areola lack sensation and function as a result of disruption to the nerves supplying the tissue.

Surgery for Risk Reduction

BCS or mastectomy is often a component of treatment for precancerous (Stage 0) diseases, such as ductal carcinoma in situ. Total mastectomy (including skin- and nipple-sparing procedures) is also offered as an option to reduce the risk of a future cancer in people with familial genetic syndromes that confer high lifetime risk for cancer (particularly high-risk mutations of *BRCA1* or *BRCA2*). The use of bilateral mastectomy has increased markedly over the past 2 decades given the increased use of genetic testing to screen for high-risk genetic mutations. In addition, a small but growing proportion of women with breast cancer who do not have known genetic risk factors are opting for removal of the unaffected breast at the time of mastectomy, a preference driven more by cancer-related worry than objective risk reduction (Ager et al., 2016).

Reconstruction After Breast Surgery

Various forms of reconstructive surgery are used to recreate the breast(s) removed during mastectomy or correct distortions in the breast after BCS. Reconstruction may be accompanied by surgery in the opposite breast (e.g., breast lift, breast reduction) to improve symmetry.

These are three of the most common general approaches:

- *Implant reconstruction*: A silicone implant, filled with saline or gel, can be placed over or under the chest muscle to replace breast tissue. Often, the first step in this approach is to gradually stretch the remaining skin over the mastectomy site using a temporary implant called a *tissue expander*. The tissue expander is filled with saline at regular intervals to increase volume over a few months until the skin accommodates the desired size and shape of implant. The temporary implant is then exchanged for the permanent one.
- *Autologous reconstruction*: The patient's own tissue can be used to reconstruct the breast after mastectomy. Many autologous procedures recreate the breast from a flap of skin, fat, and muscle removed from elsewhere in the body. Others use only a fat graft taken from elsewhere in the body.
- *Oncoplastic breast surgery*: At the time of BCS, a surgeon may be able to reposition the remaining breast tissue to reconstruct the breast without the need for additional tissue from another site.

Reconstruction can be performed at the time of mastectomy or at a later time. The type and timing of reconstruction depend on many factors, including the treatment plan (especially if radiation therapy is planned after mastectomy), the type of reconstruction desired, and patient preference for immediate versus delayed reconstruction.

Breast reconstruction is increasingly common after mastectomy. However, about half of women who receive a mastectomy forego reconstruction. Among the most commonly reported reasons to choose against reconstruction are the desire to avoid another surgery or to avoid potential surgical complications (Flitcroft et al., 2017; Manne et al., 2016). Medically underserved populations, in particular, are less likely to undergo breast reconstruction compared with women with greater access to information and resources (Zahedi et al., 2019). In the United States, most publicly and privately administered health insurance plans reimburse for reconstruction after mastectomy for breast cancer. However, access barriers, out-of-pocket costs, and indirect expenses still present obstacles to reconstructive surgery for low-income and underserved populations. Survivors with private insurance are more likely to undergo reconstruction when compared with Medicaid and Medicare beneficiaries (Siotos et al., 2020).

Side Effects and Adverse Events After Surgery

People with breast cancer commonly report fatigue, pain, and other somatic symptoms. These symptoms are less likely to be related to the cancer itself (nonmetastatic breast cancer typically causes little to no discomfort) than to side effects of treatment. Surgery, in particular, can cause neuropathic pain at the mastectomy site, musculoskeletal pain, and limited range of motion in the affected side. Removal of lymph nodes at the time of surgery can cause *lymphedema*, persistent fluid retention and swelling in the arm, which causes discomfort as well as disfigurement. Adjuvant therapies can cause a host of side effects, including fatigue (Abrahams et al., 2016), joint pain (Beckwée et al., 2017), changes in cognitive function (Janelsins et al., 2017), infertility (Christian & Gemignani, 2019), and menopausal symptoms (Hickey et al., 2005) as well as long-term health risks (Bodai & Tuso, 2015). Side effects of adjuvant therapies can affect quality of life as much as the surgery or diagnosis itself.

PSYCHOLOGICAL MALADJUSTMENT IN PEOPLE UNDERGOING SURGERY FOR BREAST CANCER

Breast cancer is a distressing experience. Large prospective studies paint an overall optimistic picture of psychological adjustment to breast cancer in women with Stage III or lower disease: Distress tends to be greatest at the time of diagnosis and initial surgery, decreases within the first year of treatment, and approaches baseline levels of distress in the general population in the several years thereafter (Bidstrup et al., 2015; Maass et al., 2015). A relatively small percentage of people with breast cancer endorse persistently high distress throughout the course of treatment, and this response is often evident before surgery (Bidstrup et al., 2015). Less is known about the trajectory of distress in metastatic breast cancer, but it is likely associated with disease progression (Lee et al., 2018).

Psychologists and mental health professionals who work with multidisciplinary cancer care teams should be aware that, in the oncology setting, "distress" tends to be defined broadly. For example, the NCCN (2021) guidelines define *distress* as "a multifactorial, unpleasant experience of a psychologic (i.e., cognitive, behavioral, emotional), social, spiritual, and/or physical nature that may interfere with the ability to cope effectively with cancer, its physical symptoms, and its treatment" (p. DIS-1). As such, "distress" functions as an umbrella term, and further assessment of specific problems is needed to formulate an appropriate clinical response.

In patients who do not have clinically significant mood and anxiety symptoms at the time of surgery, future development of depression and anxiety is uncommon. In contrast, more than one third of patients with clinically significant anxiety and depression at baseline have persistence of these problems 5 years posttreatment (Hopwood et al., 2010). However, trajectories of distress differ greatly among individuals. Younger age, low social support, and previous history of mental health conditions are risk factors for depression and anxiety 1 year or longer after diagnosis (Burgess et al., 2005).

DISTRESS SCREENING IN THE BREAST SURGERY SETTING

Universal distress screening in the surgical setting has several advantages. First, it captures nearly all patients with breast cancer, reducing reliance on clinician judgment and opportunistic screening to detect high levels of distress and unmet psychosocial needs. Second, implementing (or enhancing) distress screening is likely to have support from leaders in cancer care organizations. Distress screening allows for baseline measurement and early detection of unusually high distress, thereby facilitating early intervention.

Screening Instruments

A simple screening tool is the NCCN Distress Thermometer (NCCN, 2021), which uses a visual analog scale ranging from 0 = *no distress* to 10 = *extreme distress* to assess subjective distress in the past week. The Distress Thermometer is usually paired with a checklist that patients use to indicate various problems (i.e., practical, family, emotional, spiritual, and physical) they have experienced in the past week. A score of 4 or higher on the Distress Thermometer is a commonly accepted cut-off point for further assessment (Donovan et al., 2014). Studies that have used the Distress Thermometer and problem checklist have found that fatigue is the most frequently endorsed problem; worry, sleep disturbance, and pain are also among the most frequently endorsed problems across studies of people with breast cancer (Dabrowski et al., 2007; Head et al., 2012; McFarland et al., 2018).

An alternative to the Distress Thermometer is the Edmonton Symptom Assessment System (Bruera et al., 1991; Watanabe et al., 2012), a self-report instrument that prompts the respondent to rate each of 10 symptoms on scale ranging from 0 (e.g., *not depressed*) to 10 (e.g., *worst possible depression*). However, the scope of this instrument is less comprehensive than the problem checklist. Brief assessment tools that are specific to negative affect, such as the Hospital Anxiety and Depression Scale (Zigmond & Snaith, 1983), the Patient Health Questionnaire–9 (Kroenke & Spitzer, 2002; see also Thekkumpurath et al., 2011), and the Brief Symptom Inventory-18 (Zabora et al., 2001), can provide more detail about emotional symptoms, but their scoring is more complicated than that of the Distress Thermometer.

Practical Considerations for Implementing Distress Screening

Published studies on the clinical outcomes of distress screening have mixed results, and a small number have identified possible adverse effects of screening (Mitchell, 2013; Schouten et al., 2019). Perhaps one reason for modest clinical outcomes is that most distressed patients decline referrals and therefore do not receive further intervention. Moreover, few settings have the resources to provide high-quality, evidence-based psychological assessment and treatment. Zebrack et al. (2017) noted that adherence to use of the Distress Thermometer (NCCN, 2021) was variable and often poor, even in comprehensive cancer center settings in which screening protocols were in place.

Considerations for implementing distress screening include the following:

- Who is responsible for screening patients? Who will train and supervise clinic staff who are involved in screening?
- What thresholds will trigger a referral to psychological services?
- Who is responsible for following up with patients who screen positive?
- How will the screening process address the needs of medically underserved patients, who have greater barriers to accessing recommended services?
- What are the intended outcomes of screening, and how will the team determine whether these are being achieved?

Additional recommendations for implementing distress screening are provided in a 2014 report from the American Psychosocial Oncology Society,

Association of Oncology Social Work, and Oncology Nursing Society Joint Task Force (Pirl et al., 2014). Clearly, introducing a screening instrument into the clinic without a clear strategy to address barriers is almost certain to fail (Mitchell et al., 2011). Clinicians and clinic staff need to be engaged early in implementation to ensure ownership of the screening process and troubleshoot obstacles. Consider using a quality improvement approach, such as the plan–do–study–act model, to learn from and adapt the screening process (Bush et al., 2020). Other quality improvement models and tools are freely available from the Institute for Healthcare Improvement (see https://www.ihi.org).

ASSESSMENT OF PSYCHOLOGICAL DIFFICULTIES IN PEOPLE WITH BREAST CANCER

Breast cancer survivors who screen positive for distress or who are referred by themselves or others should be assessed primarily using a clinical interview that focuses on the presenting concern or referral question and incorporates a psychosocial history. Because many breast cancer survivors report good health before their diagnosis and may have had limited contact with mental health professionals, the psychological assessment may be the patient's first encounter with mental health care. Patients are appreciative of professionals who are familiar with breast cancer and cancer treatments so that they minimize the time and effort spent educating the clinician about their illness. If the clinician providing assessment is not affiliated with the medical care site, it is helpful to request from the referring provider some basic details, such as the date of diagnosis, type and stage of breast cancer (although this may not be known before surgery), and treatment plan.

Judicious use of questionnaires takes into consideration setting, time constraints, and the purpose of the consultation. Multidimensional, cancer-specific quality-of-life measures, such as the Functional Assessment of Cancer Therapy–Breast (Brady et al., 1997) and BREAST-Q (Pusic et al., 2009), can provide a helpful snapshot of multiple symptom or functional domains, particularly in the pre- and postsurgical settings. More focused assessment of individual symptoms is warranted when problems are severe or are a particular focus of clinical attention. Domain-specific measures of depression, anxiety, fatigue, and sleep disturbance that are appropriate for the general population are also generally appropriate for use in people with breast cancer. The Patient-Reported Outcomes Measurement Information System (Cella et al., 2007), for instance, includes several scales that have been favorably assessed in oncology populations (e.g., Flynn et al., 2013; Rothrock et al., 2019; Stone et al., 2016).

In some situations, cancer-specific questionnaires can provide more targeted clinical information. Because of the specific nature of appearance and functional concerns after treatment, cancer-specific questionnaires, such as the Body Image Scale (Hopwood et al., 2001) and subscales of the BREAST-Q (Pusic et al., 2009), are especially appropriate for assessing body image. In addition, fear of recurrence is a common source of distress in people with breast cancer and can be assessed efficiently using measures that include the Fear of Cancer Recurrence Inventory (Simard & Savard, 2009, 2015) or the Cancer Worry Scale (Custers et al., 2014).

The following sections describe several common sources of distress in people undergoing surgery for breast cancer. In general, clinicians should address each of these areas when assessing patients before breast surgery. These domains are also appropriate to assess at any other point during treatment (e.g., during adjuvant chemotherapy, during radiation therapy) or after completion of treatment if evidence of persistent distress exists.

Cancer-Related Anxiety, Worries, and Fears

Breast cancer surgery typically occurs early in the course of treatment, so patients who are assessed at this interval are likely still in the initial phase of adjustment to the diagnosis. Patients commonly voice fears of losing control, being in pain, experiencing adverse outcomes, being a burden to loved ones, and experiencing other life-altering consequences of their disease. In addition to worry about effects on their lives, patients sometimes endorse worry about anxiety itself and may have internalized the idea that stress or anxiety caused or exacerbated the cancer. Young women with metastatic disease appear to be especially vulnerable to anxiety (Park et al., 2018; Spencer et al., 2010). Although anxiety tends to subside over time, Hopwood et al. (2010) found that high anxiety immediately following surgery was a risk factor for persistent high anxiety over time. Social support is an important buffer against these adjustment difficulties and should be assessed in distressed patients.

Fear of recurrence (i.e., fear of the cancer returning) often emerges during or after treatment, and although most patients endorse fear of recurrence to some degree, high levels of fear of recurrence can lead to functional impairment. Fear of recurrence encompasses not only worry about cancer but also intrusive thoughts and hypervigilance to physical symptoms that are experienced as threatening. Young women and mothers are especially vulnerable to high fear of recurrence (Koch et al., 2014; Lebel et al., 2013).

People with high-risk genetic mutations, but no personal cancer history, also report distress and worry about developing cancer. They may describe feeling like a "time bomb" and anticipate regret for not doing everything in their control to prevent a future cancer (Brown et al., 2017). Risk-reducing mastectomy significantly reduces cancer-related worry, but at the expense of a higher risk of body image disturbance and poorer quality of life (Parker et al., 2018). Increasingly, breast cancer survivors at average risk for cancer recurrence opt for *contralateral preventive mastectomy*, removal of the opposite, unaffected breast, which is a preference that appears closely linked to higher anxiety and worry before surgery (Momoh et al., 2017). Risk factors for postmastectomy adjustment problems include opposition to surgery or lack of support from intimate partners, unclear or unrealistic expectations, and lack of information or preparation for side effects (Glassey, O'Connor et al., 2018; Rosenberg et al., 2018).

Fatigue

Fatigue is common in breast cancer survivors, but the severity and trajectory of fatigue vary considerably among individuals. A prospective study of more than 200 women with breast cancer found that about two thirds reported relatively low levels of fatigue over a period of 18 months. Survivors who reported high levels of fatigue over time did not necessarily have more advanced disease but reported higher levels of depression and sleep disturbance that are consistent with previous observations in the literature (Bower et al., 2021). The co-occurrence of fatigue, sleep problems, depression, and pain has been hypothesized to result from a common underlying inflammatory process, although data to support this hypothesis have been inconsistent, whereas psychological factors are strongly associated with subjective fatigue (Abrahams et al., 2018; Bower et al., 2018).

Fatigue may be provoked or exacerbated by adjuvant treatments, including chemotherapy and radiation therapy. In the presurgical setting, fatigue tends to be at a low point in the symptom trajectory, unless surgery is preceded by neoadjuvant chemotherapy. As such, high fatigue before surgery should alert the clinician to possible difficulties with mood and coping.

Sleep Disturbance

Sleep disturbance tends to persist or worsen over the course of breast cancer treatment but is often present before surgery. Many patients find it difficult to sleep in the days leading up to surgery or reconstruction, and after surgery, sleep may be challenging because of pain and the need to change sleeping positions, especially for prone sleepers. Insomnia before surgery is associated with more intense depression and anxiety symptoms (Van Onselen et al., 2012).

Although it is reasonable to defer screening for insomnia immediately after surgery to reduce false positives, data otherwise do not point to an ideal time for screening during treatment given a high likelihood of at least transient insomnia throughout the 12-month period after diagnosis (Bean et al., 2021; Fleming et al., 2019). Whether through questionnaire or clinical interview, assessment should differentiate long-standing sleep habits and patterns from new or recent difficulties with sleep onset or maintenance that coincide with contextual factors related to cancer treatment. A history of insomnia before diagnosis and high symptom burden in other domains are risk factors for persistent insomnia after surgery (Fleming et al., 2019).

Mood Disturbance

A high burden of somatic symptoms complicates assessment of mood disturbance in people with cancer, and if these common symptoms are not taken into account, psychologists and other mental health professionals risk overdiagnosing mood disorders. Studies of depression in cancer survivors tend to have inflated prevalence estimates because they are based on cut-off criteria for self-report measures; when structured clinical interviews and rigorous criteria are used, the estimated prevalence of depression is around 10% in breast cancer survivors (Krebber et al., 2014; Walker et al., 2013).

Typically, depression is most prevalent during the active phase of treatment and gradually declines over time. Clinically, however, it is not unusual for mood changes to have a delayed onset, becoming noticeable toward the end of primary treatment or even later. Not coincidentally, this is also a period during which some survivors perceive a withdrawal of social support, a shift in others' expectations (e.g., feeling pressured to be "back to normal"), and a sense of vulnerability that accompanies less frequent contact with the medical team (Powers et al., 2016).

Body Image and Sexual Function

Concerns about changes in appearance and function are common before and after surgery. Typical areas of dissatisfaction or concern after surgery include the appearance of a mastectomy scar, changes in the shape or symmetry of the breast(s), and loss of sensation after surgery. Adjuvant therapies may contribute to other body image concerns, such as weight gain (a common side effect of chemotherapy and hormone therapy), hair loss (from chemotherapy), and early menopause (from chemotherapy and hormone therapy; Fobair et al., 2006). Younger age and greater investment in appearance tend to be associated with greater body image–related distress (Miller et al., 2014; Teo et al., 2018). Treatment is also a significant factor in body image outcomes, with BCS generally associated with better body image outcomes compared with mastectomy followed by breast reconstruction (Fang et al., 2013; Rosenberg et al., 2020). In women who experience poorer body image after risk-reducing mastectomy, body image disturbance tends to persist in the long term, even with breast reconstruction (Bai et al., 2019).

Mood disturbance, chemotherapy sequelae, and problems with body image are among the most important risk factors for sexual dysfunction in this population (Fobair et al., 2006). Body image concerns often lead to concerns about rejection or negative social evaluation and may manifest as avoidance of sexual activity or reduced interest in sex. Women who have an intimate partner participating in their care may experience discomfort not only with appearance changes, but also the shifts in personal boundaries that come with being a care recipient (e.g., requiring help with dressing, lifting, or caring for drains or dressings after surgery). The quality of the intimate relationship can buffer these negative effects, or, when the relationship is poorly adjusted, can magnify them (Kinsinger et al., 2011; Soriano et al., 2017). Women who do not have intimate partners but desire a relationship may also feel concerned about rejection and may avoid meeting new dating partners or becoming invested in dating relationships (Shaw et al., 2018).

Suicidal Ideation

The estimated prevalence of suicidal ideation in cancer survivors varies significantly among studies, and few studies have focused exclusively on breast cancer survivors (Kolva et al., 2020). Mortality from suicide is higher in cancer survivors than in the general population, and the risk is highest in the first few years after diagnosis (Schairer et al., 2006; Zaorsky et al., 2019).

Risk factors for suicidal ideation include living alone and having a more advanced cancer stage. Similar risk factors are associated with death by suicide. In addition, socioeconomic factors, such as lower income, lower educational attainment, and unemployment, are also associated with higher risk for suicide in people with cancer (Abdel-Rahman, 2019).

FUTURE DIRECTIONS

Although current guidelines from the NCCN and other groups recommend a screening and referral approach for most care settings, there is ample room for innovation to improve the quality of care for breast surgery candidates. Routine psychological assessment may be reasonable to implement in populations at especially high risk for distress, such as adolescents and young adults as well as in young "previvors" with high-risk genetic mutations. As an example, a small qualitative study assessed 26 young women (under age 35) who did or did not receive a psychological consultation before risk-reducing bilateral mastectomy. Those who received a consultation reported feeling better prepared for surgery and were found to experience more positive body image and intimacy than those who had not (Glassey, Hardcastle, et al., 2018). Standardized psychological assessment using patient-reported outcome instruments is helpful for assessing and communicating the effect of presurgical consultation on survivors' well-being.

Ensuring that assessment of distress is responsive to the needs of diverse populations is also a priority. Single-institution studies have identified elevated rates of distress in rural (Burris & Andrykowski, 2010) and Hispanic (Fayanju et al., 2021; Gonzalez et al., 2022) breast cancer survivors, whereas mental health diagnosis and treatment after a cancer diagnosis appear to be more accessible to White, non-Hispanic patients (Chen et al., 2022). Adverse experiences with the health care system, including medical mistrust and experience of discrimination, may be more salient for minoritized populations and should be included in assessment of distress (Kano et al., 2022; Sheppard et al., 2014).

CONCLUSION

People who are undergoing surgery for breast cancer tend to be highly distressed at what is typically an early point in their treatment course. Common problems in this population include anxiety, mood disturbance, sleep disturbance, fatigue, body image concerns, and sexual problems. Often these problems come to the oncology team's attention only when distress is prolonged or severe.

Presurgical screening and assessment of psychological difficulties can improve identification of patients who could benefit from close monitoring or psychological intervention. Further efforts to make routine distress screening more efficient, equitable, and patient centered will help to further improve experiences and outcomes of breast cancer treatment.

REFERENCES

Abdel-Rahman, O. (2019). Socioeconomic predictors of suicide risk among cancer patients in the United States: A population-based study. *Cancer Epidemiology*, *63*, Article 101601. https://doi.org/10.1016/j.canep.2019.101601

Abrahams, H. J. G., Gielissen, M. F. M., Schmits, I. C., Verhagen, C. A. H. H. V. M., Rovers, M. M., & Knoop, H. (2016). Risk factors, prevalence, and course of severe fatigue after breast cancer treatment: A meta-analysis involving 12 327 breast cancer survivors. *Annals of Oncology*, *27*(6), 965–974. https://doi.org/10.1093/annonc/mdw099

Abrahams, H. J. G., Gielissen, M. F. M., Verhagen, C. A. H. H. V. M., & Knoop, H. (2018). The relationship of fatigue in breast cancer survivors with quality of life and factors to address in psychological interventions: A systematic review. *Clinical Psychology Review*, *63*, 1–11. https://doi.org/10.1016/j.cpr.2018.05.004

Ager, B., Butow, P., Jansen, J., Phillips, K.-A., Porter, D., & the CPM DA Advisory Group. (2016). Contralateral prophylactic mastectomy (CPM): A systematic review of patient reported factors and psychological predictors influencing choice and satisfaction. *The Breast*, *28*, 107–120. https://doi.org/10.1016/j.breast.2016.04.005

American Cancer Society. (2021). *Cancer facts & figures: 2021*. https://www.cancer.org/content/dam/cancer-org/research/cancer-facts-and-statistics/annual-cancer-facts-and-figures/2021/cancer-facts-and-figures-2021.pdf

American College of Surgeons Commission on Cancer. (2012). *Cancer program standards 2012: Ensuring patient-centered care* (Version 1.2.1). https://apos-society.org/wp-content/uploads/2016/06/CoCStandards.pdf

Andersen, B. L., Rowland, J. H., & Somerfield, M. R. (2015). Screening, assessment, and care of anxiety and depressive symptoms in adults with cancer: An American Society of Clinical Oncology guideline adaptation. *Journal of Oncology Practice*, *11*(2), 133–134. https://doi.org/10.1200/JOP.2014.002311

Bai, L., Arver, B., Johansson, H., Sandelin, K., Wickman, M., & Brandberg, Y. (2019). Body image problems in women with and without breast cancer 6–20 years after bilateral risk-reducing surgery—A prospective follow-up study. *The Breast*, *44*, 120–127. https://doi.org/10.1016/j.breast.2019.01.013

Bean, H. R., Diggens, J., Ftanou, M., Weihs, K. L., Stanton, A. L., & Wiley, J. F. (2021). Insomnia and fatigue symptom trajectories in breast cancer: A longitudinal cohort study. *Behavioral Sleep Medicine*, *19*(6), 814–827. https://doi.org/10.1080/15402002.2020.1869005

Beckwée, D., Leysen, L., Meuwis, K., & Adriaenssens, N. (2017). Prevalence of aromatase inhibitor-induced arthralgia in breast cancer: A systematic review and meta-analysis. *Supportive Care in Cancer*, *25*(5), 1673–1686. https://doi.org/10.1007/s00520-017-3613-z

Bidstrup, P. E., Christensen, J., Mertz, B. G., Rottmann, N., Dalton, S. O., & Johansen, C. (2015). Trajectories of distress, anxiety, and depression among women with breast cancer: Looking beyond the mean. *Acta Oncologica*, *54*(5), 789–796. https://doi.org/10.3109/0284186X.2014.1002571

Bodai, B. I., & Tuso, P. (2015). Breast cancer survivorship: A comprehensive review of long-term medical issues and lifestyle recommendations. *The Permanente Journal*, *19*(2), 48–79. https://doi.org/10.7812/TPP/14-241

Bower, J. E., Ganz, P. A., Irwin, M. R., Cole, S. W., Garet, D., Petersen, L., Asher, A., Hurvitz, S. A., & Crespi, C. M. (2021). Do all patients with cancer experience fatigue? A longitudinal study of fatigue trajectories in women with breast cancer. *Cancer, 127*(8), 1334–1344. https://doi.org/10.1002/cncr.33327

Bower, J. E., Wiley, J., Petersen, L., Irwin, M. R., Cole, S. W., & Ganz, P. A. (2018). Fatigue after breast cancer treatment: Biobehavioral predictors of fatigue trajectories. *Health Psychology, 37*(11), 1025–1034. https://doi.org/10.1037/hea0000652

Brady, M. J., Cella, D. F., Mo, F., Bonomi, A. E., Tulsky, D. S., Lloyd, S. R., Deasy, S., Cobleigh, M., & Shiomoto, G. (1997). Reliability and validity of the Functional Assessment of Cancer Therapy–Breast quality-of-life instrument. *Journal of Clinical Oncology, 15*(3), 974–986. https://doi.org/10.1200/JCO.1997.15.3.974

Brown, S. L., Whiting, D., Fielden, H. G., Saini, P., Beesley, H., Holcombe, C., Holcombe, S., Greenhalgh, L., Fairburn, L., & Salmon, P. (2017). Qualitative analysis of how patients decide that they want risk-reducing mastectomy, and the implications for surgeons in responding to emotionally-motivated patient requests. *PLOS ONE, 12*(5), Article e0178392. https://doi.org/10.1371/journal.pone.0178392

Bruera, E., Kuehn, N., Miller, M. J., Selmser, P., & Macmillan, K. (1991). The Edmonton Symptom Assessment System (ESAS): A simple method for the assessment of palliative care patients. *Journal of Palliative Care, 7*(2), 6–9. https://doi.org/10.1177/082585979100700202

Burgess, C., Cornelius, V., Love, S., Graham, J., Richards, M., & Ramirez, A. (2005). Depression and anxiety in women with early breast cancer: Five year observational cohort study. *The BMJ, 330*(7493), Article 702. https://doi.org/10.1136/bmj.38343.670868.D3

Burris, J. L., & Andrykowski, M. (2010). Disparities in mental health between rural and nonrural cancer survivors: A preliminary study. *Psycho-Oncology, 19*(6), 637–645. https://doi.org/10.1002/pon.1600

Bush, N. J., Goebel, J. R., Hardan-Khalil, K., & Matsumoto, K. (2020). Using a quality improvement model to implement distress screening in a community cancer setting. *Journal of the Advanced Practitioner in Oncology, 11*(8), 825–834. https://doi.org/10.6004/jadpro.2020.11.8.3

Cella, D., Yount, S., Rothrock, N., Gershon, R., Cook, K., Reeve, B., Ader, D., Fries, J. F., Bruce, B., & Rose, M. (2007). The Patient-Reported Outcomes Measurement Information System (PROMIS): Progress of an NIH roadmap cooperative group during its first two years. *Medical Care, 45*(5, Suppl. 1), S3–S11. https://doi.org/10.1097/01.mlr.0000258615.42478.55

Chen, W. C., Boreta, L., Braunstein, S. E., Rabow, M. W., Kaplan, L. E., Tenenbaum, J. D., Morin, O., Park, C. C., & Hong, J. C. (2022). Association of mental health diagnosis with race and all-cause mortality after a cancer diagnosis: Large-scale analysis of electronic health record data. *Cancer, 128*(2), 344–352. https://doi.org/10.1002/cncr.33903

Christian, N., & Gemignani, M. L. (2019). Issues with fertility in young women with breast cancer. *Current Oncology Reports, 21*(7), Article 58. https://doi.org/10.1007/s11912-019-0812-4

Custers, J. A., van den Berg, S. W., van Laarhoven, H. W., Bleiker, E. M., Gielissen, M. F., & Prins, J. B. (2014). The Cancer Worry Scale: Detecting fear of recurrence in breast cancer survivors. *Cancer Nursing, 37*(1), E44–E50. https://doi.org/10.1097/NCC.0b013e3182813a17

Dabrowski, M., Boucher, K., Ward, J. H., Lovell, M. M., Sandre, A., Bloch, J., Carlquist, L., Porter, M., Norman, L., & Buys, S. S. (2007). Clinical experience with the NCCN Distress Thermometer in breast cancer patients. *Journal of the National Comprehensive Cancer Network, 5*(1), 104–111. https://doi.org/10.6004/jnccn.2007.0011

Donovan, K. A., Grassi, L., McGinty, H. L., & Jacobsen, P. B. (2014). Validation of the Distress Thermometer worldwide: State of the science. *Psycho-Oncology, 23*(3), 241–250. https://doi.org/10.1002/pon.3430

Drinane, J. J., Pham, T.-H., Schalet, G., & Rezak, K. (2019). Depression is associated with worse outcomes among women undergoing breast reconstruction following mastectomy. *Journal of Plastic, Reconstructive & Aesthetic Surgery, 72*(8), 1292–1298. https://doi.org/10.1016/j.bjps.2019.03.036

Fang, S.-Y., Shu, B.-C., & Chang, Y.-J. (2013). The effect of breast reconstruction surgery on body image among women after mastectomy: A meta-analysis. *Breast Cancer Research and Treatment, 137*(1), 13–21. https://doi.org/10.1007/s10549-012-2349-1

Fayanju, O. M., Ren, Y., Stashko, I., Power, S., Thornton, M. J., Marcom, P. K., Hyslop, T., & Hwang, E. S. (2021). Patient-reported causes of distress predict disparities in time to evaluation and time to treatment after breast cancer diagnosis. *Cancer, 127*(5), 757–768. https://doi.org/10.1002/cncr.33310

Fleming, L., Randell, K., Stewart, E., Espie, C. A., Morrison, D. S., Lawless, C., & Paul, J. (2019). Insomnia in breast cancer: A prospective observational study. *Sleep, 42*(3). Advance online publication. https://doi.org/10.1093/sleep/zsy245

Flitcroft, K., Brennan, M., & Spillane, A. (2017). Making decisions about breast reconstruction: A systematic review of patient-reported factors influencing choice. *Quality of Life Research, 26*(9), 2287–2319. https://doi.org/10.1007/s11136-017-1555-z

Flynn, K. E., Reeve, B. B., Lin, L., Cyranowski, J. M., Bruner, D. W., & Weinfurt, K. P. (2013). Construct validity of the PROMIS® sexual function and satisfaction measures in patients with cancer. *Health and Quality of Life Outcomes, 11*(1), Article 40. https://doi.org/10.1186/1477-7525-11-40

Fobair, P., Stewart, S. L., Chang, S., D'Onofrio, C., Banks, P. J., & Bloom, J. R. (2006). Body image and sexual problems in young women with breast cancer. *Psycho-Oncology, 15*(7), 579–594. https://doi.org/10.1002/pon.991

Glassey, R., Hardcastle, S. J., O'Connor, M., Ives, A., kConFab Investigators, & Saunders, C. (2018). Perceived influence of psychological consultation on psychological well-being, body image, and intimacy following bilateral prophylactic mastectomy: A qualitative analysis. *Psycho-Oncology, 27*(2), 633–639. https://doi.org/10.1002/pon.4558

Glassey, R., O'Connor, M., Ives, A., Saunders, C., Hardcastle, S. J., & the kConFab Investigators. (2018). Influences on satisfaction with reconstructed breasts and intimacy in younger women following bilateral prophylactic mastectomy: A qualitative analysis. *International Journal of Behavioral Medicine, 25*(4), 390–398. https://doi.org/10.1007/s12529-018-9722-3

Gonzalez, L., Sun, C., Loscalzo, M., Clark, K., Kruper, L., Mortimer, J., & Jones, V. (2022). A cross-sectional study of distress levels in patients with newly diagnosed breast cancer: The impact of race, ethnicity, and language preference. *Annals of Surgical Oncology, 29*(2), 981–988. https://doi.org/10.1245/s10434-021-10561-6

Head, B. A., Schapmire, T. J., Keeney, C. E., Deck, S. M., Studts, J. L., Hermann, C. P., Scharfenberger, J. A., & Pfeifer, M. P. (2012). Use of the Distress Thermometer to discern clinically relevant quality of life differences in women with breast cancer.

Quality of Life Research, *21*(2), 215–223. https://doi.org/10.1007/s11136-011-9934-3

Hickey, M., Saunders, C. M., & Stuckey, B. G. (2005). Management of menopausal symptoms in patients with breast cancer: An evidence-based approach. *The Lancet Oncology*, *6*(9), 687–695. https://doi.org/10.1016/S1470-2045(05)70316-8

Hopwood, P., Fletcher, I., Lee, A., & Al Ghazal, S. (2001). A body image scale for use with cancer patients. *European Journal of Cancer*, *37*(2), 189–197. https://doi.org/10.1016/S0959-8049(00)00353-1

Hopwood, P., Sumo, G., Mills, J., Haviland, J., Bliss, J. M., & the START Trials Management Group. (2010). The course of anxiety and depression over 5 years of follow-up and risk factors in women with early breast cancer: Results from the UK Standardisation of Radiotherapy Trials (START). *The Breast*, *19*(2), 84–91. https://doi.org/10.1016/j.breast.2009.11.007

Janelsins, M. C., Heckler, C. E., Peppone, L. J., Kamen, C., Mustian, K. M., Mohile, S. G., Magnuson, A., Kleckner, I. R., Guido, J. J., Young, K. L., Conlin, A. K., Weiselberg, L. R., Mitchell, J. W., Ambrosone, C. A., Ahles, T. A., & Morrow, G. R. (2017). Cognitive complaints in survivors of breast cancer after chemotherapy compared with age-matched controls: An analysis from a nationwide, multicenter, prospective longitudinal study. *Journal of Clinical Oncology*, *35*(5), 506–514. https://doi.org/10.1200/JCO.2016.68.5826

Kano, M., Jaffe, S. A., Rieder, S., Kosich, M., Guest, D. D., Burgess, E., Hurwitz, A., Pankratz, V. S., Rutledge, T. L., Dayao, Z., & Myaskovsky, L. (2022). Improving sexual and gender minority cancer care: Patient and caregiver perspectives from a multi-methods pilot study. *Frontiers in Oncology*, *12*, Article 833195. https://doi.org/10.3389/fonc.2022.833195

Kinsinger, S. W., Laurenceau, J. P., Carver, C. S., & Antoni, M. H. (2011). Perceived partner support and psychosexual adjustment to breast cancer. *Psychology & Health*, *26*(12), 1571–1588. https://doi.org/10.1080/08870446.2010.533771

Koch, L., Bertram, H., Eberle, A., Holleczek, B., Schmid-Höpfner, S., Waldmann, A., Zeissig, S. R., Brenner, H., & Arndt, V. (2014). Fear of recurrence in long-term breast cancer survivors-still an issue. Results on prevalence, determinants, and the association with quality of life and depression from the cancer survivorship—A multi-regional population-based study. *Psycho-Oncology*, *23*(5), 547–554. https://doi.org/10.1002/pon.3452

Kolva, E., Hoffecker, L., & Cox-Martin, E. (2020). Suicidal ideation in patients with cancer: A systematic review of prevalence, risk factors, intervention and assessment. *Palliative & Supportive Care*, *18*(2), 206–219. https://doi.org/10.1017/S1478951519000610

Krebber, A. M. H., Buffart, L. M., Kleijn, G., Riepma, I. C., de Bree, R., Leemans, C. R., Becker, A., Brug, J., van Straten, A., Cuijpers, P., & Verdonck-de Leeuw, I. M. (2014). Prevalence of depression in cancer patients: A meta-analysis of diagnostic interviews and self-report instruments. *Psycho-Oncology*, *23*(2), 121–130. https://doi.org/10.1002/pon.3409

Kroenke, K., & Spitzer, R. L. (2002). The PHQ-9: A new depression diagnostic and severity measure. *Psychiatric Annals*, *32*(9), 509–515. https://doi.org/10.3928/0048-5713-20020901-06

Kuchenbaecker, K. B., Hopper, J. L., Barnes, D. R., Phillips, K. A., Mooij, T. M., Roos-Blom, M. J., Jervis, S., van Leeuwen, F. E., Milne, R. L., Andrieu, N., Goldgar,

D. E., Terry, M. B., Rookus, M. A., Easton, D. F., Antoniou, A. C., & the BRCA1 and BRCA2 Cohort Consortium. (2017). Risks of breast, ovarian, and contralateral breast cancer for *BRCA1* and *BRCA2* mutation carriers. *JAMA, 317*(23), 2402–2416. https://doi.org/10.1001/jama.2017.7112

Lazenby, M., Ercolano, E., Grant, M., Holland, J. C., Jacobsen, P. B., & McCorkle, R. (2015). Supporting Commission on Cancer–mandated psychosocial distress screening with implementation strategies. *Journal of Oncology Practice, 11*(3), e413–e420. https://doi.org/10.1200/JOP.2014.002816

Lebel, S., Beattie, S., Arès, I., & Bielajew, C. (2013). Young and worried: Age and fear of recurrence in breast cancer survivors. *Health Psychology, 32*(6), 695–705. https://doi.org/10.1037/a0030186

Lee, C. K., Hudson, M., Simes, J., Ribi, K., Bernhard, J., & Coates, A. S. (2018). When do patient reported quality of life indicators become prognostic in breast cancer? *Health and Quality of Life Outcomes, 16*(1), 13–13. https://doi.org/10.1186/s12955-017-0834-2

Maass, S. W. M. C., Roorda, C., Berendsen, A. J., Verhaak, P. F. M., & de Bock, G. H. (2015). The prevalence of long-term symptoms of depression and anxiety after breast cancer treatment: A systematic review. *Maturitas, 82*(1), 100–108. https://doi.org/10.1016/j.maturitas.2015.04.010

Manne, S. L., Topham, N., Kirstein, L., Virtue, S. M., Brill, K., Devine, K. A., Gajda, T., Frederick, S., Darabos, K., & Sorice, K. (2016). Attitudes and decisional conflict regarding breast reconstruction among breast cancer patients. *Cancer Nursing, 39*(6), 427–436. https://doi.org/10.1097/NCC.0000000000000320

McFarland, D. C., Shaffer, K. M., Tiersten, A., & Holland, J. (2018). Prevalence of physical problems detected by the Distress Thermometer and problem list in patients with breast cancer. *Psycho-Oncology, 27*(5), 1394–1403. https://doi.org/10.1002/pon.4631

Miller, S. J., Schnur, J. B., Weinberger-Litman, S. L., & Montgomery, G. H. (2014). The relationship between body image, age, and distress in women facing breast cancer surgery. *Palliative & Supportive Care, 12*(5), 363–367. https://doi.org/10.1017/S1478951513000321

Mitchell, A. J. (2013). Screening for cancer-related distress: When is implementation successful and when is it unsuccessful? *Acta Oncologica, 52*(2), 216–224. https://doi.org/10.3109/0284186X.2012.745949

Mitchell, A. J., Vahabzadeh, A., & Magruder, K. (2011). Screening for distress and depression in cancer settings: 10 lessons from 40 years of primary-care research. *Psycho-Oncology, 20*(6), 572–584. https://doi.org/10.1002/pon.1943

Momoh, A. O., Cohen, W. A., Kidwell, K. M., Hamill, J. B., Qi, J., Pusic, A. L., Wilkins, E. G., & Matros, E. (2017). Tradeoffs associated with contralateral prophylactic mastectomy in women choosing breast reconstruction: Results of a prospective multicenter cohort. *Annals of Surgery, 266*(1), 158–164. https://doi.org/10.1097/SLA.0000000000001840

National Cancer Institute. (n.d.). *Cancer stat facts: Female breast cancer*. National Institutes of Health. Retrieved July 1, 2021, from https://seer.cancer.gov/statfacts/html/breast.html

National Comprehensive Cancer Network. (2021). *NCCN clinical practice guidelines in oncology: Distress management* (Version 2.2021) [Available with free registration]. https://www.nccn.org/home

Park, E. M., Gelber, S., Rosenberg, S. M., Seah, D. S. E., Schapira, L., Come, S. E., & Partridge, A. H. (2018). Anxiety and depression in young women with metastatic breast cancer: A cross-sectional study. *Psychosomatics*, *59*(3), 251–258. https://doi.org/10.1016/j.psym.2018.01.007

Parker, P. A., Peterson, S. K., Shen, Y., Bedrosian, I., Black, D. M., Thompson, A. M., Nelson, J. C., DeSnyder, S. M., Cook, R. L., Hunt, K. K., Volk, R. J., Cantor, S. B., Dong, W., & Brewster, A. M. (2018). Prospective study of psychosocial outcomes of having contralateral prophylactic mastectomy among women with nonhereditary breast cancer. *Journal of Clinical Oncology*, *36*(25), 2630–2638. https://doi.org/10.1200/JCO.2018.78.6442

Pirl, W. F., Fann, J. R., Greer, J. A., Braun, I., Deshields, T., Fulcher, C., Harvey, E., Holland, J., Kennedy, V., Lazenby, M., Wagner, L., Underhill, M., Walker, D. K., Zabora, J., Zebrack, B., & Bardwell, W. A. (2014). Recommendations for the implementation of distress screening programs in cancer centers: Report from the American Psychosocial Oncology Society (APOS), Association of Oncology Social Work (AOSW), and Oncology Nursing Society (ONS) Joint Task Force. *Cancer*, *120*(19), 2946–2954. https://doi.org/10.1002/cncr.28750

Powers, N., Gullifer, J., & Shaw, R. (2016). When the treatment stops: A qualitative study of life post breast cancer treatment. *Journal of Health Psychology*, *21*(7), 1371–1382. https://doi.org/10.1177/1359105314553963

Pusic, A. L., Klassen, A. F., Scott, A. M., Klok, J. A., Cordeiro, P. G., & Cano, S. J. (2009). Development of a new patient-reported outcome measure for breast surgery: The BREAST-Q. *Plastic and Reconstructive Surgery*, *124*(2), 345–353. https://doi.org/10.1097/PRS.0b013e3181aee807

Rosenberg, S. M., Dominici, L. S., Gelber, S., Poorvu, P. D., Ruddy, K. J., Wong, J. S., Tamimi, R. M., Schapira, L., Come, S., Peppercorn, J. M., Borges, V. F., & Partridge, A. H. (2020). Association of breast cancer surgery with quality of life and psychosocial well-being in young breast cancer survivors. *JAMA Surgery*, *155*(11), 1035–1042. https://doi.org/10.1001/jamasurg.2020.3325

Rosenberg, S. M., Greaney, M. L., Patenaude, A. F., Sepucha, K. R., Meyer, M. E., & Partridge, A. H. (2018). "I don't want to take chances": A qualitative exploration of surgical decision making in young breast cancer survivors. *Psycho-Oncology*, *27*(6), 1524–1529. https://doi.org/10.1002/pon.4683

Rothrock, N. E., Cook, K. F., O'Connor, M., Cella, D., Smith, A. W., & Yount, S. E. (2019). Establishing clinically-relevant terms and severity thresholds for Patient-Reported Outcomes Measurement Information System® (PROMIS®) measures of physical function, cognitive function, and sleep disturbance in people with cancer using standard setting. *Quality of Life Research*, *28*(12), 3355–3362. https://doi.org/10.1007/s11136-019-02261-2

Schairer, C., Brown, L. M., Chen, B. E., Howard, R., Lynch, C. F., Hall, P., Storm, H., Pukkala, E., Anderson, A., Kaijser, M., Andersson, M., Joensuu, H., Fosså, S. D. A., Ganz, P. A., & Travis, L. B. (2006). Suicide after breast cancer: An international population-based study of 723,810 women. *Journal of the National Cancer Institute*, *98*(19), 1416–1419. https://doi.org/10.1093/jnci/djj377

Schouten, B., Avau, B., Bekkering, G. T. E., Vankrunkelsven, P., Mebis, J., Hellings, J., & Van Hecke, A. (2019). Systematic screening and assessment of psychosocial well-being and care needs of people with cancer. *Cochrane Database of Systematic Reviews*, *3*(3), Article CD012387. https://doi.org/10.1002/14651858.CD012387.pub2

Shaw, L. K., Sherman, K. A., Fitness, J., Elder, E., & the Breast Cancer Network Australia. (2018). Factors associated with romantic relationship formation difficulties in women with breast cancer. *Psycho-Oncology, 27*(4), 1270–1276. https://doi.org/10.1002/pon.4666

Sheppard, V. B., Harper, F. W., Davis, K., Hirpa, F., & Makambi, K. (2014). The importance of contextual factors and age in association with anxiety and depression in Black breast cancer patients. *Psycho-Oncology, 23*(2), 143–150. https://doi.org/10.1002/pon.3382

Simard, S., & Savard, J. (2009). Fear of Cancer Recurrence Inventory: Development and initial validation of a multidimensional measure of fear of cancer recurrence. *Supportive Care in Cancer, 17*(3), 241–251. https://doi.org/10.1007/s00520-008-0444-y

Simard, S., & Savard, J. (2015). Screening and comorbidity of clinical levels of fear of cancer recurrence. *Journal of Cancer Survivorship: Research and Practice, 9*(3), 481–491. https://doi.org/10.1007/s11764-015-0424-4

Siotos, C., Azizi, A., Assam, L., Rosson, G. D., Seal, S. M., Pollack, C. E., & Aliu, O. (2020). Breast reconstruction for Medicaid beneficiaries: A systematic review of the current evidence. *Journal of Plastic Surgery and Hand Surgery, 54*(2), 77–82. https://doi.org/10.1080/2000656X.2019.1688167

Soriano, E. C., Otto, A. K., Siegel, S. D., & Laurenceau, J. P. (2017). Partner social constraints and early-stage breast cancer: Longitudinal associations with psychosexual adjustment. *Journal of Family Psychology, 31*(5), 574–583. https://doi.org/10.1037/fam0000302

Spencer, R., Nilsson, M., Wright, A., Pirl, W., & Prigerson, H. (2010). Anxiety disorders in advanced cancer patients: Correlates and predictors of end-of-life outcomes. *Cancer, 116*(7), 1810–1819. https://doi.org/10.1002/cncr.24954

Stone, A. A., Broderick, J. E., Junghaenel, D. U., Schneider, S., & Schwartz, J. E. (2016). PROMIS fatigue, pain intensity, pain interference, pain behavior, physical function, depression, anxiety, and anger scales demonstrate ecological validity. *Journal of Clinical Epidemiology, 74*, 194–206. https://doi.org/10.1016/j.jclinepi.2015.08.029

Sung, H., Ferlay, J., Siegel, R. L., Laversanne, M., Soerjomataram, I., Jemal, A., & Bray, F. (2021). Global cancer statistics 2020: GLOBOCAN estimates of incidence and mortality worldwide for 36 cancers in 185 countries. *CA: A Cancer Journal for Clinicians, 71*(3), 209–249. https://doi.org/10.3322/caac.21660

Teo, I., Reece, G. P., Huang, S. C., Mahajan, K., Andon, J., Khanal, P., Sun, C., Nicklaus, K., Merchant, F., Markey, M. K., & Fingeret, M. C. (2018). Body image dissatisfaction in patients undergoing breast reconstruction: Examining the roles of breast symmetry and appearance investment. *Psycho-Oncology, 27*(3), 857–863. https://doi.org/10.1002/pon.4586

Thekkumpurath, P., Walker, J., Butcher, I., Hodges, L., Kleiboer, A., O'Connor, M., Wall, L., Murray, G., Kroenke, K., & Sharpe, M. (2011). Screening for major depression in cancer outpatients: The diagnostic accuracy of the 9-item Patient Health Questionnaire. *Cancer, 117*(1), 218–227. https://doi.org/10.1002/cncr.25514

Van Onselen, C., Cooper, B. A., Lee, K., Dunn, L., Aouizerat, B. E., West, C., Dodd, M., Paul, S., & Miaskowski, C. (2012). Identification of distinct subgroups of breast cancer patients based on self-reported changes in sleep disturbance. *Supportive Care in Cancer, 20*(10), 2611–2619. https://doi.org/10.1007/s00520-012-1381-3

Walker, J., Holm Hansen, C., Martin, P., Sawhney, A., Thekkumpurath, P., Beale, C., Symeonides, S., Wall, L., Murray, G., & Sharpe, M. (2013). Prevalence of depression in adults with cancer: A systematic review. *Annals of Oncology*, *24*(4), 895–900. https://doi.org/10.1093/annonc/mds575

Wang, F., Shu, X., Meszoely, I., Pal, T., Mayer, I. A., Yu, Z., Zheng, W., Bailey, C. E., & Shu, X.-O. (2019). Overall mortality after diagnosis of breast cancer in men vs women. *JAMA Oncology*, *5*(11), 1589–1596. https://doi.org/10.1001/jamaoncol.2019.2803

Watanabe, S. M., Nekolaichuk, C. L., & Beaumont, C. (2012). The Edmonton Symptom Assessment System, a proposed tool for distress screening in cancer patients: Development and refinement. *Psycho-Oncology*, *21*(9), 977–985. https://doi.org/10.1002/pon.1996

Ye, M., Du, K., Zhou, J., Zhou, Q., Shou, M., Hu, B., Jiang, P., Dong, N., He, L., Liang, S., Yu, C., Zhang, J., Ding, Z., & Liu, Z. (2018). A meta-analysis of the efficacy of cognitive behavior therapy on quality of life and psychological health of breast cancer survivors and patients. *Psycho-Oncology*, *27*(7), 1695–1703. https://doi.org/10.1002/pon.4687

Zabora, J., Brintzenhofeszoc, K., Jacobsen, P., Curbow, B., Piantadosi, S., Hooker, C., Owens, A., & Derogatis, L. (2001). A new psychosocial screening instrument for use with cancer patients. *Psychosomatics*, *42*(3), 241–246. https://doi.org/10.1176/appi.psy.42.3.241

Zahedi, S., Colvill, K., Lopez, M., & Phillips, L. G. (2019). Implications of demographics and socioeconomic factors in breast cancer reconstruction. *Annals of Plastic Surgery*, *83*(4), 388–391. https://doi.org/10.1097/SAP.0000000000001919

Zaorsky, N. G., Zhang, Y., Tuanquin, L., Bluethmann, S. M., Park, H. S., & Chinchilli, V. M. (2019). Suicide among cancer patients. *Nature Communications*, *10*(1), Article 207. https://doi.org/10.1038/s41467-018-08170-1 (Author correction published 2020, *Nature Communications*, *11*, Article 718. https://doi.org/10.1038/s41467-020-14506-7)

Zebrack, B., Kayser, K., Bybee, D., Padgett, L., Sundstrom, L., Jobin, C., & Oktay, J. (2017). A practice-based evaluation of distress screening protocol adherence and medical service utilization. *Journal of the National Comprehensive Cancer Network*, *15*(7), 903–912. https://doi.org/10.6004/jnccn.2017.0120

Zigmond, A. S., & Snaith, R. P. (1983). The Hospital Anxiety and Depression Scale. *Acta Psychiatrica Scandinavica*, *67*(6), 361–370. https://doi.org/10.1111/j.1600-0447.1983.tb09716.x

8 SOLID ORGAN TRANSPLANT

WENDY BALLIET, D. BRIAN HAVER, STACEY MAURER, AND LILLIAN CHRISTON

Although solid organ transplantation (SOT) is considered one of the exceptional medical victories of the 20th century, there is a widening gap between available organs and potential recipients. In the United States, every 9 minutes, another person is added to the transplant waitlist, and on average, 17 people die per day while waiting to receive SOT (Health Resources and Services Administration, 2021). As a result, transplant teams are often considered custodians of this limited and valued resource for patients with advanced or end-stage organ disease (ESOD). This chapter focuses on areas most applicable to the presurgical psychosocial assessment of adult SOT candidates (PPA-TC), incorporating a brief review of the distinct domains across the four most common organ transplants and associated disease states. Pretransplant psychosocial, behavioral, and cognitive factors that have been empirically linked to posttransplant outcomes are reviewed to help guide why and how to best assess adult patients being considered for liver, heart, lung, or kidney transplantation (LT, HT, LGT, KT, respectively). Guidelines for evaluating

This chapter has additional files available for download from the Resource Library tab on this book's website (https://www.apa.org/pubs/books/psychological-assessment-surgical-candidates).

https://doi.org/10.1037/0000346-009
Psychological Assessment of Surgical Candidates: Evidence-Based Procedures and Practices, R. J. Marek and A. R. Block (Editors)

these factors will assist mental health providers in optimizing transplant candidate (TC) selection and postsurgical outcomes.

BACKGROUND ON ORGAN TRANSPLANTATION AND EVALUATION

SOT is a surgical procedure in which an organ from a living or deceased donor is transferred to a person diagnosed with ESOD; it became the optimal treatment choice for ESOD in the 1960s. Many patients with ESOD live for years with their chronic illness, while others become suddenly and gravely ill; both scenarios may result in the need for a life-saving transplant.

The PPA-TC across organ groups is generally similar; however, there are differences among various ESODs to consider when conducting PPA-TC, and we review these variables as applicable. Refer to Table 8.1 for organ-specific guidelines. When performing PPA-TC, it is important to inquire about how the TC's unique physical symptoms and associated treatment related to their ESOD may be affecting their overall well-being.

Liver Transplantation

The liver is the largest solid internal organ in the body, performing critical functions including removing bacteria and toxins, preventing infection, regulating immune responses, producing bile, making proteins that help the blood clot, and processing nutrients, medications, and hormones. When it stops working correctly, many normal functions of the body break down. Cirrhosis is the irreversible scarring of the liver and is the most common reason for LT. Common etiologies of cirrhosis in the United States include alcohol-related liver disease, nonalcoholic steatohepatitis (i.e., fatty-liver disease), hepatocellular carcinoma, metabolic and genetic conditions, and viral hepatitis. LT is the best treatment option for end-stage liver disease. As liver function declines, individuals often experience physical symptoms (e.g., swelling, variceal bleeding, hepatic encephalopathy, extreme fatigue, jaundice and itchy skin, gastrointestinal disturbance) that need medical intervention, which can have negative consequences on mental health and quality of life.

Lung Transplantation

The lungs are responsible for respiration and gas exchange processes in the body. Patients may experience challenges with either obstructive or restrictive lung diseases that may lead to significant and impairing symptoms (e.g., dyspnea, cough, increased sputum production, exacerbations and infections, fatigue), affecting the quality of life. Patients may be asked to complete

TABLE 8.1. Organ-Specific Guidelines for Assessment of Transplant Candidates

Organ type	Guideline	Citation
CT/MCS	The 2018 International Society for Heart and Lung Transplantation (ISHLT), Academy of Psychosomatic Medicine, American Society of Transplantation, International Consortium of Circulatory Assist Clinicians, and Society for Transplant Social Workers Recommendations for the Psychosocial Evaluation of Adult Cardiothoracic Transplant Candidates and Candidates for Long-Term Mechanical Circulatory Support	(Dew et al., 2018)
	Consensus Document for the Selection of Lung Transplant Candidates: An Update From the International Society for Heart and Lung Transplantation	(Leard et al., 2021)
	The 2016 ISHLT Listing Criteria for Heart Transplantation: A 10-Year Update	(Mehra et al., 2016)
	The 2013 ISHLT Summary Guidelines for Mechanical Circulatory Support: Executive Summary	(Feldman et al., 2013)
Kidney	KDIGO Clinical Practice Guidelines on the Evaluation and Management of Candidates for Kidney Transplantation	(Chadban et al., 2020)
	Guidelines for Living Donor Kidney Transplantation	(British Transplantation Society & The Renal Association, 2018)
Liver	Evaluation for Liver Transplantation in Adults: 2013 Practice Guideline by the American Association for the Study of Liver Diseases and the American Society of Transplantation	(Martin et al., 2014)
	Adult Liver Transplantation: A UK Clinical Guideline—Part 1: Pre-operation [from the British Society of Gastroenterology]	(Millson et al., 2020)
	European Association of the Study of the Liver Clinical Practice Guidelines: Liver Transplantation	(European Association for the Study of the Liver, 2016)
	The Dallas Consensus Conference on Liver Transplantation for Alcohol Associated Hepatitis	(Asrani et al., 2020)

Note. CT = cardiothoracic transplantation; MCS = mechanical circulatory support.

lengthy breathing treatment routines or to use supplemental oxygen as their lung disease progresses. For patients with advanced lung disease, LGT is an effective treatment option for carefully selected candidates. Etiologies of end-stage lung diseases most commonly leading to the need for consideration of LGT include interstitial lung disease, advanced chronic obstructive pulmonary disease, cystic fibrosis, emphysema due to alpha-1 antitrypsin deficiency, pulmonary arterial hypertension, and other conditions (Chambers et al., 2019). LGT survival lags behind SOT for other ESODs (Chambers et al., 2019). The specific challenges inherent in advanced lung disease, LGT, and lower survival compared with other SOT populations underscore the importance of careful patient selection.

Heart Transplant and Long-Term Mechanical Circulatory Support Devices

The heart is responsible for blood circulation and flow throughout the body. Heart failure may occur when the heart is not able to pump blood as effectively to parts of the body as it should. Conditions leading to consideration of HT include nonischemic and ischemic cardiomyopathy, which may result in a worsened quality of life secondary to fatigue, dyspnea, chest pains, rapid or irregular heartbeats, and breathlessness. HT remains one of the most effective interventions for advanced heart failure. Other management strategies have evolved to include mechanical circulatory support devices (MCSD), such as ventricular assist devices or the total artificial heart. These can provide a long-term intervention for patients who may not be immediate HT candidates due to psychosocial or medical concerns (Melton et al., 2019). MCSDs need unique care, including frequent site dressing changes, adequate power sources, limitations to activities, including water-based activities, special precautions, management of alarms, and so forth (Grady et al., 2015). There are thus many considerations regarding candidacy selection for heart failure patients.

Kidney Transplantation

Kidneys perform several crucial functions in our bodies, including maintaining overall fluid balance and filtering minerals and waste materials from food, medications, and toxic agents. When kidney function reaches 15% less than normal, individuals meet the criteria for end-stage kidney disease (ESKD). Treatments for ESKD are limited to KT or dialysis. While a viable alternative, dialysis requires a significant time commitment and may include serious side effects. The most common indications for KT are diabetes, hypertension, glomerulonephritis, and cystic kidney disease (U.S. Department of Health & Human Services [USDHHS], 2019). KT offers improved survival outcomes and physical and psychosocial quality of life compared with dialysis (Kostro et al., 2016). The wait times for KT remain long, with only a quarter of waitlisted patients receiving a deceased-donor transplant within 5 years (USDHHS, 2019). In ESKD, waste products such as urea, salt, and extra water can build up in the blood, causing a condition called uremia. Uremia may cause fatigue and insomnia, among other distressing physical symptoms, such as dry or itchy skin, chronic pain, weight loss, nausea or vomiting, shortness of breath, and chest pain (Shirazian et al., 2017). KT remains the most performed SOT, with 22,817 KTs completed in the United States in 2020, and most individuals waiting for a transplant are currently waiting for a KT (Organ Procurement and Transplantation Network, 2021).

PRESURGICAL PSYCHOSOCIAL ASSESSMENT OF TRANSPLANT CANDIDATES

The practices for the SOT assessment include medical, surgical, and psychosocial components, which differ across transplant centers and organ groups (Skillings & Lewandowski, 2015). When the assessment is complete, a multidisciplinary committee of transplant providers meets to discuss the appropriateness for an SOT listing and then approve, defer, or decline a patient for listing. Medical criteria for being listed for SOT are well established and described by the United Network for Organ Sharing (2021; Organ Procurement and Transplantation Network [OPTN], 2021). Although transplant centers in the United States require TCs to undergo a psychosocial assessment, these assessments remain heterogenous in breadth and depth and can be performed by any mental health provider (Collins & Labott, 2007). Given the increasing demand for SOTs against a limited supply, the PPA-TC has become increasingly important for prospectively identifying areas that need intervention to maximize posttransplant outcomes.

The PPA-TC collects baseline data on the TC's psychological, cognitive, and social functioning and quality of life, which can be reassessed throughout the SOT process. The PPA-TC includes a conceptualization of the constellation of risk and protective factors for the TC, which simultaneously allows the transplant team to be good stewards of donated organs. The goal of the PPA-TC is to determine the appropriateness for SOT listing, as well as to provide recommendations and treatment targeting modifiable risk factors that can be employed before and/or after SOT.

PSYCHOSOCIAL FACTORS LIKELY ASSOCIATED WITH POOR TRANSPLANT OUTCOMES

Pretransplant psychosocial risk factors associated with adverse posttransplant outcomes include nonadherence, limited knowledge or health literacy, cognitive dysfunction, maladaptive coping, past or present mental health concerns, limited social support, and substance abuse. The TC may be at increased risk of poor clinical outcomes after transplant if risk factors are present during the PPA-TC; the more risk factors present, the higher the risk of undesirable outcomes (Maldonado et al., 2015; Rivard et al., 2005). Risk factors may be predictive of posttransplant nonadherence, increased infection and rejection rates, hospital readmissions, graft loss, posttransplant morbidity, and decreased survival (Delibasic et al., 2017; Dew et al., 2015). Mental health concerns may negatively affect SOT outcomes through various mechanisms, including nonadherence, interpersonal challenges, limited social support, self-injury, and medication interactions between psychotropic medications and immunosuppressants (Zimbrean & Emre, 2015). Maintaining current knowledge of the empirical literature is critical because research differs across organ types, transplant phases, and research methodology. The following outlines specific domains that should be integrated into the PPA-TC based on current empirical literature.

Adherence

Treatment adherence is "the active cooperation of patients with their health-care professional regarding attendance to clinics and laboratory appointments, following a specific medication schedule without deviations, following a diet and/or exercise rehabilitation plan, and the notification of problems to the treatment team" (Sher & Maldonado, 2019, p. 23). A primary cause of organ failure after SOT is patient nonadherence to their posttransplant regimen, which occurs in around 23 per 100 persons per year (Dew et al., 2007). Organ rejection can occur after SOT when the body's immune system does not recognize the transplanted organ and attempts to destroy it. To reduce the risk of rejection, SOT recipients are prescribed immunosuppressants that lower their immune response. The success of SOT depends on the recipient's ability, willingness, and commitment to manage a complex posttransplant routine, including lifelong adherence to daily medications, frequent blood draws, medical procedures, appointments, and behavior changes.

The literature indicates that pretransplant nonadherence is associated with posttransplant nonadherence and organ rejection; thus, understanding pretransplant adherence behaviors is essential to help mitigate the risk of poor outcomes (Dobbels et al., 2009; Neuberger et al., 2017; Telles-Correia et al., 2012). Numerous patient-level factors have been associated with posttransplant nonadherence, including age, gender, ethnicity, self-efficacy, self-care agency, substance abuse, socioeconomic status (SES), education, employment status, social support, and health literacy (Bailey et al., 2021; Neuberger et al., 2017). Examining the variables related to nonadherence will help develop interventions that address the individual and systems-level factors at play (Dew et al., 2007; Neuberger et al., 2017).

Rates of nonadherence to immunosuppression are highest among KT recipients, increasing the risk for acute KT rejection (Al-Sheyyab et al., 2019; Dew et al., 2007). Posttransplant nonadherence is associated with higher rates of hospital readmissions and acute rejection among KT recipients (Mohamed et al., 2021). Concomitant nonadherence to appointments and medication regimens is associated with a fourfold increased risk of graft loss after KT (Taber et al., 2017). From a systems level, a lack of cultural sensitivity by health care providers could negatively impact adherence because trust and shared decision making are correlated with improved adherence, and one-size-fits-all interventions for nonadherence are ineffective. Further, the lack of involved caregivers to report nonadherence can be problematic (Dew et al., 2007; Fine et al., 2009).

The PPA-TC should thoroughly assess the TCs adherence to recommendations made by the transplant team, and the evaluator should be knowledgeable about recommendations made to the TC. Many facets of adherence should be assessed, including attendance at appointments, active engagement in treatments (e.g., cardiopulmonary rehabilitation, dialysis, supplemental oxygen), adherence to medication regimen (including any missed or delayed dosages), and engagement in self-management behaviors (e.g., checking blood glucose). Evidence supports measuring adherence through a detailed interview and validated questionnaires or objective measures because providers tend to overestimate adherence (Neuberger et al., 2017). When assessing adherence, the evaluator must be empathic and nonconfrontational because TCs tend to minimize poor adherence; it is important for the evaluator to acknowledge the challenges associated with the complexity of recommendations. Understanding barriers to adherence, such as health literacy, medical trust, and other culture-specific variables, is critical to an unbiased assessment. A strong therapeutic alliance allows the evaluator to make recommendations that may improve candidacy rather than disqualifying candidates for a history of poor adherence.

Health Literacy

The Centers for Disease Control and Prevention defines *health literacy* as "the degree to which individuals have the ability to find, understand, and use information and services to inform health-related decisions and actions for themselves and others" (Santana et al., 2021, Table 1). Given the complexity of SOT-related health information, health literacy must be considered in the PPA-TC. Limited health literacy in TCs is associated with difficulty attending pretransplant appointments; a lower likelihood of being referred, listed, and receiving a SOT; and a greater risk of posttransplant nonadherence and graft failure (Green et al., 2013; Grubbs et al., 2009; Kazley et al., 2015; Miller-Matero et al., 2016). Low health literacy is associated with TCs who are older, are of minority status, are non-English speaking, have a lower education level, have a lower income, and are unemployed. Posttransplant, limited health literacy is implicated in higher rates of emergency department visits, hospitalizations, and mortality (Chisholm-Burns et al., 2018). Understanding unique TC factors and culture can inform the PPA-TCs and tailored interventions and address concerns about bias and equity, although a thorough discussion of inequities throughout SOT is beyond the scope of this chapter (Olbrisch, 1996).

Health literacy may be assessed through open-ended questioning of the TC's understanding of their health conditions and treatments as well as the use of validated tools. Frequently used measures to assess health literacy are the Short Test of Functional Health Literacy in Adults (R. M. Parker et al., 1995) and the Rapid Estimate of Adult Literacy in Medicine-Transplantation (Davis et al., 1993). The Knowledge Questionnaire for Renal Recipients (Urstad et al., 2011) is a validated questionnaire that assesses awareness of terms that are specific to KT, and the Decision-Making Capacity Assessment Tool (Kazley et al., 2014) was designed and validated with KTCs to assess transplant-specific health literacy and decision-making ability. The Agency for Healthcare Research and Quality has developed an evidence-based toolkit to help reduce health literacy barriers (Brega et al., 2015). Early identification of health literacy challenges allows more time for interventions (e.g., caregiver support) to mitigate risks. Reevaluation of health literacy should continue through the posttransplant period because it has an impact on posttransplant nonadherence (Serper et al., 2015).

Social Support and Caregiving

Patients with ESOD face multiple psychosocial stressors, including feeling uncertain about the future, feeling like a burden, needing help with activities of daily life, and experiencing a loss of identity; social support may ameliorate these variables. Social support has been associated with improved adherence, quality of life, health behaviors, mental health, and SOT outcomes, including a lower risk of graft failure and longer survival (Bui, Allen, et al., 2019;

Dew et al., 2018; DiMatteo, 2004; Dobbels et al., 2006; Duffy et al., 2010; Maldonado, 2019). For LGT recipients with a more challenging posttransplant course, social support may buffer against mortality (Smith et al., 2018). Limited support has been called a "critical determinant of medical non-adherence" among TCs (Dobbels et al., 2009, Discussion section, para. 3). Limited pretransplant social support has been associated with posttransplant mortality, graft loss, and risk of relapse to substance use disorders and was an independent predictor of nonadherence after SOT (Dew et al., 2008; Dobbels et al., 2009; Rivard et al., 2005; Telles-Correia et al., 2012). Importantly, the relationship of the caregiver to the TC may affect posttransplant outcomes. TCs who have spouses as caregivers have improved survival and less risk of graft failure compared with SOT recipients with other types of caregivers (e.g., adult–child; Mollberg et al., 2015). It is essential to assess the quality and ability to provide practical support beyond the mere presence of a caregiver (DiMatteo, 2004). TCs may complete objective validated measures of social support (e.g., Farmer et al., 2013; Sirri et al., 2011). The evaluator may provide feedback on improvements to existing support systems and facilitate resource sharing (Maldonado, 2019). For those with physical, psychological, or cognitive limitations that affect self-care, social support may mitigate the risk that these limitations carry.

Other Social History

It is important to assess other social factors such as SES, occupational history, exposure to trauma, and adverse childhood experiences to provide a comprehensive understanding of the TC's culture, history, and context (Dew et al., 2018; Farmer et al., 2013; Ravi et al., 2018; Rudasill et al., 2019; Tsuang et al., 2020). For instance, adverse childhood experiences elevate the risk of developing other psychological and medical or health concerns (Petruccelli et al., 2019). Understanding these factors will help develop an integrated, comprehensive conceptualization of TC strength and risk factors. Many of these factors are not modifiable by the patient alone, but PPA-TC allows for an opportunity to provide education and recommendations to the SOT team, which may combat systemic barriers that TCs may face.

Transplant Knowledge

Knowledge is a key domain of assessment for TCs; however, TCs frequently suffer from gaps in their understanding of their ESOD, resulting in decisional conflict and inability to care for themselves appropriately (Dew et al., 2018). TCs should be knowledgeable about transplant center policies and expectations as well as the risks and complications related to surgery and recovery time to optimize preparedness (Kauffman et al., 2008). Because much of SOT education occurs during the assessment where the focus is on the TC's candidacy, many TCs do not retain critical information, which is a risk factor for later nonadherence (Fine et al., 2009; Weng et al., 2017). Improved knowledge and shared decision making (e.g., via decision aids) for TCs may contribute to reduced decisional conflict and improved self-care (Blumenthal-Barby et al., 2015). Knowledge should be assessed during the PPA-TC interview, and the use of validated tools may be considered to supplement the PPA. There are decision aids for LGT (Vandemheen et al., 2009) and ventricular assist devices (Blumenthal-Barby et al., 2015), as well as measures of SOT-related knowledge (Ismail et al., 2013; Peipert et al., 2019; Schaevers et al., 2021).

Cognitive Functioning

Cognitive functioning should be assessed to identify barriers to providing informed consent for SOT and posttransplant self-management. Cognitive dysfunction may be present among TCs due to the effects of ESOD itself (e.g., hepatic encephalopathy, uremia, hypoxia) and/or premorbid cognitive or intellectual disability. Within care guidelines and consensus documents, intellectual disability and dementia are identified as relative contraindications to HT, and progressive cognitive impairment of the brain is considered an absolute contraindication to LGT (Leard et al., 2021; Mehra et al., 2016). Liver and kidney guidelines do not identify cognitive factors as absolute contraindications, though programs vary widely in their practices (Wall et al., 2020). However, programs are encouraged to avoid categorizing patients as contraindicated for SOT based solely on intellectual disability and should instead evaluate each individual, taking into consideration the interactive effects of protective and risk factors when making decisions about SOT listing (Wall et al., 2020). TCs with even severe cognitive impairments may receive benefits from SOT when they have appropriate caregiving support in place to promote posttransplant adherence (Galante et al., 2010; Samelson-Jones et al., 2012).

Cognitive functioning is relevant to consider across ESOD patients being evaluated for transplant. Better cognitive functioning is associated with higher self-efficacy, postsurgical adherence, and improved quality of life among patients who received a ventricular assist device (Casida et al., 2017) and with reduced risk of all-cause mortality after controlling for SES, psychiatric comorbidities, etiology, and disease severity among LT patients (Madan et al., 2015). Patients with ESKD with cognitive impairments experience a lower likelihood of being placed on KT waitlists, and for those without diabetes, cognitive impairment is associated with increased mortality when on the KT waitlist (Chu et al., 2020). Pretransplant cognitive dysfunction is associated with lower posttransplant adherence, increased all-cause graft loss, and higher mortality (Gelb et al., 2010; Smith et al., 2014; Thomas et al., 2019). Individuals with cognitive impairments may need additional supports in place as part of the transplant process to have success with pre- and posttransplant management.

Outside of premorbid cognitive conditions, cognitive changes are common among liver transplant candidates (LTCs) due to the effects of their ESOD. To illustrate, hepatic encephalopathy (HE) is cognitive dysfunction (impairments in response inhibition, learning, and working memory) resulting from liver insufficiency or portal shunting and occurs in up to 70% of LTCs (Bajaj et al., 2010; Teperman, 2013; Vilstrup et al., 2014). HE symptoms present on a spectrum, including impaired cognition, disorientation and confusion, personality and behavior changes, psychosis, and even altered consciousness. HE may be transient or persistent, and although overt HE is typically evident, subtle HE likely necessitates neurocognitive testing to diagnose because even minimal HE can cause self-care tasks to be more difficult and increase the risk for motor vehicle accidents (Bajaj et al., 2009; Vilstrup et al., 2014). Therefore, it is recommended that HE is assessed using cognitive assessments that evaluate executive functioning, processing speed, attention, and concentration. Results substantiating impairments can help the LTC's hepatologist to choose the appropriate course of HE treatment.

When evaluating the cognition of TCs, objective assessment measures are necessary to accurately identify cognitive impairment because clinician perception of cognitive impairment is frequently inaccurate (Gupta et al., 2018). Depending on the setting and specific concerns about the TC, cognition may be assessed in a number of ways, ranging from brief screeners such as the Montreal Cognitive Assessment (Szymkowicz et al., 2021) to multidomain measures such as the Repeatable Battery of Neuropsychological Status (Mooney et al., 2007), or a full battery of neuropsychological assessments tailored to the TC (Lacerda et al., 2008; Roman, 2018). Providing feedback from cognitive testing and making recommendations (e.g., communication and compensatory strategies) to TCs and their caregiver(s) during the PPAs may reduce posttransplant nonadherence (Cheng et al., 2012).

Coping

Coping is defined as any effort used to minimize distress in the context of a particular stressor (Amoyal et al., 2016). Active coping has been associated with better health outcomes and higher quality of life in TCs, and maladaptive coping, including avoidance and defensiveness, has been associated with nonadherence after SOT, worse mental health, poorer psychological adjustment, and lower quality of life among SOT candidates and recipients (Burker et al., 2005; Olbrisch et al., 2002; Pisanti et al., 2017; Sher & Maldonado, 2019; Swanson et al., 2018). In LGTCs, lower levels of resilience are associated with pretransplant death or delisting, and higher negative affect is associated with death on the waiting list (Bui et al., 2020; Pennington et al., 2020). Coping may be modifiable through psychological intervention, which may mitigate the risk for worse outcomes after SOT. Therefore, a thorough assessment of TCs' coping strategies and past adaptation to stressors is completed as part of the PPA-TC; standardized measures can augment the clinical interview in understanding the TC's coping style (e.g., Müller et al., 2015; Swanson et al., 2018).

Depression and Anxiety

Individuals with ESOD often experience a slow decline in physical and cognitive functioning, which can negatively affect the quality of life. Mental health concerns are common among TCs across organ types and throughout SOT stages, with depression and anxiety occurring at higher rates in the SOT population than in the general population, and are the most frequently studied mental health concerns (Dobbels et al., 2001, 2006). The uncertainty that TCs face, intensified by the fear of being ineligible for SOT listing, and the real anxieties about posttransplant life are often magnified by premorbid mental health issues such as anxiety, depression, and substance use disorders (SUD; Corbett et al., 2013; Corruble et al., 2011; Olbrisch et al., 2002). Studies of patients with ESOD have found that symptoms of depression are present in 20% of patients with kidney (on dialysis, this increases to 39%; Shirazian et al., 2017), liver, or heart disease (Buganza-Torio et al., 2019; Delibasic et al., 2017; Kop, 2010) and up to 48% of patients with lung disease (Dobbels et al., 2006), which significantly increases the risk of posttransplant mortality (Dew et al., 2018, 2015). LTCs are at 3 times the risk for a suicide attempt compared with healthy controls (Le Strat et al., 2015), and HTCs with a historical suicide attempt (or attempts) are at increased risk of infection and reduced survival (Owen et al., 2006). A meta-analysis found that pretransplant depression predicted posttransplant depression and increased risk of posttransplant mortality, with depression being determined with diagnostic assessments or standardized symptoms scales (Dew et al., 2015). This effect is hypothesized in part to be through behavioral pathways, including depression contributing to poorer medical adherence (Cukor et al., 2009; Delibasic et al., 2017), reduced physical activity (Dew et al., 2018; Kop et al., 2011), substance abuse (Kop, 2010), and potential dysregulation in neurohormones, autonomic nervous system function, or inflammatory processes (Kop et al., 2011; Martelli et al., 2019). These biobehavioral processes may pose an increased risk for infections, complications, rehospitalization, graft rejection, and/or mortality (Dew et al., 2018).

PPA for TCs should consider assessing how potential stigma related to diagnosis (i.e., SUD), a decline in the quality of life, multiple hospitalizations, functional decline, and changes to social support may all affect mood symptoms. Such discussion and demonstration of understanding ESOD medical sequelae may help build rapport and lower defenses with the TC, thereby obtaining more honest disclosure of past and current mood states.

Serious Mental Illness

Given the low prevalence of serious mental illness (SMI; i.e., symptoms of schizophrenia, schizoaffective disorder, bipolar disorder, major depression with psychotic features, and other psychotic disorders) in the general and SOT population, the empirical literature on SMI and SOT is sparse, with no consensus on the effect of pretransplant SMI on SOT outcomes. There is some evidence that if symptoms negatively affect a TC's ability to manage their care or impact their caregiving plan, it may negatively affect clinical outcomes (Dew & DiMartini, 2005; Dew et al., 2018). However, the research also suggests that if the SMI is well controlled and a strong support system is in place, these TCs may fare as well as SOT recipients without an SMI (Coffman & Crone, 2002; Zimbrean & Emre, 2015). The PPA-TC with SMI should assess for triggers to previous psychotic episodes, adherence, social support, and the time of the last episode. SMI should not be an absolute contraindication to SOT (Cahn-Fuller & Parent, 2017; OPTN Ethics Committee, 2021); however, early detection, accomplished through PPA-TC, and adherence to recommended mental health treatment may improve SOT outcomes (Chadban et al., 2020).

Personality Disorders

Personality traits and dimensions have the potential to influence all aspects of a person's life, including how they navigate SOT. Personality disorders (i.e., personality characteristics that are significantly disruptive or maladaptive) are estimated to occur at roughly the same rate in the SOT population as in the general population (Dobbels et al., 2001). TCs may need additional support to prevent their interpersonal style from impairing their relationship with their caregivers and transplant team (Dobbels et al., 2006; Kumnig & Jowsey-Gregoire, 2015). Interventions to manage personality disorders in TCs include education and caregiver (and potentially SOT team) engagement, with the goal of mitigating the consequences of poor interpersonal functioning (Dobbels et al., 2000; Stilley et al., 2005). Personality concerns may be determined through the clinical interview and the use of relevant standardized psychological assessments of personality.

Substance Use and Abuse

SUDs are complex, as these disorders disrupt the brain and one's ability to control and/or modify social, emotional, and cognitive behavior. Posttransplant relapse to alcohol, tobacco, and/or other substances of abuse can result in direct and/or indirect harm to the new organ, graft rejection, medical complications, nonadherence, and increased use of medical care and stress on the SOT team as a whole (Dew et al., 2007; Olbrisch et al., 2002; R. Parker et al., 2013). Guidelines suggest that TCs with concern for SUD should undergo further assessment by a provider who specializes in PPA-TCs (R. Parker et al., 2013). Early identification of past or present SUD is critical because treatment is generally recommended to reduce the risk of relapse and improve posttransplant outcomes (Chadban et al., 2020). Depending on the type of ESOD and the transplant center's specific policies, alcohol, tobacco, and illicit drug use (including cannabis) may be absolute or relative contraindications to SOT. The evaluator should be knowledgeable about these policies at their specific center. Gathering biomarkers such as ethyl glucuronide and phosphatidylethanol for alcohol, urine or serum drug screens, and nicotine urine or serum screens can help confirm TC reports (Fleming et al., 2017), and evaluators should obtain collateral information (e.g., spouse; Beresford & Lucey, 2018). KT candidates may not be able to produce the urine needed for lab screening (Ward et al., 2014); as such, it is advisable to request blood serum samples with KTCs.

Alcohol

Alcohol abuse has been identified as a risk factor for multiple health conditions, including those leading to ESOD (Dobbels et al., 2019). Research on alcohol use in SOT patients tends to focus on LT patients; however, the effects of posttransplant alcohol relapse on transplant outcomes can be significant across organ groups (Owen et al., 2006). Approaching the assessment of alcohol use can be challenging due to the tendency for impression management and defensive responding (Ruchinskas et al., 2006). When asking about alcohol use during the PPA-TC, additional rationale, time, and effort made for rapport building can help the evaluator obtain more honest responses. Risk factors associated with relapse to alcohol that should be assessed include limited social stability, alcohol abuse among first-degree relatives, repeated failed alcohol treatments, poor adherence to medical care, polysubstance abuse, and coexisting mental disorders (Dew et al., 2008; Rodrigue et al., 2013). Understanding the risk factors, scope, and severity of alcohol use can help connect the TC to the appropriate level of treatment required for lifelong abstinence. TCs with SUDs may be in denial, underreport, or underestimate substance use, hoping to be listed for a life-saving intervention, making accurate assessment challenging. Consequently, mental health providers are best suited to assess for SUD and risk for posttransplant relapse during PPA-TC. Evaluators should use nonjudgmental language to ask detailed questions about the TC's history of SUD regardless of disease etiology.

Alcohol-Related Liver Disease

Alcohol-related liver disease (ARLD) is now the most common indication for LT (Cholankeril & Ahmed, 2018; Kwong et al., 2021). LTCs with ARLD may have low insight into their alcohol use disorder and may be reluctant to engage in treatment, often focusing more on their medical treatments and physical well-being (Mellinger et al., 2018; Weinrieb et al., 2001). Although most LTCs with ARLD seem genuinely committed to lifelong alcohol abstinence, the data suggest that up to 50% of LTCs with ARLD relapse following LT (Dew et al., 2008; DiMartini et al., 2006; Pageaux et al., 2003). Preliminary research conducted at one transplant center found temporal trends in relapse rate following LT (confirmed via biomarker testing) related to the COVID-19 pandemic. This pilot study found the risk of relapse increased from 4.3% prepandemic (2018–2020) to 18.8% for the cut point of April 2020 to 2021 (Torosian et al., 2022). Post-LT alcohol relapse may have serious consequences, including rejection, fibrosis, graft loss, nonadherence to medical care, rehospitalizations, and poorer survival (Conjeevaram et al., 1999; DiMartini et al., 2010; Pageaux et al., 2003; Rice et al., 2013). Sustained alcohol use post-LT is the strongest predictor of post-LT mortality, associated with a fivefold increased risk of death compared with abstinent LT recipients (Lee et al., 2018). Assessment should include a standard diagnostic assessment of alcohol use disorder and assessment of specific risk factors that may increase the risk of recidivism to alcohol post-LT, as described in key references (i.e., Lee et al., 2019; Lombardo-Quezada et al., 2019; Rodrigue et al., 2013).

Alcohol-Associated Hepatitis

Alcohol-associated hepatitis (AAH) is a subset of ARLD characterized by acute jaundice in the setting of chronic heavy alcohol use and is associated with high short-term mortality (75% to 90% within 2 months of onset) when patients do not respond to steroid treatment (Bui, Braun, et al., 2019; Lee et al., 2018). In recent years, LT for AAH has become more acceptable among highly selected patients, given the high mortality rate without LT and generally good preliminary outcomes. Nonetheless, LT for AAH remains controversial as it is typically preceded by recent alcohol consumption with little to no period of sobriety. When conducting PPA for AAH, it is essential to know the nuances in this unique circumstance, specifically as it relates to risk factors associated with recidivism following LT. The most common assessment tool used at the time of this writing is the Sustained Alcohol Use Post-LT score, which assesses the number of drinks per day before hospitalization, history of non-THC illicit substance use, alcohol-related legal issues, and past rehabilitation attempts to derive scores that yield positive and negative predictive values (see Lee et al., 2019). We suspect additional tools will be available as more LT for AAH are completed and associated research is conducted. Additional considerations for PPA-TC within this subgroup include a stronger focus on obtaining collateral information from medical providers and the patient's support system, a thorough explanation of post-LT expectations (typically involving intensive alcohol use disorder treatment) using the teach-back method to confirm the understanding of LTC and caregivers, and use of a post-LT agreement signed by the patient and providers. A thorough review is beyond the scope of this chapter; refer to Table 8.1 for a review of various guidelines and consensus conferences (Asrani et al., 2020; Lee et al., 2018).

Patients with ARLD have special assessment considerations. First, clinicians should routinely use validated tools (see Table 8.2) to assess relapse risk, which should be applied in a standardized fashion across TCs with ARLD. Further, patient reports on abstinence pre- and posttransplant should be

TABLE 8.2. Assessment Tools for Risk to Recidivism to Alcohol Post-LT

Measure	Reference	Cohort
Alcohol Relapse Risk Assessment	(Rodrigue et al., 2013)	LT recipients (all etiologies)
High-Risk Alcoholism Relapse Score	(Lombardo-Quezada et al., 2019)	LT recipients with AUD diagnosis
Sustained Alcohol Use Post-Liver Transplant Score	(Lee et al., 2019)	LT recipients with AAH, no length of sobriety
Hopkins Psychosocial Scale	(Lee et al., 2017)	LT recipients with AAH, no length of sobriety

Note. AAH = alcohol-associated hepatitis; AUD = alcohol use disorder; LT = liver transplant.

obtained regularly by interview with trained clinicians and corroborated with routine random biological marker testing. Recommended biomarkers include phosphatidylethanol and ethyl glucuronide. Carbohydrate-deficient transferrin should be avoided in LT patients because this test may be better thought of as indicating the degree of liver impairment and may not accurately portray recent alcohol use.

Tobacco

Pretransplant tobacco use is related to a greater risk of early rejection, allograft loss, and patient death following SOT (Corbett et al., 2012; Dew et al., 2008; Nogueira et al., 2010; Sher & Maldonado, 2019). For instance, for LT recipients, smokers had a 79% higher risk of dying than never smokers or those who quit before LT (López-Lazcano et al., 2020). Shorter periods of tobacco abstinence before SOT are associated with a higher risk of relapse after SOT (Duerinckx et al., 2016). Early intervention is recommended to promote abstinence at the time of SOT. Tobacco use contributes to respiratory diseases and is related to a range of cardiovascular diseases (USDHHS, 2014). Active tobacco use is a contraindication to LGT and is a relative contraindication to HT (Mehra et al., 2016). Tobacco use increases the risk for cardiovascular events and cancer—two main causes of mortality among LT and KT recipients (Hurst et al., 2011; Li et al., 2017). The PPA-TC should assess past and current tobacco use (cigarettes, dip/chew/snuff, pipe tobacco, hookah, vaping, Juul, E-juice, dripping). Vaporizing tobacco with tetrahydrocannabinol has led to an increase in E-cigarette/vaping-associated lung injury in the United States, which for some has necessitated LGT (Jacobs et al., 2020; Nemeh et al., 2021). Understanding the volume, frequency, and behaviors related to tobacco use aids in diagnosis and treatment planning to reduce posttransplant risks.

Cannabis

Cannabis use among TCs remains controversial, and there is no consensus among transplant centers on the acceptability of cannabis use, which, in the United States, parallels the wide range of legal policies regarding cannabis use across states. Medical risks related to cannabis use among SOT patients include cardiovascular, pulmonary, cognitive, and infectious complications. There is some evidence that cannabis use posttransplant increases the risk for malignancy, cannabis–drug interactions, and infection (e.g., aspergillosis; Melaragno et al., 2021). An estimated 0.5% to 10% of TCs use cannabis products (Alhamad et al., 2019; Ranney et al., 2009), making it the most commonly used illicit substance (per federal law) in this population (Majumder & Sarkar, 2020). While more research is needed on the effects of cannabis on SOT outcomes, it has been suggested that "it is reasonable to ask patients not to use substances that can impair outcomes after transplantation or, at a minimum, compel modified use in a way that could also support good post-transplant care and subsequent outcomes," which may include medicinal marijuana (Allen & Ambardekar, 2016, para. 8; Sher & Maldonado, 2019). Cannabis use after SOT has been significantly associated with death-censored graft failure in KT recipients and was associated with twice the risk of graft failure (including death censored), all-cause graft loss, and death up to 2 years after SOT (Alhamad et al., 2019; Vaitla et al., 2021). Thus, the PPA-TC should assess past and current cannabis use among TCs to provide recommendations regarding the need for abstinence, which may be most salient to outcomes after SOT.

Prescribed Opioids

TCs are commonly prescribed opioid pain medications, which may come with certain risks. Opioid prescription rates the year before SOT are 43.1% among KTCs (Lentine et al., 2018) and 40% among HTCs (Lentine et al., 2019); high levels of posttransplant opioid use have been associated with increased risk of death and/or graft loss (Lentine et al., 2019). Higher morphine equivalent levels pretransplant are found to result in the highest risk of death and graft loss after SOT (Lentine et al., 2019; Randall et al., 2017). Distinguishing between opioid use and misuse requires a review of prescription records and early refills, a review of state databases of controlled substances and drug screen reports, and patient, provider, and caregiver input.

Other Substances of Abuse

Although research on the relationship between illicit drug use and SOT outcomes is sparse, illicit drug use has been associated with worse post-transplant adherence, although the impact on posttransplant survival rates and other posttransplant outcomes is less clear (Majumder & Sarkar, 2020). In patients with ESKD, illicit drug use was associated with increased mortality and disease progression before transplant (Bundy et al., 2018). Gathering information about the type, frequency, and amount of illicit substance used and other drug use behaviors can help to create an individualized treatment plan to mitigate potential risks of poor SOT outcomes.

PSYCHOMETRIC TOOLS FOR PPA-TC

Unfortunately, the literature examining psychometrics of commonly used measures in PPA-TCs is sparse, with no broadband instruments of psychosocial functioning normed among TCs. The Millon Behavioral Medicine

Diagnostic Instrument (Millon et al., 2001), Minnesota Multiphasic Personality Inventory–2 (Butcher et al., 1989), and Personality Assessment Inventory (Morey, 1991, 1996) have been used in the assessment of TCs and may provide useful information on mental health concerns, substance use, adherence behaviors, and social support, but further research is needed to determine the predictive value of these instruments in regard to posttransplant outcomes (Nghiem et al., 2020). Narrowband or domain-specific measures, such as the Beck Depression Inventory–II (BDI-II; Beck et al., 1996), Patient Health Questionnaire–9 (Kroenke et al., 2002), Hospital Anxiety and Depression Scale (Zigmond & Snaith, 1983), and Center for Epidemiologic Studies Depression Scale (Radloff, 1977) have been validated in KTCs, with the BDI having the most support (Kondo et al., 2020; Nghiem et al., 2020). Validation studies suggest a higher cutoff score should be used in TCs compared with the general population to show the greatest specificity and sensitivity (Cohen et al., 2007; Shirazian et al., 2017). Given the paucity of literature on the psychometric tools used with TCs, using measures that have norms and good psychometric properties in other medical settings is suggested until the evidence base develops further (Block & Marek, 2020; Nghiem et al., 2020).

Standardized Psychosocial Transplant Candidacy Assessment Interview Tools

Psychosocial SOT-specific assessment interview and rating tools have been developed to help mental health providers evaluate TCs. Tools include the Stanford Integrated Psychosocial Assessment for Transplant (Maldonado et al., 2015), Transplant Evaluation Rating Scale (Twillman et al., 1993), and Psychosocial Assessment of Candidates for Transplantation (Olbrisch et al., 2002).

A standardized approach to pretransplant assessments has several strengths. First and foremost, a standardized approach based on current empirical evidence can support the ethical standards of equity and justice by consistently applying clear standards across patients and transplant centers, concerns highlighted by the OPTN Ethics Committee (2021). Standardized assessments were developed with research in mind (e.g., Transplant Evaluation Rating Scale and the Psychosocial Assessment of Candidates for Transplantation) and can facilitate future understanding of pretransplant psychosocial risk factors that may affect posttransplant outcomes. Using a standardized tool can also help the multitude of providers that form a transplant team develop and use a shared language and framework for understanding a patient's unique risks and needs.

Despite the admirable goals of standardized instruments, there are several limitations to this approach. Primarily, the current research base has limited prospective studies that adequately identify pretransplant psychosocial predictors of posttransplant outcomes. As such, these standardized measures may not adequately capture the most important risks to posttransplant outcomes. Furthermore, any standardized measure would need to be routinely updated to maintain an evidence-based standardization with the frequently evolving research. It is notable as well that each of these standardized instruments may be intended for use across multiple organ types but lack clear psychometrics for each of these distinct populations. Although standardized instruments may serve to display and communicate psychosocial information relevant to transplant, such as a patient's modifiable versus unmodifiable risk factors, the burden remains on the clinician to maintain and implement their knowledge of the current research to guide the clinical interview, conceptualization, and consultation and communication with the transplant team.

Health Disparities Among Patients With End-Stage Kidney Disease

Health disparities among patients with ESKD and access to KT are significant in the United States. The prevalence of ESKD is 3.7 times greater in Black patients, who are less likely to be waitlisted and receive a KT, compared with White patients with ESKD, even after controlling for SES and medical comorbidities (Centers for Disease Control, 2021). Suggestions to address this gap are systemic, including addressing provider bias, distrust of medical providers, health literacy, and financial barriers to SOT (Harding et al., 2017; Patzer & Pastan, 2013). The PPA of KTCs should thoroughly assess for modifiable factors that contribute to these disparities. In addition, mental health providers are uniquely positioned to understand the biopsychosocial factors impacting a patient's experience in the health care system and can provide feedback to SOT teams about ways to improve cultural sensitivity and patient communication.

CONCLUSION

Conducting PPA-TCs requires the careful and thorough assessment of patient functioning associated with posttransplant outcomes. For each TC, a careful conceptualization of the constellation of risk is critical versus reporting on isolated risk factors. PPA-TC promotes the opportunity to develop interventions and mitigate risks, aiding SOT teams in identifying the best TCs for the limited number of donor organs available. Evaluators should be educated on the current research and guidelines related to PPA-TC; the contents of this chapter can provide a useful framework for conducting the PPA-TC.

REFERENCES

Alhamad, T., Koraishy, F. M., Lam, N. N., Katari, S., Naik, A. S., Schnitzler, M. A., Xiao, H., Axelrod, D. A., Dharnidharka, V. R., Randall, H., Ouseph, R., Segev, D. L., Brennan, D. C., Devraj, R., Kasiske, B. L., & Lentine, K. L. (2019). Cannabis dependence or abuse in kidney transplantation: Implications for posttransplant outcomes. *Transplantation*, *103*(11), 2373–2382. https://doi.org/10.1097/TP.0000000000002599

Allen, L. A., & Ambardekar, A. V. (2016). Hashing it out over cannabis: Moving toward a standard guideline on substance use for cardiac transplantation eligibility that includes marijuana. *Circulation: Heart Failure*, *9*(7), e003330. Advance online publication. https://doi.org/10.1161/CIRCHEARTFAILURE.116.003330

Al-Sheyyab, A., Binari, L., Shwetar, M., Ramos, E., Kapp, M. E., Bala, S., Wilson, N., Forbes, R. C., Helderman, J. H., Abdel-Kader, K., & Concepcion, B. P. (2019). Association of medication non-adherence with short-term allograft loss after the treatment of severe acute kidney transplant rejection. *BMC Nephrology*, *20*(1), 373. https://doi.org/10.1186/s12882-019-1563-z

Amoyal, N., Fernandez, A. C., Ng, R., & Fehon, D. C. (2016). Measuring coping behavior in liver transplant candidates: A psychometric analysis of the brief COPE. *Progress in Transplantation*, *26*(3), 277–285. https://doi.org/10.1177/1526924816655253

Asrani, S. K., Trotter, J., Lake, J., Ahmed, A., Bonagura, A., Cameron, A., DiMartini, A., Gonzalez, S., Im, G., Martin, P., Mathurin, P., Mellinger, J., Rice, J. P., Shah, V. H., Terrault, N., Wall, A., Winder, S., & Klintmalm, G. (2020). Meeting report: The Dallas Consensus Conference on Liver Transplantation for Alcohol Associated Hepatitis. *Liver Transplantation*, *26*(1), 127–140. https://doi.org/10.1002/lt.25681

Bailey, P., Vergis, N., Allison, M., Riddell, A., & Massey, E. (2021). Psychosocial evaluation of candidates for Solid Organ Transplantation. *Transplantation*, *105*(12), e292–e302. Advance online publication. https://doi.org/10.1097/TP.0000000000003732

Bajaj, J. S., Saeian, K., Schubert, C. M., Hafeezullah, M., Franco, J., Varma, R. R., Gibson, D. P., Hoffmann, R. G., Stravitz, R. T., Heuman, D. M., Sterling, R. K., Shiffman, M., Topaz, A., Boyett, S., Bell, D., & Sanyal, A. J. (2009). Minimal hepatic encephalopathy is associated with motor vehicle crashes: The reality beyond the driving test. *Hepatology*, *50*(4), 1175–1183. https://doi.org/10.1002/hep.23128

Bajaj, J. S., Schubert, C. M., Heuman, D. M., Wade, J. B., Gibson, D. P., Topaz, A., Saeian, K., Hafeezullah, M., Bell, D. E., Sterling, R. K., Stravitz, R. T., Luketic, V., White, M. B., & Sanyal, A. J. (2010). Persistence of cognitive impairment after resolution of overt hepatic encephalopathy. *Gastroenterology*, *138*(7), 2332–2340. https://doi.org/10.1053/j.gastro.2010.02.015

Beck, A. T., Steer, R. A., & Brown, G. K. (1996). *Manual for the Beck Depression Inventory–II*. Psychological Corporation.

Beresford, T. P., & Lucey, M. R. (2018). Towards standardizing the alcoholism evaluation of potential liver transplant recipients. *Alcohol and Alcoholism*, *53*(2), 135–144. https://doi.org/10.1093/alcalc/agx104

Block, A. R., & Marek, R. J. (2020). Presurgical psychological evaluation: Risk factor identification and mitigation. *Journal of Clinical Psychology in Medical Settings*, *27*(2), 396–405. https://doi.org/10.1007/s10880-019-09660-0

Blumenthal-Barby, J. S., Kostick, K. M., Delgado, E. D., Volk, R. J., Kaplan, H. M., Wilhelms, L. A., McCurdy, S. A., Estep, J. D., Loebe, M., & Bruce, C. R. (2015). Assessment of patients' and caregivers' informational and decisional needs for left ventricular assist device placement: Implications for informed consent and shared decision-making. *The Journal of Heart and Lung Transplantation, 34*(9), 1182–1189. https://doi.org/10.1016/j.healun.2015.03.026

Brega, A. G., Barnard, J., Mabachi, N. M., Weiss, B. D., DeWalt, D. A., Brach, C., Cifuentes, M., Albright, K., & West, D. R. (2015). *AHRQ Health Literacy Universal Precautions Toolkit* (AHRQ Publication No. 15-0023-EF). Agency for Healthcare Research and Quality.

British Transplantation Society & The Renal Association. (2018). *Guidelines for living donor kidney transplantation*. British Transplantation Society. https://bts.org.uk/wp-content/uploads/2018/07/FINAL_LDKT-guidelines_June-2018.pdf

Buganza-Torio, E., Mitchell, N., Abraldes, J. G., Thomas, L., Ma, M., Bailey, R. J., & Tandon, P. (2019). Depression in cirrhosis—A prospective evaluation of the prevalence, predictors and development of a screening nomogram. *Alimentary Pharmacology & Therapeutics, 49*(2), 194–201. https://doi.org/10.1111/apt.15068

Bui, Q. M., Allen, L. A., LeMond, L., Brambatti, M., & Adler, E. (2019). Psychosocial evaluation of candidates for heart transplant and ventricular assist devices: Beyond the current consensus. *Circulation: Heart Failure, 12*(7), e006058. https://doi.org/10.1161/CIRCHEARTFAILURE.119.006058

Bui, Q. M., Braun, O. O., Brambatti, M., Gernhofer, Y. K., Hernandez, H., Pretorius, V., & Adler, E. (2019). The value of Stanford integrated psychosocial assessment for transplantation (SIPAT) in prediction of clinical outcomes following left ventricular assist device (LVAD) implantation. *Heart & Lung, 48*(2), 85–89. https://doi.org/10.1016/j.hrtlng.2018.08.011

Bui, Y. T., Hathcock, M. A., Benzo, R. P., Budev, M. M., Chandrashekaran, S., Erasmus, D. B., Lease, E. D., Levine, D. J., Thompson, K. L., Johnson, B. K., Jowsey-Gregoire, S. G., & Kennedy, C. C. (2020). Evaluating resilience as a predictor of outcomes in lung transplant candidates. *Clinical Transplantation, 34*(10), e14056. https://doi.org/10.1111/ctr.14056

Bundy, J. D., Bazzano, L. A., Xie, D., Cohan, J., Dolata, J., Fink, J. C., Hsu, C. Y., Jamerson, K., Lash, J., Makos, G., Steigerwalt, S., Wang, X., Mills, K. T., Chen, J., He, J., & the CRIC Study Investigators. (2018). Self-reported tobacco, alcohol, and illicit drug use and progression of chronic kidney disease. *Clinical Journal of the American Society of Nephrology, 13*(7), 993–1001. https://doi.org/10.2215/CJN.11121017

Burker, E. J., Evon, D. M., Marroquin Loiselle, M., Finkel, J. B., & Mill, M. R. (2005). Coping predicts depression and disability in heart transplant candidates. *Journal of Psychosomatic Research, 59*(4), 215–222. https://doi.org/10.1016/j.jpsychores.2005.06.055

Butcher, J. N., Dahlstrom, W. G., Graham, J. R., Tellegen, A., & Kaemmer, B. (1989). *The Minnesota Multiphasic Personality Inventory–2 (MMPI-2): Manual for administration and scoring*. University of Minnesota Press.

Cahn-Fuller, K. L., & Parent, B. (2017). Transplant eligibility for patients with affective and psychotic disorders: A review of practices and a call for justice. *BMC Medical Ethics, 18*(1), 72. https://doi.org/10.1186/s12910-017-0235-4

Casida, J. M., Wu, H. S., Abshire, M., Ghosh, B., & Yang, J. J. (2017). Cognition and adherence are self-management factors predicting the quality of life of adults living with a left ventricular assist device. *The Journal of Heart and Lung Transplantation, 36*(3), 325–330. https://doi.org/10.1016/j.healun.2016.08.023

Centers for Disease Control and Prevention. (2021). *Chronic Kidney Disease Surveillance System*. https://nccd.cdc.gov/ckd/detail.aspx?QNum=Q89&Strat=CKD+Stage%2C+Age

Chadban, S. J., Ahn, C., Axelrod, D. A., Foster, B. J., Kasiske, B. L., Kher, V., Kumar, D., Oberbauer, R., Pascual, J., Pilmore, H. L., Rodrigue, J. R., Segev, D. L., Sheerin, N. S., Tinckam, K. J., Wong, G., & Knoll, G. A. (2020). KDIGO clinical practice guideline on the evaluation and management of candidates for kidney transplantation. *Transplantation, 104*(4S1). https://doi.org/10.1097/TP.0000000000003136

Chambers, D. C., Cherikh, W. S., Harhay, M. O., Hayes, D., Jr., Hsich, E., Khush, K. K., Meiser, B., Potena, L., Rossano, J. W., Toll, A. E., Singh, T. P., Sadavarte, A., Zuckermann, A., Stehlik, J., & the International Society for Heart and Lung Transplantation. (2019). The International Thoracic Organ Transplant Registry of the International Society for Heart and Lung Transplantation: Thirty-sixth adult lung and heart–lung transplantation Report—2019; Focus theme: Donor and recipient size match. *The Journal of Heart and Lung Transplantation, 38*(10), 1042–1055. https://doi.org/10.1016/j.healun.2019.08.001

Cheng, C. Y., Lin, B. Y., Chang, K. H., Shu, K. H., & Wu, M. J. (2012). Awareness of memory impairment increases the adherence to immunosuppressants in kidney transplant recipients. *Transplantation Proceedings, 44*(3), 746–748. https://doi.org/10.1016/j.transproceed.2011.11.030

Chisholm-Burns, M. A., Spivey, C. A., & Pickett, L. R. (2018). Health literacy in solid-organ transplantation: A model to improve understanding. *Patient Preference and Adherence, 12*, 2325–2338. https://doi.org/10.2147/PPA.S183092

Cholankeril, G., & Ahmed, A. (2018). Alcoholic liver disease replaces hepatitis C virus infection as the leading indication for liver transplantation in the United States. *Clinical Gastroenterology and Hepatology, 16*(8), 1356–1358. https://doi.org/10.1016/j.cgh.2017.11.045

Chu, N. M., Shi, Z., Haugen, C. E., Norman, S. P., Gross, A. L., Brennan, D. C., Carlson, M. C., Segev, D. L., & McAdams-DeMarco, M. A. (2020). Cognitive function, access to kidney transplantation, and waitlist mortality among kidney transplant candidates with or without diabetes. *American Journal of Kidney Diseases, 76*(1), 72–81. https://doi.org/10.1053/j.ajkd.2019.10.014

Coffman, K. L., & Crone, C. (2002). Rational guidelines for transplantation in patients with psychotic disorders. *Current Opinion in Organ Transplantation, 7*(4), 385–388. https://doi.org/10.1097/00075200-200212000-00015

Cohen, S. D., Norris, L., Acquaviva, K., Peterson, R. A., & Kimmel, P. L. (2007). Screening, diagnosis, and treatment of depression in patients with end-stage renal disease. *Clinical Journal of the American Society of Nephrology, 2*(6), 1332–1342. https://doi.org/10.2215/CJN.03951106

Collins, C. A., & Labott, S. M. (2007). Psychological assessment of candidates for solid organ transplantation. *Professional Psychology, Research and Practice, 38*(2), 150–157. https://doi.org/10.1037/0735-7028.38.2.150

Conjeevaram, H. S., Hart, J., Lissoos, T. W., Schiano, T. D., Dasgupta, K., Befeler, A. S., Millis, J. M., & Baker, A. L. (1999). Rapidly progressive liver injury and fatal alcoholic hepatitis occurring after liver transplantation in alcoholic patients. *Transplantation, 67*(12), 1562–1568. https://doi.org/10.1097/00007890-199906270-00010

Corbett, C., Armstrong, M. J., & Neuberger, J. (2012). Tobacco smoking and solid organ transplantation. *Transplantation*, *94*(10), 979–987. https://doi.org/10.1097/TP.0b013e318263ad5b

Corbett, C., Armstrong, M. J., Parker, R., Webb, K., & Neuberger, J. M. (2013). Mental health disorders and solid-organ transplant recipients. *Transplantation*, *96*(7), 593–600. https://doi.org/10.1097/TP.0b013e31829584e0

Corruble, E., Barry, C., Varescon, I., Durrbach, A., Samuel, D., Lang, P., Castaing, D., Charpentier, B., & Falissard, B. (2011). Report of depressive symptoms on waiting list and mortality after liver and kidney transplantation: A prospective cohort study. *BMC Psychiatry*, *11*(1), 182. https://doi.org/10.1186/1471-244X-11-182

Cukor, D., Rosenthal, D. S., Jindal, R. M., Brown, C. D., & Kimmel, P. L. (2009). Depression is an important contributor to low medication adherence in hemodialyzed patients and transplant recipients. *Kidney International*, *75*(11), 1223–1229. https://doi.org/10.1038/ki.2009.51

Davis, T. C., Long, S. W., Jackson, R. H., Mayeaux, E. J., George, R. B., Murphy, P. W., & Crouch, M. A. (1993). Rapid estimate of adult literacy in medicine: A shortened screening instrument. *Family Medicine*, *25*(6), 391–395. https://www.ncbi.nlm.nih.gov/pubmed/8349060

Delibasic, M., Mohamedali, B., Dobrilovic, N., & Raman, J. (2017). Pre-transplant depression as a predictor of adherence and morbidities after orthotopic heart transplantation. *Journal of Cardiothoracic Surgery*, *12*(1), 62. https://doi.org/10.1186/s13019-017-0626-0

Dew, M. A., & DiMartini, A. F. (2005). Psychological disorders and distress after adult cardiothoracic transplantation. *The Journal of Cardiovascular Nursing*, *20*(5, Suppl.), S51–S66. https://doi.org/10.1097/00005082-200509001-00007

Dew, M. A., DiMartini, A. F., De Vito Dabbs, A., Myaskovsky, L., Steel, J., Unruh, M., Switzer, G. E., Zomak, R., Kormos, R. L., & Greenhouse, J. B. (2007). Rates and risk factors for nonadherence to the medical regimen after adult solid organ transplantation. *Transplantation*, *83*(7), 858–873. https://doi.org/10.1097/01.tp.0000258599.65257.a6

Dew, M. A., DiMartini, A. F., Dobbels, F., Grady, K. L., Jowsey-Gregoire, S. G., Kaan, A., Kendall, K., Young, Q. R., Abbey, S. E., Butt, Z., Crone, C. C., De Geest, S., Doligalski, C. T., Kugler, C., McDonald, L., Ohler, L., Painter, L., Petty, M. G., Robson, D., . . . Zimbrean, P. C. (2018). The 2018 ISHLT/APM/AST/ICCAC/STSW recommendations for the psychosocial evaluation of adult cardiothoracic transplant candidates and candidates for long-term mechanical circulatory support. *Psychosomatics*, *59*(5), 415–440. https://doi.org/10.1016/j.psym.2018.04.003

Dew, M. A., DiMartini, A. F., Steel, J., De Vito Dabbs, A., Myaskovsky, L., Unruh, M., & Greenhouse, J. (2008). Meta-analysis of risk for relapse to substance use after transplantation of the liver or other solid organs. *Liver Transplantation*, *14*(2), 159–172. https://doi.org/10.1002/lt.21278

Dew, M. A., Rosenberger, E. M., Myaskovsky, L., DiMartini, A. F., DeVito Dabbs, A. J., Posluszny, D. M., Steel, J., Switzer, G. E., Shellmer, D. A., & Greenhouse, J. B. (2015). Depression and anxiety as risk factors for morbidity and mortality after organ transplantation: A systematic review and meta-analysis. *Transplantation*, *100*(5), 988–1003. https://doi.org/10.1097/TP.0000000000000901

DiMartini, A., Day, N., Dew, M. A., Javed, L., Fitzgerald, M. G., Jain, A., Fung, J. J., & Fontes, P. (2006). Alcohol consumption patterns and predictors of use following liver transplantation for alcoholic liver disease. *Liver Transplantation*, *12*(5), 813–820. https://doi.org/10.1002/lt.20688

DiMartini, A., Dew, M. A., Day, N., Fitzgerald, M. G., Jones, B. L., deVera, M. E., & Fontes, P. (2010). Trajectories of alcohol consumption following liver transplantation. *American Journal of Transplantation*, *10*(10), 2305–2312. https://doi.org/10.1111/j.1600-6143.2010.03232.x

DiMatteo, M. R. (2004). Social support and patient adherence to medical treatment: A meta-analysis. *Health Psychology*, *23*(2), 207–218. https://doi.org/10.1037/0278-6133.23.2.207

Dobbels, F., De Geest, S., Cleemput, I., Fischler, B., Kesteloot, K., Vanhaecke, J., & Vanrenterghem, Y. (2001). Psychosocial and behavioral selection criteria for solid organ transplantation. *Progress in Transplantation*, *11*(2), 121–132. https://doi.org/10.1177/152692480101100208

Dobbels, F., Denhaerynck, K., Klem, M. L., Sereika, S. M., De Geest, S., De Simone, P., Berben, L., Binet, I., Burkhalter, H., Drent, G., Duerinckx, N., Engberg, S. J., Glass, T., Gordon, E., Kirsch, M., Kugler, C., Lerret, S., Rossmeissl, A., Russell, C., . . . de Almeida, S. S. (2019). Correlates and outcomes of alcohol use after single solid organ transplantation: A systematic review and meta-analysis. *Transplantation Reviews*, *33*(1), 17–28. https://doi.org/10.1016/j.trre.2018.09.003

Dobbels, F., Put, C., & Vanhaecke, J. (2000). Personality disorders: A challenge for transplantation. *Progress in Transplantation*, *10*(4), 226–232. https://doi.org/10.1177/152692480001000406

Dobbels, F., Vanhaecke, J., Dupont, L., Nevens, F., Verleden, G., Pirenne, J., & De Geest, S. (2009). Pretransplant predictors of posttransplant adherence and clinical outcome: An evidence base for pretransplant psychosocial screening. *Transplantation*, *87*(10), 1497–1504. https://doi.org/10.1097/TP.0b013e3181a440ae

Dobbels, F., Verleden, G., Dupont, L., Vanhaecke, J., & De Geest, S. (2006). To transplant or not? The importance of psychosocial and behavioural factors before lung transplantation. *Chronic Respiratory Disease*, *3*(1), 39–47. https://doi.org/10.1191/1479972306cd082ra

Duerinckx, N., Burkhalter, H., Engberg, S. J., Kirsch, M., Klem, M.-L., Sereika, S. M., De Simone, P., De Geest, S., & Dobbels, F. (2016). Correlates and outcomes of posttransplant smoking in solid organ transplant recipients: A systematic literature review and meta-analysis. *Transplantation*, *100*(11), 2252–2263. https://doi.org/10.1097/TP.0000000000001335

Duffy, J. P., Kao, K., Ko, C. Y., Farmer, D. G., McDiarmid, S. V., Hong, J. C., Venick, R. S., Feist, S., Goldstein, L., Saab, S., Hiatt, J. R., & Busuttil, R. W. (2010). Long-term patient outcome and quality of life after liver transplantation: Analysis of 20-year survivors. *Annals of Surgery*, *252*(4), 652–661. https://doi.org/10.1097/SLA.0b013e3181f5f23a

European Association for the Study of the Liver. (2016). EASL clinical practice guidelines: Liver transplantation. *Journal of Hepatology*, *64*(2), 433–485. https://doi.org/10.1016/j.jhep.2015.10.006

Farmer, S. A., Grady, K. L., Wang, E., McGee, E. C., Jr., Cotts, W. G., & McCarthy, P. M. (2013). Demographic, psychosocial, and behavioral factors associated with survival after heart transplantation. *The Annals of Thoracic Surgery*, *95*(3), 876–883. https://doi.org/10.1016/j.athoracsur.2012.11.041

Feldman, D., Pamboukian, S. V., Teuteberg, J. J., Birks, E., Lietz, K., Moore, S. A., Morgan, J. A., Arabia, F., Bauman, M. E., Buchholz, H. W., Deng, M., Dickstein, M. L., El-Banayosy, A., Elliot, T., Goldstein, D. J., Grady, K. L., Jones, K., Hryniewicz, K., John, R., . . . Rogers, J., & the International Society for Heart and Lung Transplantation. (2013). The 2013 International Society for Heart and Lung Transplantation guidelines for mechanical circulatory support: Executive summary. *The Journal of Heart and Lung Transplantation*, *32*(2), 157–187. https://doi.org/10.1016/j.healun.2012.09.013

Fine, R. N., Becker, Y., De Geest, S., Eisen, H., Ettenger, R., Evans, R., Rudow, D. L., McKay, D., Neu, A., Nevins, T., Reyes, J., Wray, J., & Dobbels, F. (2009). Nonadherence consensus conference summary report. *American Journal of Transplantation*, *9*(1), 35–41. https://doi.org/10.1111/j.1600-6143.2008.02495.x

Fleming, M. F., Smith, M. J., Oslakovic, E., Lucey, M. R., Vue, J. X., Al-Saden, P., & Levitsky, J. (2017). Phosphatidylethanol detects moderate-to-heavy alcohol use in liver transplant recipients. *Alcoholism, Clinical and Experimental Research*, *41*(4), 857–862. https://doi.org/10.1111/acer.13353

Galante, N. Z., Dib, G. A., & Medina-Pestana, J. O. (2010). Severe intellectual disability does not preclude renal transplantation. *Nephrology, Dialysis, Transplantation*, *25*(8), 2753–2757. https://doi.org/10.1093/ndt/gfq105

Gelb, S. R., Shapiro, R. J., & Thornton, W. J. (2010). Predicting medication adherence and employment status following kidney transplant: The relative utility of traditional and everyday cognitive approaches. *Neuropsychology*, *24*(4), 514–526. https://doi.org/10.1037/a0018670

Grady, K. L., Magasi, S., Hahn, E. A., Buono, S., McGee, E. C., Jr., & Yancy, C. (2015). Health-related quality of life in mechanical circulatory support: Development of a new conceptual model and items for self-administration. *The Journal of Heart and Lung Transplantation*, *34*(10), 1292–1304. https://doi.org/10.1016/j.healun.2015.04.003

Green, J. A., Mor, M. K., Shields, A. M., Sevick, M. A., Arnold, R. M., Palevsky, P. M., Fine, M. J., & Weisbord, S. D. (2013). Associations of health literacy with dialysis adherence and health resource utilization in patients receiving maintenance hemodialysis. *American Journal of Kidney Diseases*, *62*(1), 73–80. https://doi.org/10.1053/j.ajkd.2012.12.014

Grubbs, V., Gregorich, S. E., Perez-Stable, E. J., & Hsu, C. Y. (2009). Health literacy and access to kidney transplantation. *Clinical Journal of the American Society of Nephrology*, *4*(1), 195–200. https://doi.org/10.2215/CJN.03290708

Gupta, A., Thomas, T. S., Klein, J. A., Montgomery, R. N., Mahnken, J. D., Johnson, D. K., Drew, D. A., Sarnak, M. J., & Burns, J. M. (2018). Discrepancies between perceived and measured cognition in kidney transplant recipients: Implications for clinical management. *Nephron*, *138*(1), 22–28. https://doi.org/10.1159/000481182

Harding, K., Mersha, T. B., Pham, P. T., Waterman, A. D., Webb, F. A., Vassalotti, J. A., & Nicholas, S. B. (2017). Health disparities in kidney transplantation for African Americans. *American Journal of Nephrology*, *46*(2), 165–175. https://doi.org/10.1159/000479480

Health Resources and Services Administration. (2021, April 2021). *Organ donation statistics*. https://www.organdonor.gov/statistics-stories/statistics.html

Hurst, F. P., Altieri, M., Patel, P. P., Jindal, T. R., Guy, S. R., Sidawy, A. N., Agodoa, L. Y., Abbott, K. C., & Jindal, R. M. (2011). Effect of smoking on kidney transplant outcomes: Analysis of the United States Renal Data System. *Transplantation*, *92*(10), 1101–1107. https://doi.org/10.1097/TP.0b013e3182336095

Ismail, S. Y., Timmerman, L., Timman, R., Luchtenburg, A. E., Smak Gregoor, P. J., Nette, R. W., van den Dorpel, R. M., Zuidema, W. C., Weimar, W., Massey, E. K., & Busschbach, J. J. (2013). A psychometric analysis of the Rotterdam Renal Replacement Knowledge-Test (R3K-T) using item response theory. *Transplant International*, *26*(12), 1164–1172. https://doi.org/10.1111/tri.12188

Jacobs, E. T., Dean, D. J., Aaron, C. K., Tilford, B. D., Schneider, J. S., Clark, J. A., & King, A. M. (2020). First double lung transplant secondary to suspected e-cigarette vaping-associated lung injury. *Journal of Medical Toxicology*, *16*(2), 2.

Kauffman, H. M., Woodle, E. S., Cole, E. H., Paykin, C., & the National Kidney Foundation. (2008). Transplant recipient's knowledge of posttransplant malignancy risk: Implications for educational programs. *Transplantation*, *85*(7), 928–933. https://doi.org/10.1097/TP.0b013e31816a105b

Kazley, A. S., Hund, J. J., Simpson, K. N., Chavin, K., & Baliga, P. (2015). Health literacy and kidney transplant outcomes. *Progress in Transplantation*, *25*(1), 85–90. https://doi.org/10.7182/pit2015463

Kazley, A. S., Jordan, J., Simpson, K. N., Chavin, K., Rodrigue, J., & Baliga, P. (2014). Development and testing of a disease-specific health literacy measure in kidney transplant patients. *Progress in Transplantation*, *24*(3), 263–270. https://doi.org/10.7182/pit2014958

Kondo, K., Antick, J. R., Ayers, C. K., Kansagara, D., & Chopra, P. (2020). Depression screening tools for patients with kidney failure: A systematic review. *Clinical Journal of the American Society of Nephrology*, *15*(12), 1785–1795. https://doi.org/10.2215/CJN.05540420

Kop, W. J. (2010). Role of psychological factors in the clinical course of heart transplant patients. *The Journal of Heart and Lung Transplantation*, *29*(3), 257–260. https://doi.org/10.1016/j.healun.2009.10.013

Kop, W. J., Synowski, S. J., & Gottlieb, S. S. (2011). Depression in heart failure: Biobehavioral mechanisms. *Heart Failure Clinics*, *7*(1), 23–38. https://doi.org/10.1016/j.hfc.2010.08.011

Kostro, J. Z., Hellmann, A., Kobiela, J., Skóra, I., Lichodziejewska-Niemierko, M., Dębska-Slizień, A., & Sledziński, Z. (2016). Quality of life After kidney transplantation: A prospective study. *Transplantation Proceedings*, *48*(1), 50–54. https://doi.org/10.1016/j.transproceed.2015.10.058

Kroenke, K., & Spitzer, R. L. (2002). The PHQ-9: A new depression diagnostic and severity measure. *Psychiatric Annals*, *32*(9), 509–515. https://doi.org/10.3928/0048-5713-20020901-06

Kumnig, M., & Jowsey-Gregoire, S. (2015). Preoperative psychological evaluation of transplant patients: Challenges and solutions. *Transplant Research and Risk Management*, 35. Advance online publication. https://doi.org/10.2147/TRRM.S59268

Kwong, A. J., Kim, W. R., Lake, J. R., Smith, J. M., Schladt, D. P., Skeans, M. A., Noreen, S. M., Foutz, J., Booker, S. E., Cafarella, M., Snyder, J. J., Israni, A. K., & Kasiske, B. L. (2021). OPTN/SRTR 2019 annual data report: Liver. *American Journal of Transplantation*, *21*(S2, Suppl. 2), 208–315. https://doi.org/10.1111/ajt.16494

Lacerda, S. S., Guimaro, M. S., Prade, C. V., Ferraz-Neto, B. H., Karam, C. H., & Andreoli, P. B. (2008). Neuropsychological assessment in kidney and liver transplantation candidates. *Transplantation Proceedings, 40*(3), 729–731. https://doi.org/10.1016/j.transproceed.2008.02.042

Le Strat, Y., Le Foll, B., & Dubertret, C. (2015). Major depression and suicide attempts in patients with liver disease in the United States. *Liver International, 35*(7), 1910–1916. https://doi.org/10.1111/liv.12612

Leard, L. E., Holm, A. M., Valapour, M., Glanville, A. R., Attawar, S., Aversa, M., Campos, S. V., Christon, L. M., Cypel, M., Dellgren, G., Hartwig, M. G., Kapnadak, S. G., Kolaitis, N. A., Kotloff, R. M., Patterson, C. M., Shlobin, O. A., Smith, P. J., Solé, A., Solomon, M., . . . Ramos, K. J. (2021). Consensus document for the selection of lung transplant candidates: An update from the International Society for Heart and Lung Transplantation. *The Journal of Heart and Lung Transplantation, 40*(11), 1349–1379. https://doi.org/10.1016/j.healun.2021.07.005

Lee, B. P., Chen, P. H., Haugen, C., Hernaez, R., Gurakar, A., Philosophe, B., Dagher, N., Moore, S. A., Li, Z., & Cameron, A. M. (2017). Three-year results of a pilot program in early liver transplantation for severe alcoholic hepatitis. *Annals of Surgery, 265*(1), 20–29. https://doi.org/10.1097/SLA.0000000000001831

Lee, B. P., Mehta, N., Platt, L., Gurakar, A., Rice, J. P., Lucey, M. R., Im, G. Y., Therapondos, G., Han, H., Victor, D. W., Fix, O. K., Dinges, L., Dronamraju, D., Hsu, C., Voigt, M. D., Rinella, M. E., Maddur, H., Eswaran, S., Hause, J., . . . Terrault, N. A. (2018). Outcomes of early liver transplantation for patients with severe alcoholic hepatitis. *Gastroenterology, 155*(2), 422–430.e1. https://doi.org/10.1053/j.gastro.2018.04.009

Lee, B. P., Vittinghoff, E., Hsu, C., Han, H., Therapondos, G., Fix, O. K., Victor, D. W., Dronamraju, D., Im, G. Y., Voigt, M. D., Rice, J. P., Lucey, M. R., Eswaran, S., Chen, P. H., Li, Z., Maddur, H., & Terrault, N. A. (2019). Predicting low risk for sustained alcohol use after early liver transplant for acute alcoholic hepatitis: The sustained alcohol use post-liver transplant score. *Hepatology, 69*(4), 1477–1487. https://doi.org/10.1002/hep.30478

Lentine, K. L., Lam, N. N., Naik, A. S., Axelrod, D. A., Zhang, Z., Dharnidharka, V. R., Hess, G. P., Segev, D. L., Ouseph, R., Randall, H., Alhamad, T., Devraj, R., Gadi, R., Kasiske, B. L., Brennan, D. C., & Schnitzler, M. A. (2018). Prescription opioid use before and after kidney transplant: Implications for posttransplant outcomes. *American Journal of Transplantation, 18*(12), 2987–2999. https://doi.org/10.1111/ajt.14714

Lentine, K. L., Shah, K. S., Kobashigawa, J. A., Xiao, H., Zhang, Z., Axelrod, D. A., Lam, N. N., Segev, D. L., McAdams-DeMarco, M. A., Randall, H., Hess, G. P., Yuan, H., Vest, L. S., Kasiske, B. L., & Schnitzler, M. A. (2019). Prescription opioid use before and after heart transplant: Associations with posttransplant outcomes. *American Journal of Transplantation, 19*(12), 3405–3414. https://doi.org/10.1111/ajt.15565

Li, Q., Wang, Y., Ma, T., Liu, X., Wang, B., Wu, Z., Lv, Y., & Wu, R. (2017). Impact of cigarette smoking on early complications after liver transplantation: A single-center experience and a meta-analysis. *PLOS ONE, 12*(5), Article e0178570. https://doi.org/10.1371/journal.pone.0178570

Lombardo-Quezada, J., Colmenero, J., López-Pelayo, H., Gavotti, C., Lopez, A., Crespo, G., Lopez, E., Gual, A., Lligoña, A., & Navasa, M. (2019). Prediction of alcohol relapse among liver transplant candidates with less than 6 months of abstinence using the high-risk alcoholism relapse score. *Liver Transplantation, 25*(8), 1142–1154.

López-Lazcano, A. I., Gual, A., Colmenero, J., Caballería, E., Lligoña, A., Navasa, M., Crespo, G., López, E., & López-Pelayo, H. (2020). Active smoking before liver transplantation in patients with alcohol use disorder: Risk factors and outcomes. *Journal of Clinical Medicine, 9*(9), 2710. Advance online publication. https://doi.org/10.3390/jcm9092710

Madan, A., Borckardt, J. J., Balliet, W. E., Barth, K. S., Delustro, L. M., Malcolm, R. M., Koch, D., Willner, I., Baliga, P., & Reuben, A. (2015). Neurocognitive status is associated with all-cause mortality among psychiatric, high-risk liver transplant candidates and recipients. *International Journal of Psychiatry in Medicine, 49*(4), 279–295. https://doi.org/10.1177/0091217415589304

Majumder, P., & Sarkar, S. (2020). A review of the prevalence of illicit substance use in solid-organ transplant candidates and the effects of illicit substance use on solid-organ transplant treatment outcomes. *Cureus, 12*(7), Article e8986. https://doi.org/10.7759/cureus.8986

Maldonado, J. R. (2019). Why it is important to consider social support when assessing organ transplant candidates? *The American Journal of Bioethics, 19*(11), 1–8. https://doi.org/10.1080/15265161.2019.1671689

Maldonado, J. R., Sher, Y., Lolak, S., Swendsen, H., Skibola, D., Neri, E., David, E. E., Sullivan, C., & Standridge, K. (2015). The Stanford Integrated Psychosocial Assessment for Transplantation: A prospective study of medical and psychosocial outcomes. *Psychosomatic Medicine, 77*(9), 1018–1030. https://doi.org/10.1097/PSY.0000000000000241

Martelli, V., Mathur, S., Wickerson, L., Gottesman, C., Helm, D., Singer, L. G., & Rozenberg, D. (2019). Impaired cardiac autonomic response in lung transplant patients: A retrospective cohort study. *Clinical Transplantation, 33*(7), Article e13612. https://doi.org/10.1111/ctr.13612

Martin, P., DiMartini, A., Feng, S., Brown, R., Jr., & Fallon, M. (2014). Evaluation for liver transplantation in adults: 2013 practice guideline by the American Association for the Study of Liver Diseases and the American Society of Transplantation. *Hepatology, 59*(3), 1144–1165. https://doi.org/10.1002/hep.26972

Mehra, M. R., Canter, C. E., Hannan, M. M., Semigran, M. J., Uber, P. A., Baran, D. A., Danziger-Isakov, L., Kirklin, J. K., Kirk, R., Kushwaha, S. S., Lund, L. H., Potena, L., Ross, H. J., Taylor, D. O., Verschuuren, E. A. M., Zuckermann, A., & the International Society for Heart Lung Transplantation (ISHLT) Infectious Diseases, Pediatric and Heart Failure and Transplantation Councils. (2016). The 2016 International Society for Heart Lung Transplantation listing criteria for heart transplantation: A 10-year update. *The Journal of Heart and Lung Transplantation, 35*(1), 1–23. https://doi.org/10.1016/j.healun.2015.10.023

Melaragno, J. I., Bowman, L. J., Park, J. M., Lourenco, L. M., Doligalski, C. T., Brady, B. L., Descourouez, J. L., Chandran, M. M., Nickels, M. W., & Page, R. L., II. (2021). The clinical conundrum of cannabis: Current practices and recommendations for transplant clinicians: An opinion of the immunology/transplantation PRN of the American College of Clinical Pharmacy. *Transplantation, 105*(2), 291–299. https://doi.org/10.1097/TP.0000000000003309

Mellinger, J. L., Scott Winder, G., DeJonckheere, M., Fontana, R. J., Volk, M. L., Lok, A. S. F., & Blow, F. C. (2018). Misconceptions, preferences and barriers to alcohol use disorder treatment in alcohol-related cirrhosis. *Journal of Substance Abuse Treatment*, *91*, 20–27. https://doi.org/10.1016/j.jsat.2018.05.003

Melton, N., Soleimani, B., & Dowling, R. (2019). Current role of the total artificial heart in the management of advanced heart failure. *Current Cardiology Reports*, *21*(11), 142. https://doi.org/10.1007/s11886-019-1242-5

Miller-Matero, L. R., Bryce, K., Hyde-Nolan, M. E., Dykhuis, K. E., Eshelman, A., & Abouljoud, M. (2016). Health literacy status affects outcomes for patients referred for transplant. *Psychosomatics*, *57*(5), 522–528. https://doi.org/10.1016/j.psym.2016.04.001

Millon T., Antoni M. H., Millon C., Meagher S., & Grossman S. (2001). *Test manual for the Millon Behavioral Medicine Diagnostic (MBMD)*. National Computer Services.

Millson, C., Considine, A., Cramp, M. E., Holt, A., Hubscher, S., Hutchinson, J., Jones, K., Leithead, J., Masson, S., Menon, K., Mirza, D., Neuberger, J., Prasad, R., Pratt, A., Prentice, W., Shepherd, L., Simpson, K., Thorburn, D., Westbrook, R., & Tripathi, D. (2020). Adult liver transplantation: A UK clinical guideline—Part 1: Pre-operation. *Frontline Gastroenterology*, *11*(5), 375–384. https://doi.org/10.1136/flgastro-2019-101215

Mohamed, M., Soliman, K., Pullalarevu, R., Kamel, M., Srinivas, T., Taber, D., & Posadas Salas, M. A. (2021). Non-adherence to appointments is a strong predictor of medication non-adherence and outcomes in kidney transplant recipients. *The American Journal of the Medical Sciences*, *362*(4), 381–386. Advance online publication. https://doi.org/10.1016/j.amjms.2021.05.011

Mollberg, N. M., Farjah, F., Howell, E., Ortiz, J., Backhus, L., & Mulligan, M. S. (2015). Impact of primary caregivers on long-term outcomes after lung transplantation. *The Journal of Heart and Lung Transplantation*, *34*(1), 59–64. https://doi.org/10.1016/j.healun.2014.09.022

Mooney, S., Hasssanein, T. I., Hilsabeck, R. C., Ziegler, E. A., Carlson, M., Maron, L. M., Perry, W., & the UCSD Hepatology Neurobehavioral Research Program. (2007). Utility of the Repeatable Battery for the Assessment of Neuropsychological Status (RBANS) in patients with end-stage liver disease awaiting liver transplant. *Archives of Clinical Neuropsychology*, *22*(2), 175–186. https://doi.org/10.1016/j.acn.2006.12.005

Morey, L. C. (1991). *Personality Assessment Inventory professional manual*. Psychological Assessment Resources.

Morey, L. C. (1996). *An interpretive guide to the Personality Assessment Inventory*. Psychological Assessment Resources.

Müller, H. H., Englbrecht, M., Wiesener, M. S., Titze, S., Heller, K., Groemer, T. W., Schett, G., Eckardt, K. U., Kornhuber, J., & Maler, J. M. (2015). Depression, anxiety, resilience and coping pre and post kidney transplantation—Initial findings from the Psychiatric Impairments in Kidney Transplantation (PI-KT) study. *PLOS ONE*, *10*(11), Article e0140706. https://doi.org/10.1371/journal.pone.0140706

Nemeh, H., Coba, V., Chulkov, M., Gupta, A., Yeldo, N., Chamogeorgakis, T., Tanaka, D., Allenspach, L., Simanovski, J., & Shanti, C. (2021). Lung transplantation for the treatment of vaping-induced, irreversible, end-stage lung injury. *The Annals of Thoracic Surgery*, *111*(5), e353–e355. https://doi.org/10.1016/j.athoracsur.2020.07.097

Neuberger, J. M., Bechstein, W. O., Kuypers, D. R., Burra, P., Citterio, F., De Geest, S., Duvoux, C., Jardine, A. G., Kamar, N., Kramer, B. K., Metselaar, H. J., Nevens, F., Pirenne, J., Rodriguez-Peralvarez, M. L., Samuel, D., Schneeberger, S., Seron, D., Trunecka, P., Tisone, G., & van Gelder, T. (2017). Practical recommendations for long-term management of modifiable risks in kidney and liver transplant recipients: A guidance report and clinical checklist by the Consensus on Managing Modifiable Risk in Transplantation (COMMIT) group. *Transplantation*, *101*(4S Suppl. 2), S1–S56. https://doi.org/10.1097/TP.0000000000001651

Nghiem, D. M., Gomez, J., Gloston, G. F., Torres, D. S., & Marek, R. J. (2020). Psychological assessment instruments for use in liver and kidney transplant evaluations: Scarcity of evidence and recommendations. *Journal of Personality Assessment*, *102*(2), 183–195. https://doi.org/10.1080/00223891.2019.1694527

Nogueira, J. M., Haririan, A., Jacobs, S. C., Cooper, M., & Weir, M. R. (2010). Cigarette smoking, kidney function, and mortality after live donor kidney transplant. *American Journal of Kidney Diseases*, *55*(5), 907–915. https://doi.org/10.1053/j.ajkd.2009.10.058

Olbrisch, M. E. (1996). Ethical issues in psychological evaluation of patients for organ transplant surgery. *Rehabilitation Psychology*, *41*(1), 53–71. https://doi.org/10.1037/0090-5550.41.1.53

Olbrisch, M. E., Benedict, S. M., Ashe, K., & Levenson, J. L. (2002). Psychological assessment and care of organ transplant patients. *Journal of Consulting and Clinical Psychology*, *70*(3), 771–783. https://doi.org/10.1037/0022-006X.70.3.771

Organ Procurement and Transplantation Network. (2021). *OPTN Policies*. https://optn.transplant.hrsa.gov/governance/policies/

Organ Procurement and Transplantation Network Ethics Committee. (2021). *Revise general considerations in assessment for transplant candidacy*. https://optn.transplant.hrsa.gov/governance/public-comment/revise-general-considerations-in-assessment-for-transplant-candidacy/

Owen, J. E., Bonds, C. L., & Wellisch, D. K. (2006). Psychiatric evaluations of heart transplant candidates: Predicting post-transplant hospitalizations, rejection episodes, and survival. *Psychosomatics*, *47*(3), 213–222. https://doi.org/10.1176/appi.psy.47.3.213

Pageaux, G. P., Bismuth, M., Perney, P., Costes, V., Jaber, S., Possoz, P., Fabre, J. M., Navarro, F., Blanc, P., Domergue, J., Eledjam, J. J., & Larrey, D. (2003). Alcohol relapse after liver transplantation for alcoholic liver disease: Does it matter? *Journal of Hepatology*, *38*(5), 629–634. https://doi.org/10.1016/S0168-8278(03)00088-6

Parker, R., Armstrong, M. J., Corbett, C., Day, E. J., & Neuberger, J. M. (2013). Alcohol and substance abuse in solid-organ transplant recipients. *Transplantation*, *96*(12), 1015–1024. https://doi.org/10.1097/TP.0b013e31829f7579

Parker, R. M., Baker, D. W., Williams, M. V., & Nurss, J. R. (1995). The test of functional health literacy in adults: A new instrument for measuring patients' literacy skills. *Journal of General Internal Medicine*, *10*(10), 537–541. https://doi.org/10.1007/BF02640361

Patzer, R. E., & Pastan, S. O. (2013). Measuring the disparity gap: Quality improvement to eliminate health disparities in kidney transplantation. *American Journal of Transplantation*, *13*(2), 247–248. https://doi.org/10.1111/ajt.12060

Peipert, J. D., Hays, R. D., Kawakita, S., Beaumont, J. L., & Waterman, A. D. (2019). Measurement characteristics of the knowledge assessment of renal transplantation. *Transplantation*, *103*(3), 565–572. https://doi.org/10.1097/TP.0000000000002349

Pennington, K. M., Benzo, R. P., Schneekloth, T. D., Budev, M., Chandrashekaran, S., Erasmus, D. B., Lease, E. D., Levine, D. J., Thompson, K., Stevens, E., Novotny, P. J., & Kennedy, C. C. (2020). Impact of affect on lung transplant candidate outcomes. *Progress in Transplantation*, *30*(1), 13–21. https://doi.org/10.1177/1526924819892921

Petruccelli, K., Davis, J., & Berman, T. (2019). Adverse childhood experiences and associated health outcomes: A systematic review and meta-analysis. *Child Abuse & Neglect*, *97*, 104127. https://doi.org/10.1016/j.chiabu.2019.104127

Pisanti, R., Lombardo, C., Luszczynska, A., Poli, L., Bennardi, L., Giordanengo, L., Berloco, P. B., & Violani, C. (2017). Appraisal of transplant-related stressors, coping strategies, and psychosocial adjustment following kidney transplantation. *Stress and Health*, *33*(4), 437–447. https://doi.org/10.1002/smi.2727

Radloff, L. S. (1977). The CES-D Scale: A self-report depression scale for research in the general population. *Applied Psychological Measurement*, *1*, 385–401. https://doi.org/10.1080/00380237.2009.10571345

Randall, H. B., Alhamad, T., Schnitzler, M. A., Zhang, Z., Ford-Glanton, S., Axelrod, D. A., Segev, D. L., Kasiske, B. L., Hess, G. P., Yuan, H., Ouseph, R., & Lentine, K. L. (2017). Survival implications of opioid use before and after liver transplantation. *Liver Transplantation*, *23*(3), 305–314. https://doi.org/10.1002/lt.24714

Ranney, D. N., Acker, W. B., Al-Holou, S. N., Ehrlichman, L., Lee, D. S., Lewin, S. A., Nguyen, C., Peterson, S. F., Sell, K., Kubus, J., Reid, D., & Englesbe, M. J. (2009). Marijuana use in potential liver transplant candidates. *American Journal of Transplantation*, *9*(2), 280–285. https://doi.org/10.1111/j.1600-6143.2008.02468.x

Ravi, Y., Lella, S. K., Copeland, L. A., Zolfaghari, K., Grady, K., Emani, S., & Sai-Sudhakar, C. B. (2018). Does recipient work status pre-transplant affect post-heart transplant survival? A United Network for Organ Sharing database review. *The Journal of Heart and Lung Transplantation*, *37*(5), 604–610. https://doi.org/10.1016/j.healun.2018.01.1307

Rice, J. P., Eickhoff, J., Agni, R., Ghufran, A., Brahmbhatt, R., & Lucey, M. R. (2013). Abusive drinking after liver transplantation is associated with allograft loss and advanced allograft fibrosis. *Liver Transplantation*, *19*(12), 1377–1386. https://doi.org/10.1002/lt.23762

Rivard, A. L., Hellmich, C., Sampson, B., Bianco, R. W., Crow, S. J., & Miller, L. W. (2005). Preoperative predictors for postoperative problems in heart transplantation: Psychiatric and psychosocial considerations. *Progress in Transplantation*, *15*(3), 276–282. https://doi.org/10.1177/152692480501500312

Rodrigue, J. R., Hanto, D. W., & Curry, M. P. (2013). The Alcohol Relapse Risk Assessment: A scoring system to predict the risk of relapse to any alcohol use after liver transplant. *Progress in Transplantation*, *23*(4), 310–318. https://doi.org/10.7182/pit2013604

Roman, D. D. (2018). The role of neuropsychology on organ transplant teams. *Archives of Clinical Neuropsychology*, *33*(3), 339–343. https://doi.org/10.1093/arclin/acx127

Ruchinskas, R. A., Combs, C. J., Riley, K. C., & Broshek, D. K. (2006). Defensive responding on the MMPI-2 in pre-surgical candidates. *Journal of Clinical Psychology in Medical Settings*, *13*(4), 435–439. https://doi.org/10.1007/s10880-006-9044-5

Rudasill, S. E., Iyengar, A., Kwon, O. J., Sanaiha, Y., Dobaria, V., & Benharash, P. (2019). Recipient working status is independently associated with outcomes in heart and lung transplantation. *Clinical Transplantation*, *33*(2), Article e13462.

Samelson-Jones, E., Mancini, D. M., & Shapiro, P. A. (2012). Cardiac transplantation in adult patients with mental retardation: Do outcomes support consensus guidelines? *Psychosomatics*, *53*(2), 133–138. https://doi.org/10.1016/j.psym.2011.12.011

Santana, S., Brach, C., Harris, L., Ochiai, E., Blakey, C., Bevington, F., Kleinman, D., & Pronk, N. (2021). Updating health literacy for healthy people 2030: Defining its importance for a new decade in public health. *Journal of Public Health Management and Practice*, *27*(Suppl. 6), S258–S264. Advance online publication. https://doi.org/10.1097/PHH.0000000000001324

Schaevers, V., De Bondt, K., Duerinckx, N., Berentsen, S., De Vos, M., Stulens, S., De Castro, C. F., Vandenbossche, V., Vos, R., & Dobbels, F. (2021). Development, validation and implementation of an instrument to measure knowledge in transplant recipients. *The Journal of Heart and Lung Transplantation*, *40*(4), S310. Advance online publication. https://doi.org/10.1016/j.healun.2021.01.878

Serper, M., Patzer, R. E., Reese, P. P., Przytula, K., Koval, R., Ladner, D. P., Levitsky, J., Abecassis, M. M., & Wolf, M. S. (2015). Medication misuse, nonadherence, and clinical outcomes among liver transplant recipients. *Liver Transplantation*, *21*(1), 22–28. https://doi.org/10.1002/lt.24023

Sher, Y., & Maldonado, J. R. (Eds.). (2019). *Psychosocial care of end-stage organ disease and transplant patients*. Springer. https://doi.org/10.1007/978-3-319-94914-7

Shirazian, S., Grant, C. D., Aina, O., Mattana, J., Khorassani, F., & Ricardo, A. C. (2017). Depression in chronic kidney disease and end-stage renal disease: Similarities and differences in diagnosis, epidemiology, and management. *Kidney International Reports*, *2*(1), 94–107. https://doi.org/10.1016/j.ekir.2016.09.005

Sirri, L., Magelli, C., & Grandi, S. (2011). Predictors of perceived social support in long-term survivors of cardiac transplant: The role of psychological distress, quality of life, demographic characteristics and clinical course. *Psychology & Health*, *26*(1), 77–94. https://doi.org/10.1080/08870440903377339

Skillings, J. L., & Lewandowski, A. N. (2015). Team-based biopsychosocial care in solid organ transplantation. *Journal of Clinical Psychology in Medical Settings*, *22*(2–3), 113–121. https://doi.org/10.1007/s10880-015-9428-5

Smith, P. J., Blumenthal, J. A., Carney, R. M., Freedland, K. E., O'Hayer, C. V. F., Trulock, E. P., Martinu, T., Schwartz, T. A., Hoffman, B. M., Koch, G. G., Davis, R. D., & Palmer, S. M. (2014). Neurobehavioral functioning and survival following lung transplantation. *Chest*, *145*(3), 604–611. https://doi.org/10.1378/chest.12-2127

Smith, P. J., Snyder, L. D., Palmer, S. M., Hoffman, B. M., Stonerock, G. L., Ingle, K. K., Saulino, C. K., & Blumenthal, J. A. (2018). Depression, social support, and clinical outcomes following lung transplantation: A single-center cohort study. *Transplant International*, *31*(5), 495–502. https://doi.org/10.1111/tri.13094

Stilley, C. S., Dew, M. A., Pilkonis, P., Bender, A., McNulty, M., Christensen, A., McCurry, K. R., & Kormos, R. L. (2005). Personality characteristics among cardiothoracic transplant recipients. *General Hospital Psychiatry*, *27*(2), 113–118. https://doi.org/10.1016/j.genhosppsych.2004.11.005

Swanson, A., Geller, J., DeMartini, K., Fernandez, A., & Fehon, D. (2018). Active coping and perceived social support mediate the relationship between physical health and resilience in liver transplant candidates. *Journal of Clinical Psychology in Medical Settings*, *25*(4), 485–496. https://doi.org/10.1007/s10880-018-9559-6

Szymkowicz, S. M., May, P. E., Weeks, J. W., O'Connell, D., & Nelson Sheese, A. L. (2021). Psychometric properties of the Montreal Cognitive Assessment (MoCA) in inpatient liver transplant candidates. *Applied Neuropsychology: Adult*. Advance online publication. https://doi.org/10.1080/23279095.2021.1986510

Taber, D. J., Fleming, J. N., Fominaya, C. E., Gebregziabher, M., Hunt, K. J., Srinivas, T. R., Baliga, P. K., McGillicuddy, J. W., & Egede, L. E. (2017). The impact of health care appointment non-adherence on graft outcomes in kidney transplantation. *American Journal of Nephrology*, *45*(1), 91–98. https://doi.org/10.1159/000453554

Telles-Correia, D., Barbosa, A., Mega, I., & Monteiro, E. (2012). Psychosocial predictors of adherence after liver transplant in a single transplant center in Portugal. *Progress in Transplantation*, *22*(1), 91–94. https://doi.org/10.7182/pit2012569

Teperman, L. W. (2013). Impact of pretransplant hepatic encephalopathy on liver posttransplantation outcomes. *International Journal of Hepatology*, *2013*, Article 952828. Advance online publication. https://doi.org/10.1155/2013/952828

Thomas, A. G., Ruck, J. M., Shaffer, A. A., Haugen, C. E., Ying, H., Warsame, F., Chu, N., Carlson, M. C., Gross, A. L., Norman, S. P., Segev, D. L., & McAdams-DeMarco, M. (2019). Kidney transplant outcomes in recipients with cognitive impairment: A national registry and prospective cohort study. *Transplantation*, *103*(7), 1504–1513. https://doi.org/10.1097/TP.0000000000002431

Torosian, K., Delebecque, F., Liu, A., Arellano, D., Dave, S., Schnickel, G., & Ajmera, V. (2022). Social determinants of health and biochemical alcohol relapse in alcohol-associated liver disease. *American Journal of Transplantation*, *22*(Suppl. 3). https://atcmeetingabstracts.com/abstract/social-determinants-of-health-and-biochemical-alcohol-relapse-in-alcohol-associated-liver-disease/

Tsuang, W. M., Arrigain, S., Lopez, R., Snair, M., Budev, M., & Schold, J. D. (2020). Patient travel distance and post lung transplant survival in the United States: A cohort study. *Transplantation*, *104*(11), 2365–2372. https://doi.org/10.1097/TP.0000000000003129

Twillman, R. K., Manetto, C., Wellisch, D. K., & Wolcott, D. L. (1993). The Transplant Evaluation Rating Scale: A revision of the psychosocial levels system for evaluating organ transplant candidates. *Psychosomatics*, *34*(2), 144–153. https://doi.org/10.1016/S0033-3182(93)71905-2

United Network for Organ Sharing. (2021). *History of transplantation*. https://unos.org/transplant/history/

Urstad, K. H., Andersen, M. H., Oyen, O., Moum, T., & Wahl, A. K. (2011). Patients' level of knowledge measured five days after kidney transplantation. *Clinical Transplantation*, *25*(4), 646–652. https://doi.org/10.1111/j.1399-0012.2010.01355.x

U.S. Department of Health and Human Services. (2014). *The health consequences of smoking—50 years of progress: A report of the Surgeon General*. https://www.ncbi.nlm.nih.gov/books/NBK179276/

U.S. Department of Health and Human Services. (2019). *OPTN/SRTR 2019 annual data report*. https://srtr.transplant.hrsa.gov/annual_reports/Default.aspx

Vaitla, P. K., Thongprayoon, C., Hansrivijit, P., Kanduri, S. R., Kovvuru, K., Rivera, F. H. C., Cato, L. D., Garla, V., Watthanasuntorn, K., Wijarnpreecha, K., Chewcharat, A., Aeddula, N. R., Bathini, T., Koller, F. L., Matemavi, P., & Cheungpasitporn, W.

(2021). Epidemiology of cannabis use and associated outcomes among kidney transplant recipients: A meta-analysis. *Journal of Evidence-Based Medicine, 14*(2), 90–96. https://doi.org/10.1111/jebm.12401

Vandemheen, K. L., O'Connor, A., Bell, S. C., Freitag, A., Bye, P., Jeanneret, A., Berthiaume, Y., Brown, N., Wilcox, P., Ryan, G., Brager, N., Rabin, H., Morrison, N., Gibson, P., Jackson, M., Paterson, N., Middleton, P., & Aaron, S. D. (2009). Randomized trial of a decision aid for patients with cystic fibrosis considering lung transplantation. *American Journal of Respiratory and Critical Care Medicine, 180*(8), 761–768. https://doi.org/10.1164/rccm.200903-0421OC

Vilstrup, H., Amodio, P., Bajaj, J., Cordoba, J., Ferenci, P., Mullen, K. D., Weissenborn, K., & Wong, P. (2014). Hepatic encephalopathy in chronic liver disease: 2014 Practice Guideline by the American Association for the Study of Liver Diseases and the European Association for the Study of the Liver. *Hepatology, 60*(2), 715–735. https://doi.org/10.1002/hep.27210

Wall, A., Lee, G. H., Maldonado, J., & Magnus, D. (2020). Genetic disease and intellectual disability as contraindications to transplant listing in the United States: A survey of heart, kidney, liver, and lung transplant programs. *Pediatric Transplantation, 24*(7), Article e13837. https://doi.org/10.1111/petr.13837

Ward, M. B., Hackenmueller, S. A., & Strathmann, F. G. (2014). Pathology consultation on urine compliance testing and drug abuse screening. *American Journal of Clinical Pathology, 142*(5), 586–593. https://doi.org/10.1309/AJCPZ0DS4QLYNCQG

Weinrieb, R. M., Van Horn, D. H., McLellan, A. T., Volpicelli, J. R., Calarco, J. S., & Lucey, M. R. (2001). Drinking behavior and motivation for treatment among alcohol-dependent liver transplant candidates. *Journal of Addictive Diseases, 20*(2), 105–119. https://doi.org/10.1300/J069v20n02_09

Weng, F. L., Peipert, J. D., Holland, B. K., Brown, D. R., & Waterman, A. D. (2017). A clustered randomized trial of an educational intervention during transplant evaluation to increase knowledge of living donor kidney transplant. *Progress in Transplantation, 27*(4), 377–385. https://doi.org/10.1177/1526924817732021

Zigmond, A. S., & Snaith, R. P. (1983). The Hospital Anxiety and Depression Scale. *Acta Psychiatrica Scandinavica, 67*(6), 361–370. https://doi.org/10.1111/j.1600-0447.1983.tb09716.x

Zimbrean, P., & Emre, S. (2015). Patients with psychotic disorders in solid-organ transplant. *Progress in Transplantation, 25*(4), 289–296. https://doi.org/10.7182/pit2015296

9 DEEP BRAIN STIMULATION FOR PARKINSON'S DISEASE AND DEPRESSION

JENNIFER A. FOLEY

Electricity has long been used to treat medical disorders. Physicians in ancient Greece considered thunderbolts to be the "ultimate sacred weapon" and experimented with medical applications of electrical current (Tsoucalas & Sgantzos, 2016, p. 199). In early dynastic Egypt, "electric catfish of the Nile" were used to treat migraine (Finger & Piccolino, 2011, p. 19), and, in 46 A.D., Roman physician Scribonius Largus wrote about the use of electric rays for the treatment of headache (Kellaway, 1946).

Now, in the 21st century, deep brain stimulation (DBS) is routinely used to treat a range of medical conditions—most commonly disabling movement disorders, such as Parkinson's disease (PD). More recently, DBS has also been applied to intractable psychiatric illnesses, such as major depression. In PD, its success relies heavily on the appropriate selection of candidates: If selected well, DBS can lead to marked improvements in motor function. The success rates and selection criteria for its use in depression are less well known. In this chapter, I discuss the application of DBS to these two common and life-limiting medical conditions, present an evidence-based approach to presurgical psychological assessment of patients with PD, and consider use of DBS as a future treatment for intractable depression.

https://doi.org/10.1037/0000346-010
Psychological Assessment of Surgical Candidates: Evidence-Based Procedures and Practices, R. J. Marek and A. R. Block (Editors)

DEEP BRAIN STIMULATION

In DBS, stereotactically implanted electrodes provide chronic, high-frequency electrical stimulation to specific neuroanatomical targets (Lozano et al., 2019). The electrodes are connected to a pulse generator and implanted under the clavicle. Postoperative programming of this implanted pulse generator fine-tunes the stimulation parameters to achieve beneficial motor effects.

Although its precise mechanisms remain debated (see Lee et al., 2019, for a review), in general, DBS is thought to have effects at the ionic, protein, cellular, and network levels, which combine to produce changes in behavior (McIntyre & Anderson, 2016). Electrical stimulation of polarized electrodes releases charged ions into the extracellular space. The resulting electrical field stimulates a transmembrane voltage change, opening axonal voltage-gated sodium channels—constituted by proteins—and causing an action potential. This affects cells by triggering synaptic release of neurotransmitters and post-synaptic potentials in efferent target neurons, altering activity patterns at a brain network level (Jakobs et al., 2019; Lozano et al., 2019; McIntyre & Anderson, 2016).

DEEP BRAIN STIMULATION FOR PARKINSON'S DISEASE

First described by James Parkinson in 1817 as "the shaking palsy," PD is a neurodegenerative condition that causes symptoms of resting tremor, rigidity, bradykinesia, and postural instability. It progresses relentlessly to cause increasing motor disability and additional nonmotor symptoms of hallucinations and dementia. Pathologically, it is characterized by degeneration of nigrostriatal dopaminergic neurons and the presence of Lewy bodies in surviving neurons (Aarsland et al., 2017). Although Parkinson himself hoped for identification of a treatment by which "the progress of the disease may be stopped" (Parkinson, 1817, pp. 56–57), there remains no cure, and treatments provide only symptomatic relief.

Neurosurgery was the first treatment available for PD. Starting in 1921, bilateral rhizotomy was used to reduce tremor but with only partial success (Speelman & Bosch, 1998). By 1947, stereotactic devices for human neurosurgery and accompanying brain atlases had been developed (Spiegel et al., 1947), enabling precise targeting of deep brain structures and resulting in better outcomes and fewer side effects (Speelman & Bosch, 1998). However, following the discovery of the "miracle drug" levodopa in the 1960s (Cotzias et al., 1967, 1969), neurosurgery was mostly abandoned in favor of the new, inexpensive, noninvasive, and seemingly effective drug treatment. By the 1980s, the long-term effects of levodopa had become apparent: sudden symptom breakthrough and the emergence of dyskinesias, involuntary choreiform movements (Gardner, 2013).

In 1987, Benabid et al. published studies of patients with drug-resistant tremor who had been successfully treated using chronic, high-frequency stimulation of the ventral intermediate nucleus (Vim) of the thalamus. The discovery of this novel technique coincided with the development of a new scale for the quantification of PD symptom severity: the Unified Parkinson's Disease Rating Scale (Fahn, 1987). This enabled standardization of patient outcomes and comparison of the improvement associated with different stimulation sites and settings. International, multicenter clinical trials were funded to explore the benefit of DBS for the treatment of PD. In 1991, Benabid et al. reported empirically chosen Vim stimulation parameters for optimal motor outcomes. A few years later, they reported similar improvements following stimulation of other deep brain locations: the subthalamic nucleus (STN; Benabid et al., 1994) and internal globus pallidus (GPi; Krack et al., 1998). These were subsequently confirmed by an international, multicenter clinical trial (Obeso et al., 2001), and the U.S. Food and Drug Administration soon approved DBS for PD for all three neuroanatomical sites: (a) Vim, (b) STN, and (c) GPi.

Currently, DBS for PD is provided across North America, Australia, the United Kingdom, and Europe. Multicenter clinical trials have provided evidence that DBS treatment for PD is superior to best medical therapy, with enduring improvements in motor control and quality of life (e.g., Deuschl et al., 2006; Weaver et al., 2009). Data also show improvements in activities of daily living, lasting for up to at least 5 years after surgery (Krack et al., 2003). Typically, DBS is offered when the motor symptoms are refractory to less invasive therapies (Limousin & Foltynie, 2019).

There is a better understanding of the relative benefits associated with different DBS sites. It is mostly agreed that the benefits of targeting Vim are limited to its effects on dopamine-refractory tremor, whereas both STN and GPi stimulation reduce dopamine-responsive tremor, rigidity, and bradykinesia (see Lozano, 2000, for a review). STN and GPi DBS also reduce symptom breakthrough and dyskinesias (Pollak et al., 2002). The relative merits of STN and GPi stimulation are more contentious. Initially, STN DBS was considered superior to GPi DBS for reducing tremor, rigidity, and bradykinesia as well as enabling greater reductions in dopaminergic medication following surgery (Krack et al., 1998). In contrast, GPi DBS was thought to be superior for reducing dyskinesias (Krack et al., 1998). Follow-up data now suggest that STN and GPi DBS offer equivocal motor benefits (Follett et al., 2010; J. K. Wong et al., 2019), but STN DBS leads to better symptom control in *off periods*, when dopaminergic medications are not helping (see Limousin & Foltynie, 2019, for a review).

There is also a better understanding of the risks associated with DBS (Bronstein et al., 2011). A meta-analysis by Kleiner-Fisman et al. (2006) revealed the most common immediate surgical complications include transient confusion (15.6%), intracranial hemorrhage (3.9%), infection (1.7%), and seizures (1.5%). Aside from these, potential long-term motor and nonmotor side effects thought to be more common after STN DBS (Rodriguez-Oroz et al., 2005). Motor side effects include adverse events affecting speech (9.3%) as well as gait and balance (4.0%; Kleiner-Fisman et al., 2006). One review found speech articulation and phonation to be particularly affected by STN DBS (Aldridge et al., 2016), with the majority of patients reporting slurred speech that affects social interaction and quality of life (Wertheimer et al., 2014). Patients also suffer more falls when treated with DBS than with best medical therapy, often causing significant injuries necessitating hospitalization (Weaver et al., 2009).

Nonmotor side effects can occur, too, with risk of negative consequences for cognition (17.1%; Aviles-Olmos et al., 2014), mood (6.8%; Kleiner-Fisman et al., 2006) and behavior (5.4%; Kleiner-Fisman et al., 2006). Next, I discuss these effects in detail.

Effect of DBS on Cognition

The cognitive profile of PD is executive dysfunction and cognitive slowing, reflecting fronto-subcortical dysfunction (Sawamoto et al., 2002). Additional deficits in visual perception betray the involvement of the posterior cortex, heralding the onset of PD dementia (Williams-Gray et al., 2009).

In general, DBS is thought to be relatively benign (Aviles-Olmos et al., 2014), with no increased risk of dementia (see Limousin & Foltynie, 2019). However, negative cognitive consequences can occur after DBS surgery, particularly after STN DBS surgery (Wang et al., 2016). These include (usually transient) postoperative confusion (Kleiner-Fisman et al., 2006), permanent global cognitive decline (Aybek et al., 2007), and subtle deficits affecting frontal and subcortical cognitive functions (Combs et al., 2015; Wang et al., 2016). Interestingly, these cognitive sequelae do not seem to vary with stimulation settings, suggesting that the surgery itself may be the trigger for cognitive change (Leimbach et al., 2020) possibly because of interference with frontal cortical–subcortical loops (Schroeder et al., 2003).

Postoperative Confusion and Global Cognitive Decline

Postoperative confusion is documented in around 15.6% of STN DBS patients (Kleiner-Fisman et al., 2006). It usually resolves within a few days but can affect cognitive function and disease prognosis (see Li et al., 2021, for a review). It has been associated with larger ventricles, older age, longer disease duration, and more medical comorbidities (Strapasson et al., 2019) as well as greater cognitive impairment (Li et al., 2021). Permanent global cognitive decline is less common, affecting around 9.4% of patients with STN DBS (Aybek et al., 2007) and its risk factors include older age, particularly older than 70 years (Smeding et al., 2011), and greater cognitive impairment (Lang & Widner, 2002; Smeding et al., 2011).

Preoperative Risk Factors

These findings suggest that the presence of presurgical cognitive deficits should be treated as a red flag when selecting candidates for DBS. Indeed, it has been suggested that any cognitive deficits at baseline should serve as exclusion for surgery (Lang & Widner, 2002). However, most patients with PD will demonstrate some degree of cognitive impairment affecting executive functions and cognitive speed. Moreover, cognitive decline in PD is insidious so that it remains unclear what level of cognitive impairment is acceptable for DBS. This is important for assessing not only risk of cognitive side effects, but also capacity to provide informed consent to such elective invasive procedures and ability to comply with postsurgical device management.

My colleagues and I (Foley et al., 2018) explored cognitive impairment further in a sample of PD patients treated with DBS (Foley et al., 2018). One of the 40 patients demonstrated permanent global cognitive decline following STN DBS. Retrospective analysis of the baseline cognitive profile revealed that this patient performed flawlessly on the Mini-Mental State Examination (MMSE; Folstein et al., 1975) and passed two of the four tests of executive function. However, the patient had cognitive deficits that extended beyond executive function to involve language and visual perception, suggesting more advanced cognitive impairment. At age 68 years, the patient was also significantly older than the group mean. Although the results of this single case may not be generalizable, our findings support earlier reports that the presence of more encompassing cognitive deficits, affecting language or visual processing at baseline, constitute a significant risk factor for poorer cognitive outcome (Foley et al., 2018), particularly in older patients (Smeding et al., 2011). This risk may be even higher in patients with lower "cognitive reserve" (Stern, 2009, p. 2016)—that is, those with lower levels of premorbid efficiency and flexibility of cognitive processing—who are more vulnerable to cognitive decline (Woods et al., 2002).

There are reports of permanent global decline occurring in the absence of baseline cognitive deficits, but closer examination reveals that the preoperative cognitive testing was limited to screening measures (e.g., the MMSE) or measures of executive function only, precluding accurate interpretation of the wider cognitive profile (Krack et al., 2003; York et al., 2008). Such a limited approach to presurgical patient assessment was recommended by the Consensus on Deep Brain Stimulation for Parkinson's Disease (Lang et al., 2006). This consensus stated that DBS candidates should undergo assessment of cognition using the MMSE and that only those with borderline scores be referred for neuropsychological evaluation. However, the MMSE, originally designed to assess cognition in psychiatric patients (Folstein et al., 1975), fails to assess the two cognitive domains most commonly affected by PD: (a) executive function and (b) cognitive speed. Thus, the MMSE is inappropriate as a screen of cognitive function in PD.

Reliance on screening measures also fails to consider premorbid abilities. A screening measure may return a false negative for those with high premorbid ability in whom there is already evidence of significant cognitive decline, but that decline is not detectable using insensitive screening measures. It may also result in a false positive for those with low premorbid ability who, despite low scores, demonstrate no evidence of cognitive decline.

The Core Assessment Program for Surgical Interventional Therapies in Parkinson's Disease (Defer et al., 1999) recommended that, in addition to a screening measure, candidates should undergo a more expansive presurgical cognitive assessment. However, the recommended assessment focuses entirely on executive functions and memory, with no measure of visual perception or language. Thus, this limited assessment does not allow for the detection of more advanced cognitive decline. Accordingly, this cognitive assessment has been demonstrated to be insufficiently sensitive (Puy et al., 2018).

Postoperative Deficits in Specific Cognitive Domains

In contrast to these relatively rare global changes in cognition, subtler deficits in specific cognitive domains are more commonly observed (Combs et al., 2015). Meta-analyses have revealed a moderate decline in verbal fluency alongside small declines in cognitive speed, memory, attention, and executive functions (Combs et al., 2015). The decline in verbal fluency is significantly greater than that observed in PD patients who did not proceed with DBS, confirming it as a consequence of DBS (Zangaglia et al., 2012). Verbal fluency decline significantly affects communication satisfaction (Tröster et al., 2017) and is associated with lower quality of life (Parsons et al., 2006).

Preoperative Risk Factors

Few studies have sought to identify baseline risk factors of postoperative decline in verbal fluency. In a study of 28 DBS patients, my colleagues and I (Foley et al., 2017) found that greater decline in verbal fluency was associated with higher levels of apathy at baseline and greater decline in cognitive speed. A meta-review found apathy to rise significantly after DBS, even after controlling for the effects of medication (Zoon et al., 2021). This led us to speculate that DBS disruption of frontal cortical–subcortical loops may impair the frontal executive function of "energization" (Stuss, 2011, p. 759), resulting in a triad of deficits: (a) reduced verbal fluency, (b) slowed cognitive speed, and (c) increased apathy (Foley et al., 2017).

Aside from its implications for verbal fluency, apathy also has a significant effect on subjective outcome of DBS. Maier et al. (2013) found preoperative apathy was the most significant predictor of dissatisfaction with DBS, despite a significant improvement in motor symptoms (Maier et al., 2016). These patients, who also had higher depression scores, actually had better motor functioning before DBS. Interestingly, they often had unrealistic expectations of DBS, namely, "improvement of mental state," "more socializing," or "improvement of partnership," none of which improves with DBS (Maier et al., 2013, p. 1276). These expectations, although inappropriate for DBS, likely reflect the negative effect that PD can have on mood and relationship functioning as well as illustrate the importance of assessing and acting on candidates' expectations of surgery.

Effect of DBS on Mood

Around 40% of people with PD experience significant anxiety or depression (Gallagher & Schrag, 2012). This likely reflects the unique combination of disease-specific disruption to dopaminergic (Vriend et al., 2014), serotonergic, and noradrenergic neurotransmitter pathways (Politis & Loane, 2011; Remy et al., 2005) as well as the psychological effect of the motor symptoms and associated disability (Timmer et al., 2017).

Several studies have found mood to improve after DBS, representing a small-to-medium effect size (Cartmill et al., 2021; Combs et al., 2015), with rare reports of a transient euphoria (Cartmill et al., 2021). A meta-analysis found these effects on mood to be independent of any changes in quality of life or motor control, raising the possibility that they are a direct consequence of DBS on the limbic system (Cartmill et al., 2021).

Paradoxically, there are also reports of worsened depression and a greatly increased risk of suicide (Giannini et al., 2019). Deterioration in mood can be associated with rapid lowering of dopaminergic medication after DBS, but this tends to be short term (Cartmill et al., 2021). Risk factors for longer lasting depression and suicidal behavior include preoperative depression, psychiatric medication use, previous suicidal behavior, and family psychiatric history (Giannini et al., 2019). This intuitive finding supports the notion of DBS as a stressful life event by which those with lower levels of psychological resilience are more vulnerable to feeling overwhelmed. Greater executive dysfunction is also noted as a risk factor (Giannini et al., 2019), suggesting an interplay between greater mood dysfunction and lower inhibitory control and problem-solving abilities.

Thus, preoperative screening of DBS candidates must include careful assessment of a number of factors. Alongside a comprehensive cognitive assessment, the clinician needs to assess previous mental health history, focusing on current and previous experience of mood disorder and suicidality, and family mental health history.

Effect of DBS on Behavior

It is now well recognized that alongside the anticipated improvements in motor control, dopaminergic medication can also lead to changes in behavior, with a greatly increased risk of impulse control disorders (ICDs) of hypersexuality, compulsive gambling, overspending, or binge eating. These complications occur in up to 20% of patients but often present subclinically and are not admitted by the patient or detected by clinicians until after significant harm has occurred (S. H. Wong & Steiger, 2007). It is thought that these behavioral symptoms reflect the uneven pattern of dopaminergic loss in the striatum and desensitization of dopamine D2 autoreceptors, whereby dopaminergic therapy results in an "overdose" of dopamine in the ventral striatum and connected limbic areas (Cools, 2006).

Treatment for ICDs usually involves reducing dopaminergic medication. Accordingly, ICDs tend to reduce after DBS (Abbes et al., 2018). Although there are reports of de novo ICDs after DBS, these tend to be transient (Abbes et al., 2018).

PRESURGICAL PSYCHOLOGICAL ASSESSMENT OF CANDIDATES

Careful patient selection is required to mitigate risk for cognition, mood, and behavior decline (Saint-Cyr & Albanese, 2006). Therefore, presurgical psychological assessment of candidates should include a comprehensive cognitive assessment to detect the presence and extent of any presurgical cognitive decline or markers of advanced cognitive decline and as measured against premorbid level of intellectual function:

- **cognitive screen:** using a measure that includes assessments of executive functioning and cognitive speed, such as the Mattis Dementia Rating Scale (Mattis, 1988)
- **current level of intellectual functioning:** using measures of IQ, such as the Wechsler Adult Intelligence Scale–IV (Wechsler, 2008)
- **premorbid level of intellectual functioning:** estimated informally by educational and occupational history, and formally using reading tests, such as the Test of Premorbid Functioning (Wechsler, 2011)

The presurgical psychological assessment should also include measures of individual cognitive domains to determine the wider cognitive profile as well as include measures of visual perception and language:

- **memory:** using measures of verbal and nonverbal recognition and recall, such as subtests from the Recognition Memory Test (Warrington, 1984), Doors and People (Baddeley et al., 1994), or Wechsler Memory Scale (Wechsler, 2010), to ensure profile is not amnestic and thus atypical for PD
- **language:** using measures of naming, such as the Graded Naming Test (McKenna & Warrington, 1983)
- **visual perception:** using measures such as the Silhouettes subtest from the Visual Object and Space Perception battery (Warrington & James, 1991)
- **executive function:** using measures of verbal fluency (phonemic and semantic; Delis et al., 2001) among other measures, such as the Stroop Neuropsychological Screening Test (Trennery et al., 1989) and the Hayling Sentence Completion Test from the Hayling and Brixton Tests (Burgess & Shallice, 1997)
- **cognitive speed:** using a measure such as the processing speed index from the Wechsler Adult Intelligence Scale–IV (Wechsler, 2008)

Current mental state, previous mental health history, and expectations of surgery should be thoroughly assessed:

- **apathy:** using measures such as the Apathy Evaluation Scale (Marin et al., 1991)
- **depression and anxiety:** using measures such as the Hospital Anxiety and Depression Scale (Zigmond & Snaith, 1983)

- **previous episodes of low mood or anxiety necessitating treatment:** assessing during clinical interview
- **previous suicidality:** assessing during clinical interview
- **family history of mental ill health:** assessing during clinical interview

Behavioral symptoms of ICDs should be assessed using a formal measure, such as the Questionnaire for Impulsive-Compulsive Disorders in Parkinson's Disease (Weintraub et al., 2009). The specific measures chosen should be suitable for the population to be tested, with the individual measures chosen after considering any relevant cultural or linguistic factors.

The presence of presurgical cognitive deficits that reflect a severe decline from premorbid level of intellectual functioning or that extend beyond executive function to involve language and visual perception should be considered a red flag for DBS because of increased risks of postsurgical cognitive decline. Presurgical apathy is likely to mitigate any benefits in motor symptoms, whereas presurgical depression, particularly in those with greater executive dysfunction or unrealistic expectations of surgery, increases risk of postsurgical suicidal behavior. Similarly, those with greater history of adversity, personal or family history of mental health issues, or lower social or emotional support may need closer monitoring postsurgery. Lowering of dopaminergic medication should be done gradually and particularly carefully in those with greater risk of suicidal behavior.

DEEP BRAIN STIMULATION FOR MAJOR DEPRESSION

One of the oldest known surgical practices is *trepanation*, or boring into the skull for therapeutic purposes. From at least the 12th century, it is thought to have been used as a treatment for mental illness, as depicted later in Hieronymus Bosch's (ca. 1501–1505) painting of *The Extraction of the Stone of Madness* (also known as *The Cure of Folly*), despite only limited understanding of the underlying neurobiology. Although trepanation had mostly died out by the Renaissance, psychosurgery resurfaced in the 19th century. Advances in functional localization enabled identification of areas associated with mental illness, and specific loci of cortex were ablated as treatment (Cleary et al., 2015). Thus dawned the era of the prefrontal leucotomy—later renamed lobotomy—that subsequently became a popular therapy for disabling mental illness, winning Egas Moniz, one of its pioneers, a Nobel Prize. At the same time, electricity was also being used to treat mental illness in electroconvulsive therapy and early attempts at stimulation (Krauss et al., 2021).

More recently, specific neural circuits within the limbic lobe have been identified as targets for DBS for the treatment of various psychiatric disorders, including obsessive-compulsive disorder (Blomstedt et al., 2013), Tourette's disorder (Schrock et al., 2015), anorexia (Sobstyl et al., 2019), and intractable depression (Cleary et al., 2015). Because psychiatric disease remains the number one cause of disability in the world, a safe and efficacious surgical treatment offers an alluringly quick fix (Cleary et al., 2015).

Early open-label studies hailed DBS as an effective treatment for intractable depression (see Kisely et al., 2018, for a review), which brought the successes without the seizures and cognitive side effects of ablative therapies (Delaloye & Holtzheimer, 2014). Indeed, one study targeting the subcallosal cingulate white matter found that most symptoms of depression improved in 10 of the 20 patients treated (Lozano et al., 2008). Later randomized controlled trials brought more equivocal findings, with no significant benefit relative to sham stimulation (e.g., Holtzheimer et al., 2017), and some adverse events, including suicidal behavior (Hitti et al., 2020). There are also some reports of negative consequences for cognition, particularly in those who are older (Kubu et al., 2017).

DBS for severe and intractable depression also brings several ethical issues (Grant et al., 2014). These include questions about how to define success. Should DBS be used to abolish all negative affect, and what mood should be aimed for? It also raises issues about how to determine candidates' capacity to consent. Studies have shown that candidates with depression often have decision-making deficits and fail to understand the purpose of the invasive surgery (see Cleary et al., 2015). These concerns echo louder in the aftermath of early psychosurgery backlashes.

As such, DBS for depression remains an experimental procedure yet to be approved by the U.S. Food and Drug Administration. Clinical trials continue to research its benefits, and it is likely that it will be approved for at least a subset of patients in the future. Whether it will then be covered by insurance companies remains to be seen. However, as psychologists and mental health professionals, we will need to consider how best to assess candidates' cognitive and emotional competence for providing informed consent and their ability to cope with surgery. This likely will require comprehensive assessment of cognition and mental health as well as include measures of available social support and risk of suicide. We will need to work with colleagues to balance these important preoperative factors in trade-off with any expected gains and to protect those who are too vulnerable from harm resulting from surgery or inability to care for themselves postoperatively (Grant et al., 2014).

CONCLUSION

Since its first use in 1987, DBS has been used as a medical treatment for PD. International, multicenter clinical trials have investigated its benefit and developed empirically chosen stimulation parameters for optimal motor outcomes. Follow-up data have revealed long-term benefits and side effects, quantifying the risk of negative consequences for cognition, mood, and behavior. This has enabled the development of an evidence-based approach to presurgical psychological assessment of candidates.

In contrast, the application of DBS for intractable psychiatric illness, such as major depression, is still in its infancy and is used only as an experimental procedure. Although initial open-label studies have hailed success, more recent randomized controlled trials have been more equivocal. In the absence of long-term studies, there is no consensus over its benefits and side effects, raising several ethical issues and questions about how best to select candidates for surgery. However, the field continues to develop at a rapid pace, and psychologists and mental health professionals can expect that, in the future, this technology will come to be used in combination with other therapies to provide personalized treatments. We hope that these advances will offer dramatic improvements in quality of life for people with treatment-resistant depression, similar to those observed in PD.

REFERENCES

Aarsland, D., Creese, B., Politis, M., Chaudhuri, K. R., Ffytche, D. H., Weintraub, D., & Ballard, C. (2017). Cognitive decline in Parkinson disease. *Nature Reviews: Neurology*, *13*(4), 217–231. https://doi.org/10.1038/nrneurol.2017.27

Abbes, M., Lhommée, E., Thobois, S., Klinger, H., Schmitt, E., Bichon, A., Castrioto, A., Xie, J., Fraix, V., Kistner, A., Pélissier, P., Seigneuret, É., Chabardès, S., Mertens, P., Broussolle, E., Moro, E., & Krack, P. (2018). Subthalamic stimulation and neuropsychiatric symptoms in Parkinson's disease: Results from a long-term follow-up cohort study. *Journal of Neurology, Neurosurgery, & Psychiatry*, *89*(8), 836–843. https://doi.org/10.1136/jnnp-2017-316373

Aldridge, D., Theodoros, D., Angwin, A., & Vogel, A. P. (2016). Speech outcomes in Parkinson's disease after subthalamic nucleus deep brain stimulation: A systematic review. *Parkinsonism & Related Disorders*, *33*, 3–11. https://doi.org/10.1016/j.parkreldis.2016.09.022

Aviles-Olmos, I., Kefalopoulou, Z., Tripoliti, E., Candelario, J., Akram, H., Martinez-Torres, I., Jahanshahi, M., Foltynie, T., Hariz, M., Zrinzo, L., & Limousin, P. (2014). Long-term outcome of subthalamic nucleus deep brain stimulation for Parkinson's disease using an MRI-guided and MRI-verified approach. *Journal of Neurology, Neurosurgery, & Psychiatry*, *85*(12), 1419–1425. https://doi.org/10.1136/jnnp-2013-306907

Aybek, S., Gronchi-Perrin, A., Berney, A., Chiuvé, S. C., Villemure, J. G., Burkhard, P. R., & Vingerhoets, F. J. (2007). Long-term cognitive profile and incidence of dementia after STN-DBS in Parkinson's disease. *Movement Disorders*, *22*(7), 974–981. https://doi.org/10.1002/mds.21478

Baddeley, A. D., Emslie, H., & Nimmo-Smith, I. (1994). *Doors and People: A test of visual and verbal recall and recognition*. Thames Valley Test Company.

Benabid, A. L., Pollak, P., Gervason, C., Hoffmann, D., Gao, D. M., Hommel, M., Perret, J. E., & de Rougemont, J. (1991). Long-term suppression of tremor by chronic stimulation of the ventral intermediate thalamic nucleus. *The Lancet*, *337*(8738), 403–406. https://doi.org/10.1016/0140-6736(91)91175-T

Benabid, A. L., Pollak, P., Gross, C., Hoffmann, D., Benazzouz, A., Gao, D. M., Laurent, A., Gentil, M., & Perret, J. (1994). Acute and long-term effects of subthalamic nucleus stimulation in Parkinson's disease. *Stereotactic and Functional Neurosurgery*, *62*(1–4), 76–84. https://doi.org/10.1159/000098600

Benabid, A. L., Pollak, P., Louveau, A., Henry, S., & de Rougemont, J. (1987). Combined (thalamotomy and stimulation) stereotactic surgery of the VIM thalamic nucleus for bilateral Parkinson disease. *Applied Neurophysiology*, *50*(1–6), 344–346. https://doi.org/10.1159/000100803

Blomstedt, P., Sjöberg, R. L., Hansson, M., Bodlund, O., & Hariz, M. I. (2013). Deep brain stimulation in the treatment of obsessive-compulsive disorder. *World Neurosurgery*, *80*(6), e245–e253. https://doi.org/10.1016/j.wneu.2012.10.006

Bosch, H. (ca. 1501–1505). *The extraction of the stone of madness ["The cure of folly"]* [Painting]. Museo del Prado [Prado National Museum], Madrid, Spain. https://www.museodelprado.es/coleccion/obra-de-arte/la-extraccion-de-la-piedra-de-la-locura/313db7a0-f9bf-49ad-a242-67e95b14c5a2?searchMeta=extraction%20stone%20of%20madness

Bronstein, J. M., Tagliati, M., Alterman, R. L., Lozano, A. M., Volkmann, J., Stefani, A., Horak, F. B., Okun, M. S., Foote, K. D., Krack, P., Pahwa, R., Henderson, J. M., Hariz, M. I., Bakay, R. A., Rezai, A., Marks, W. J., Jr., Moro, E., Vitek, J. L., Weaver, F. M., . . . DeLong, M. R. (2011). Deep brain stimulation for Parkinson disease: An expert consensus and review of key issues. *Archives of Neurology*, *68*(2), 165–165. https://doi.org/10.1001/archneurol.2010.260

Burgess, P. W., & Shallice, T. (1997). *The Hayling and Brixton Tests*. Thames Valley Test Company.

Cartmill, T., Skvarc, D., Bittar, R., McGillivray, J., Berk, M., & Byrne, L. K. (2021). Deep brain stimulation of the subthalamic nucleus in Parkinson's disease: A meta-analysis of mood effects. *Neuropsychology Review*. Advance online publication. https://doi.org/10.1007/s11065-020-09467-z

Cleary, D. R., Ozpinar, A., Raslan, A. M., & Ko, A. L. (2015). Deep brain stimulation for psychiatric disorders: Where we are now. *Neurosurgical Focus*, *38*(6), Article E2. https://doi.org/10.3171/2015.3.FOCUS1546

Combs, H. L., Folley, B. S., Berry, D. T., Segerstrom, S. C., Han, D. Y., Anderson-Mooney, A. J., Walls, B. D., & van Horne, C. (2015). Cognition and depression following deep brain stimulation of the subthalamic nucleus and globus pallidus pars internus in Parkinson's disease: A meta-analysis. *Neuropsychology Review*, *25*(4), 439–454. https://doi.org/10.1007/s11065-015-9302-0

Cools, R. (2006). Dopaminergic modulation of cognitive function-implications for L-DOPA treatment in Parkinson's disease. *Neuroscience and Biobehavioral Reviews*, *30*(1), 1–23. https://doi.org/10.1016/j.neubiorev.2005.03.024

Cotzias, G. C., Papavasiliou, P. S., & Gellene, R. (1969). Modification of Parkinsonism—Chronic treatment with L-dopa. *The New England Journal of Medicine, 280*(7), 337–345. https://doi.org/10.1056/NEJM196902132800701

Cotzias, G. C., Van Woert, M. H., & Schiffer, L. M. (1967). Aromatic amino acids and modification of parkinsonism. *The New England Journal of Medicine, 276*(7), 374–379. https://doi.org/10.1056/NEJM196702162760703

Defer, G. L., Widner, H., Marié, R. M., Rémy, P., & Levivier, M. (1999). Core Assessment Program for Surgical Interventional Therapies in Parkinson's Disease (CAPSIT-PD). *Movement Disorders, 14*(4), 572–584. https://doi.org/10.1002/1531-8257(199907)14:4<572::AID-MDS1005>3.0.CO;2-C

Delaloye, S., & Holtzheimer, P. E. (2014). Deep brain stimulation in the treatment of depression. *Dialogues in Clinical Neuroscience, 16*(1), 83–91. https://doi.org/10.31887/DCNS.2014.16.1/sdelaloye

Delis, D. C., Kaplan, E., & Kramer, J. H. (2001). *Delis-Kaplan Executive Function System*. Psychological Corporation.

Deuschl, G., Schade-Brittinger, C., Krack, P., Volkmann, J., Schäfer, H., Bötzel, K., Daniels, C., Deutschländer, A., Dillmann, U., Eisner, W., Gruber, D., Hamel, W., Herzog, J., Hilker, R., Klebe, S., Kloß, M., Koy, J., Krause, M., Kupsch, A., . . . Voges, J. (2006). A randomized trial of deep-brain stimulation for Parkinson's disease. *The New England Journal of Medicine, 355*(9), 896–908. https://doi.org/10.1056/NEJMoa060281

Fahn, S. R. L. E. (1987). Unified Parkinson's Disease Rating Scale. In S. Fahn, C. D. Marsden, M. Goldstein, & D. B. Calne (Eds.), *Recent developments in Parkinson's disease* (Vol. 2, pp. 53–163, 293–304). Macmillan Healthcare Information.

Finger, S., & Piccolino, M. (2011). *The shocking history of electric fishes: From ancient epochs to the birth of modern neurophysiology*. Oxford University Press. https://doi.org/10.1093/acprof:oso/9780195366723.001.0001

Foley, J. A., Foltynie, T., Limousin, P., & Cipolotti, L. (2018). Standardised neuropsychological assessment for the selection of patients undergoing DBS for Parkinson's disease. *Parkinson's Disease, 2018*, Article 4328371. https://doi.org/10.1155/2018/4328371

Foley, J. A., Foltynie, T., Zrinzo, L., Hyam, J. A., Limousin, P., & Cipolotti, L. (2017). Apathy and reduced speed of processing underlie decline in verbal fluency following DBS. *Behavioural Neurology, 2017*, Article 7348101. https://doi.org/10.1155/2017/7348101

Follett, K. A., Weaver, F. M., Stern, M., Hur, K., Harris, C. L., Luo, P., Marks, W. J., Jr., Rothlind, J., Sagher, O., Moy, C., Pahwa, R., Burchiel, K., Hogarth, P., Lai, E. C., Duda, J. E., Holloway, K., Samii, A., Horn, S., Bronstein, J. M., . . . Reda, D. J. (2010). Pallidal versus subthalamic deep-brain stimulation for Parkinson's disease. *The New England Journal of Medicine, 362*(22), 2077–2091. https://doi.org/10.1056/NEJMoa0907083

Folstein, M. F., Folstein, S. E., & McHugh, P. R. (1975). "Mini-mental state": A practical method for grading the cognitive state of patients for the clinician. *Journal of Psychiatric Research, 12*(3), 189–198. https://doi.org/10.1016/0022-3956(75)90026-6

Gallagher, D. A., & Schrag, A. (2012). Psychosis, apathy, depression and anxiety in Parkinson's disease. *Neurobiology of Disease, 46*(3), 581–589. https://doi.org/10.1016/j.nbd.2011.12.041

Gardner, J. (2013). A history of deep brain stimulation: Technological innovation and the role of clinical assessment tools. *Social Studies of Science*, *43*(5), 707–728. https://doi.org/10.1177/0306312713483678

Giannini, G., Francois, M., Lhommée, E., Polosan, M., Schmitt, E., Fraix, V., Castrioto, A., Ardouin, C., Bichon, A., Pollak, P., Benabid, A.-L., Seigneuret, E., Chabardes, S., Wack, M., Krack, P., & Moro, E. (2019). Suicide and suicide attempts after subthalamic nucleus stimulation in Parkinson disease. *Neurology*, *93*(1), e97–e105. https://doi.org/10.1212/WNL.0000000000007665

Grant, R. A., Halpern, C. H., Baltuch, G. H., O'Reardon, J. P., & Caplan, A. (2014). Ethical considerations in deep brain stimulation for psychiatric illness. *Journal of Clinical Neuroscience*, *21*(1), 1–5. https://doi.org/10.1016/j.jocn.2013.04.004

Hitti, F. L., Yang, A. I., Cristancho, M. A., & Baltuch, G. H. (2020). Deep brain stimulation is effective for treatment-resistant depression: A meta-analysis and meta-regression. *Journal of Clinical Medicine*, *9*(9), Article 2796. https://doi.org/10.3390/jcm9092796

Holtzheimer, P. E., Husain, M. M., Lisanby, S. H., Taylor, S. F., Whitworth, L. A., McClintock, S., Slavin, K. V., Berman, J., McKhann, G. M., Patil, P. G., Rittberg, B. R., Abosch, A., Pandurangi, A. K., Holloway, K. L., Lam, R. W., Honey, C. R., Neimat, J. S., Henderson, J. M., DeBattista, C., . . . Mayberg, H. S. (2017). Subcallosal cingulate deep brain stimulation for treatment-resistant depression: A multisite, randomised, sham-controlled trial. *The Lancet Psychiatry*, *4*(11), 839–849. https://doi.org/10.1016/S2215-0366(17)30371-1

Jakobs, M., Fomenko, A., Lozano, A. M., & Kiening, K. L. (2019). Cellular, molecular, and clinical mechanisms of action of deep brain stimulation—A systematic review on established indications and outlook on future developments. *EMBO Molecular Medicine*, *11*(4), Article e9575. https://doi.org/10.15252/emmm.201809575

Kellaway, P. (1946). The part played by electric fish in the early history of bioelectricity and electrotherapy. *Bulletin of the History of Medicine*, *20*(2), 112–137. https://www.jstor.org/stable/44441034

Kisely, S., Li, A., Warren, N., & Siskind, D. (2018). A systematic review and meta-analysis of deep brain stimulation for depression. *Depression and Anxiety*, *35*(5), 468–480. https://doi.org/10.1002/da.22746

Kleiner-Fisman, G., Herzog, J., Fisman, D. N., Tamma, F., Lyons, K. E., Pahwa, R., Lang, A. E., & Deuschl, G. (2006). Subthalamic nucleus deep brain stimulation: Summary and meta-analysis of outcomes. *Movement Disorders*, *21*(S14), S290–S304. https://doi.org/10.1002/mds.20962

Krack, P., Batir, A., Van Blercom, N., Chabardes, S., Fraix, V., Ardouin, C., Koudsie, A., Limousin, P. D., Benazzouz, A., LeBas, J. F., Benabid, A.-L., & Pollak, P. (2003). Five-year follow-up of bilateral stimulation of the subthalamic nucleus in advanced Parkinson's disease. *The New England Journal of Medicine*, *349*(20), 1925–1934. https://doi.org/10.1056/NEJMoa035275

Krack, P., Pollak, P., Limousin, P., Hoffmann, D., Xie, J., Benazzouz, A., & Benabid, A. L. (1998). Subthalamic nucleus or internal pallidal stimulation in young onset Parkinson's disease. *Brain*, *121*(3), 451–457. https://doi.org/10.1093/brain/121.3.451

Krauss, J. K., Lipsman, N., Aziz, T., Boutet, A., Brown, P., Chang, J. W., Davidson, B., Grill, W. M., Hariz, M. I., Horn, A., Schulder, M., Mammis, A., Tass, P. A., Volkmann, J., & Lozano, A. M. (2021). Technology of deep brain stimulation: Current status and future directions. *Nature Reviews: Neurology*, *17*(2), 75–87. https://doi.org/10.1038/s41582-020-00426-z

Kubu, C. S., Brelje, T., Butters, M. A., Deckersbach, T., Malloy, P., Moberg, P., Tröster, A. I., Williamson, E., Baltuch, G. H., Bhati, M. T., Carpenter, L. L., Dougherty, D. D., Howland, R. H., Rezai, A. R., & Malone, D. A., Jr. (2017). Cognitive outcome after ventral capsule/ventral striatum stimulation for treatment-resistant major depression. *Journal of Neurology, Neurosurgery, & Psychiatry*, *88*(3), 262–265. https://doi.org/10.1136/jnnp-2016-313803

Lang, A. E., Houeto, J. L., Krack, P., Kubu, C., Lyons, K. E., Moro, E., Ondo, W., Pahwa, R., Poewe, W., Tröster, A. I., Uitti, R., & Voon, V. (2006). Deep brain stimulation: Preoperative issues. *Movement Disorders*, *21*(S14), S171–S196. https://doi.org/10.1002/mds.20955

Lang, A. E., & Widner, H. (2002). Deep brain stimulation for Parkinson's disease: Patient selection and evaluation. *Movement Disorders*, *17*(S3), S94–S101. https://doi.org/10.1002/mds.10149

Lee, D. J., Lozano, C. S., Dallapiazza, R. F., & Lozano, A. M. (2019). Current and future directions of deep brain stimulation for neurological and psychiatric disorders. *Journal of Neurosurgery*, *131*(2), 333–342. https://doi.org/10.3171/2019.4.JNS181761

Leimbach, F., Atkinson-Clement, C., Wilkinson, L., Cheung, C., & Jahanshahi, M. (2020). Dissociable effects of subthalamic nucleus deep brain stimulation surgery and acute stimulation on verbal fluency in Parkinson's disease. *Behavioural Brain Research*, *388*, Article 112621. https://doi.org/10.1016/j.bbr.2020.112621

Li, H., Han, S., & Feng, J. (2021). Delirium after deep brain stimulation in Parkinson's disease. *Parkinson's Disease*, *2021*, Article 8885386. https://doi.org/10.1155/2021/8885386

Limousin, P., & Foltynie, T. (2019). Long-term outcomes of deep brain stimulation in Parkinson disease. *Nature Reviews: Neurology*, *15*(4), 234–242. https://doi.org/10.1038/s41582-019-0145-9

Lozano, A. M. (2000). Vim thalamic stimulation for tremor. *Archives of Medical Research*, *31*(3), 266–269. https://doi.org/10.1016/S0188-4409(00)00081-3

Lozano, A. M., Lipsman, N., Bergman, H., Brown, P., Chabardes, S., Chang, J. W., Matthews, K., McIntyre, C. C., Schlaepfer, T. E., Schulder, M., Temel, Y., Volkmann, J., & Krauss, J. K. (2019). Deep brain stimulation: Current challenges and future directions. *Nature Reviews: Neurology*, *15*(3), 148–160. https://doi.org/10.1038/s41582-018-0128-2

Lozano, A. M., Mayberg, H. S., Giacobbe, P., Hamani, C., Craddock, R. C., & Kennedy, S. H. (2008). Subcallosal cingulate gyrus deep brain stimulation for treatment-resistant depression. *Biological Psychiatry*, *64*(6), 461–467. https://doi.org/10.1016/j.biopsych.2008.05.034

Maier, F., Lewis, C. J., Horstkoetter, N., Eggers, C., Dembek, T. A., Visser-Vandewalle, V., Kuhn, J., Zurowski, M., Moro, E., Woopen, C., & Timmermann, L. (2016). Subjective perceived outcome of subthalamic deep brain stimulation in Parkinson's disease one year after surgery. *Parkinsonism & Related Disorders*, *24*, 41–47. https://doi.org/10.1016/j.parkreldis.2016.01.019

Maier, F., Lewis, C. J., Horstkoetter, N., Eggers, C., Kalbe, E., Maarouf, M., Kuhn, J., Zurowski, M., Moro, E., Woopen, C., & Timmermann, L. (2013). Patients' expectations of deep brain stimulation, and subjective perceived outcome related to clinical measures in Parkinson's disease: A mixed-method approach. *Journal of Neurology, Neurosurgery, & Psychiatry*, *84*(11), 1273–1281. https://doi.org/10.1136/jnnp-2012-303670

Marin, R. S., Biedrzycki, R. C., & Firinciogullari, S. (1991). Reliability and validity of the Apathy Evaluation Scale. *Psychiatry Research*, *38*(2), 143–162. https://doi.org/10.1016/0165-1781(91)90040-V

Mattis, S. (1988). *Dementia Rating Scale*. Psychological Assessment Resources.

McIntyre, C. C., & Anderson, R. W. (2016). Deep brain stimulation mechanisms: The control of network activity via neurochemistry modulation. *Journal of Neurochemistry*, *139*(Suppl. 1), 338–345. https://doi.org/10.1111/jnc.13649

McKenna, P., & Warrington, E. K. (1983). *The Graded Naming Test*. NFER-Nelson.

Obeso, J. A., Olanow, C. W., Rodriguez-Oroz, M. C., Krack, P., Kumar, R., Lang, A. E., & the Deep-Brain Stimulation for Parkinson's Disease Study Group. (2001). Deep-brain stimulation of the subthalamic nucleus or the pars interna of the globus pallidus in Parkinson's disease. *The New England Journal of Medicine*, *345*(13), 956–963. https://doi.org/10.1056/NEJMoa000827

Parkinson, J. (1817). *An essay on the shaking palsy*. Sherwood, Neely, and Jones.

Parsons, T. D., Rogers, S. A., Braaten, A. J., Woods, S. P., & Tröster, A. I. (2006). Cognitive sequelae of subthalamic nucleus deep brain stimulation in Parkinson's disease: A meta-analysis. *The Lancet Neurology*, *5*(7), 578–588. https://doi.org/10.1016/S1474-4422(06)70475-6

Politis, M., & Loane, C. (2011). Serotonergic dysfunction in Parkinson's disease and its relevance to disability. *The Scientific World Journal*, *11*, Article 172893. https://doi.org/10.1100/2011/172893

Pollak, P., Fraix, V., Krack, P., Moro, E., Mendes, A., Chabardes, S., Koudsie, A., & Benabid, A. L. (2002). Treatment results: Parkinson's disease. *Movement Disorders*, *17*(S3), S75–S83. https://doi.org/10.1002/mds.10146

Puy, L., Tir, M., Lefranc, M., Yaïche, H., Godefroy, O., & Krystkowiak, P. (2018). Acute dementia after deep brain stimulation in Parkinson disease. *World Neurosurgery*, *119*, 63–65. https://doi.org/10.1016/j.wneu.2018.07.197

Remy, P., Doder, M., Lees, A., Turjanski, N., & Brooks, D. (2005). Depression in Parkinson's disease: Loss of dopamine and noradrenaline innervation in the limbic system. *Brain*, *128*(6), 1314–1322. https://doi.org/10.1093/brain/awh445

Rodriguez-Oroz, M. C., Obeso, J. A., Lang, A. E., Houeto, J. L., Pollak, P., Rehncrona, S., Kulisevsky, J., Albanese, A., Volkmann, J., Hariz, M. I., Quinn, N. P., Speelman, J. D., Guridi, J., Zamarbide, I., Gironell, A., Molet, J., Pascual-Sedano, B., Pidoux, B., Bonnet, A. M., . . . Van Blercom, N. (2005). Bilateral deep brain stimulation in Parkinson's disease: A multicentre study with 4 years follow-up. *Brain*, *128*(10), 2240–2249. https://doi.org/10.1093/brain/awh571

Saint-Cyr, J. A., & Albanese, A. (2006). STN DBS in PD: Selection criteria for surgery should include cognitive and psychiatric factors. *Neurology*, *66*(12), 1799–1800. https://doi.org/10.1212/01.wnl.0000227468.17113.07

Sawamoto, N., Honda, M., Hanakawa, T., Fukuyama, H., & Shibasaki, H. (2002). Cognitive slowing in Parkinson's disease: A behavioral evaluation independent of motor slowing. *The Journal of Neuroscience*, *22*(12), 5198–5203. https://doi.org/10.1523/JNEUROSCI.22-12-05198.2002

Schrock, L. E., Mink, J. W., Woods, D. W., Porta, M., Servello, D., Visser-Vandewalle, V., Silburn, P. A., Foltynie, T., Walker, H. C., Shahed-Jimenez, J., Savica, R., Klassen, B. T.,

Machado, A. G., Foote, K. D., Zhang, J. G., Hu, W., Ackermans, L., Temel, Y., Mari, Z., . . . Okun, M. S. (2015). Tourette syndrome deep brain stimulation: A review and updated recommendations. *Movement Disorders, 30*(4), 448–471. https://doi.org/10.1002/mds.26094

Schroeder, U., Kuehler, A., Lange, K. W., Haslinger, B., Tronnier, V. M., Krause, M., Pfister, R., Boecker, H., & Ceballos-Baumann, A. O. (2003). Subthalamic nucleus stimulation affects a frontotemporal network: A PET study. *Annals of Neurology, 54*(4), 445–450. https://doi.org/10.1002/ana.10683

Smeding, H. M., Speelman, J. D., Huizenga, H. M., Schuurman, P. R., & Schmand, B. (2011). Predictors of cognitive and psychosocial outcome after STN DBS in Parkinson's disease. *Journal of Neurology, Neurosurgery, & Psychiatry, 82*(7), 754–760. https://doi.org/10.1136/jnnp.2007.140012

Sobstyl, M., Stapińska-Syniec, A., Sokół-Szawłowska, M., & Kupryjaniuk, A. (2019). Deep brain stimulation for the treatment of severe intractable anorexia nervosa. *British Journal of Neurosurgery, 33*(6), 601–607. https://doi.org/10.1080/02688697.2019.1667484

Speelman, J. D., & Bosch, D. A. (1998). Resurgence of functional neurosurgery for Parkinson's disease: A historical perspective. *Movement Disorders, 13*(3), 582–588. https://doi.org/10.1002/mds.870130336

Spiegel, E. A., Wycis, H. T., Marks, M., & Lee, A. J. (1947). Stereotaxic apparatus for operations on the human brain. *Science, 106*(2754), 349–350. https://doi.org/10.1126/science.106.2754.349

Stern, Y. (2009). Cognitive reserve. *Neuropsychologia, 47*(10), 2015–2028. https://doi.org/10.1016/j.neuropsychologia.2009.03.004

Strapasson, A. C. P., Martins Antunes, Á. C., Petry Oppitz, P., Dalsin, M., & de Mello Rieder, C. R. (2019). Postoperative confusion in patients with Parkinson disease undergoing deep brain stimulation of the subthalamic nucleus. *World Neurosurgery, 125*, e966–e971. https://doi.org/10.1016/j.wneu.2019.01.216

Stuss, D. T. (2011). Functions of the frontal lobes: Relation to executive functions. *Journal of the International Neuropsychological Society, 17*(5), 759–765. https://doi.org/10.1017/S1355617711000695

Timmer, M. H. M., van Beek, M. H. C. T., Bloem, B. R., & Esselink, R. A. J. (2017). What a neurologist should know about depression in Parkinson's disease. *Practical Neurology, 17*(5), 359–368. https://doi.org/10.1136/practneurol-2017-001650

Trennery, M. R., Crosson, B., DeBoe, J., & Lebere, W. R. (1989). *Stroop Neuropsychological Screening Test*. Psychological Assessment Resources.

Tröster, A. I., Jankovic, J., Tagliati, M., Peichel, D., & Okun, M. S. (2017). Neuropsychological outcomes from constant current deep brain stimulation for Parkinson's disease. *Movement Disorders, 32*(3), 433–440. https://doi.org/10.1002/mds.26827

Tsoucalas, G., & Sgantzos, M. (2016). Electric current to cure arthritis and cephalaea in ancient Greek medicine. *Mediterranean Journal of Rheumatology, 27*(4), 198–203. https://doi.org/10.31138/mjr.27.4.198

Vriend, C., Raijmakers, P., Veltman, D. J., van Dijk, K. D., van der Werf, Y. D., Foncke, E. M., Smit, J. H., Berendse, H. W., & van den Heuvel, O. A. (2014). Depressive symptoms in Parkinson's disease are related to reduced [^{123}I]FP-CIT binding in the caudate nucleus. *Journal of Neurology, Neurosurgery, & Psychiatry, 85*(2), 159–164. https://doi.org/10.1136/jnnp-2012-304811

Wang, J. W., Zhang, Y. Q., Zhang, X. H., Wang, Y. P., Li, J. P., & Li, Y. J. (2016). Cognitive and psychiatric effects of STN versus GPi deep brain stimulation in Parkinson's disease: A meta-analysis of randomized controlled trials. *PLoS One, 11*(6), Article e0156721. https://doi.org/10.1371/journal.pone.0156721

Warrington, E. K. (1984). *Recognition Memory Test: RMT*. NFER-Nelson.

Warrington, E. K., & James, M. (1991). *The Visual Object and Space Perception Battery*. Thames Valley Test Company.

Weaver, F. M., Follett, K., Stern, M., Hur, K., Harris, C., Marks, W. J., Jr., Rothlind, J., Sagher, O., Reda, D., Moy, C. S., Pahwa, R., Burchiel, K., Hogarth, P., Lai, E. C., Duda, J. E., Holloway, K., Samii, A., Horn, S., Bronstein, J., . . . Huang, G. D. (2009). Bilateral deep brain stimulation vs best medical therapy for patients with advanced Parkinson disease: A randomized controlled trial. *Journal of the American Medical Association, 301*(1), 63–73. https://doi.org/10.1001/jama.2008.929

Wechsler, D. (2008). *Wechsler Adult Intelligence Scale* (4th ed.). Psychological Corporation.

Wechsler, D. (2010). *Wechsler Memory Scale* (4th ed.). Psychological Corporation.

Wechsler, D. (2011). *Test of Premorbid Functioning*. Psychological Corporation.

Weintraub, D., Hoops, S., Shea, J. A., Lyons, K. E., Pahwa, R., Driver-Dunckley, E. D., Adler, C. H., Potenza, M. N., Miyasaki, J., Siderowf, A. D., Duda, J. E., Hurtig, H. I., Colcher, A., Horn, S. S., Stern, M. B., & Voon, V. (2009). Validation of the Questionnaire for Impulsive-Compulsive Disorders in Parkinson's Disease. *Movement Disorders, 24*(10), 1461–1467. https://doi.org/10.1002/mds.22571

Wertheimer, J., Gottuso, A. Y., Nuno, M., Walton, C., Duboille, A., Tuchman, M., & Ramig, L. (2014). The impact of STN deep brain stimulation on speech in individuals with Parkinson's disease: The patient's perspective. *Parkinsonism & Related Disorders, 20*(10), 1065–1070. https://doi.org/10.1016/j.parkreldis.2014.06.010

Williams-Gray, C. H., Evans, J. R., Goris, A., Foltynie, T., Ban, M., Robbins, T. W., Brayne, C., Kolachana, B. S., Weinberger, D. R., Sawcer, S. J., & Barker, R. A. (2009). The distinct cognitive syndromes of Parkinson's disease: 5 year follow-up of the CamPaIGN cohort. *Brain, 132*(11), 2958–2969. https://doi.org/10.1093/brain/awp245

Wong, J. K., Cauraugh, J. H., Ho, K. W. D., Broderick, M., Ramirez-Zamora, A., Almeida, L., Wagle Shukla, A., Wilson, C. A., de Bie, R. M., Weaver, F. M., Kang, N., & Okun, M. S. (2019). STN vs. GPi deep brain stimulation for tremor suppression in Parkinson disease: A systematic review and meta-analysis. *Parkinsonism & Related Disorders, 58*, 56–62. https://doi.org/10.1016/j.parkreldis.2018.08.017

Wong, S. H., & Steiger, M. J. (2007). Pathological gambling in Parkinson's disease. *BMJ, 334*(7598), 810–811. https://doi.org/10.1136/bmj.39176.363958.80

Woods, S. P., Fields, J. A., & Tröster, A. I. (2002). Neuropsychological sequelae of subthalamic nucleus deep brain stimulation in Parkinson's disease: A critical review. *Neuropsychology Review, 12*(2), 111–126. https://doi.org/10.1023/A:1016806711705

York, M. K., Dulay, M., Macias, A., Levin, H. S., Grossman, R., Simpson, R., & Jankovic, J. (2008). Cognitive declines following bilateral subthalamic nucleus deep brain stimulation for the treatment of Parkinson's disease. *Journal of Neurology, Neurosurgery, & Psychiatry, 79*(7), 789–795. https://doi.org/10.1136/jnnp.2007.118786

Zangaglia, R., Pasotti, C., Mancini, F., Servello, D., Sinforiani, E., & Pacchetti, C. (2012). Deep brain stimulation and cognition in Parkinson's disease: An eight-year follow-up study. *Movement Disorders*, *27*(9), 1192–1194. https://doi.org/10.1002/mds.25047

Zigmond, A. S., & Snaith, R. P. (1983). The Hospital Anxiety and Depression Scale. *Acta Psychiatrica Scandinavica*, *67*(6), 361–370. https://doi.org/10.1111/j.1600-0447.1983.tb09716.x

Zoon, T. J. C., van Rooijen, G., Balm, G. M. F. C., Bergfeld, I. O., Daams, J. G., Krack, P., Denys, D. A. J. P., & de Bie, R. M. A. (2021). Apathy induced by subthalamic nucleus deep brain stimulation in Parkinson's disease: A meta-analysis. *Movement Disorders*, *36*(2), 317–326. https://doi.org/10.1002/mds.28390

10 GYNECOLOGIC SURGERY

ANDREA BRADFORD

Benign gynecologic conditions, such as uterine fibroids, endometriosis, and pelvic organ prolapse, are highly prevalent and adversely affect quality of life (Marsh et al., 2018; Nnoaham et al., 2011; Pynnä et al., 2021). Cancers of the female reproductive tract are less common but are likely to have far-reaching effects on health and quality of life. Although nonsurgical treatments are, in some cases, able to reduce or prevent the need for surgery, surgery remains a mainstay in the treatment of both benign and malignant gynecologic conditions. Negative psychosocial outcomes occur in only a small proportion of patients who undergo elective procedures for benign disease. Nevertheless, this minority represents a large number of women, given the large overall number who are treated for gynecologic disease.

In addition to the potential physical, social, emotional, and financial toll of surgery, gynecologic procedures are unique in that they specifically target reproductive organs. Surgery for gynecologic disorders may provide relief of pain and other bothersome symptoms, but it is potentially at the expense of other outcomes that reduce quality of life. Removal of reproductive organs may be associated with feelings of loss, especially in younger women and

https://doi.org/10.1037/0000346-011
Psychological Assessment of Surgical Candidates: Evidence-Based Procedures and Practices, R. J. Marek and A. R. Block (Editors)

women who have not completed desired childbearing (Canada & Schover, 2012; Carter et al., 2005). However, such reactions are not universal nor are they necessarily typical. Concerns about sustaining a sexual relationship, managing pain, and maintaining mood and well-being are also important factors to consider in psychosocial adjustment after gynecologic surgery.

This chapter reviews the prevalence of common psychological problems encountered after gynecologic surgery, risk factors for these psychological sequelae, and practical suggestions for presurgical psychological assessment (PPA) in this diverse patient population. The focus of this chapter is on hysterectomy; *salpingo-oophorectomy*, the removal of an ovary and its fallopian tube; and radical surgeries for gynecologic cancers. Obstetric and reproductive procedures, including cesarean section, pregnancy termination, and assisted reproduction interventions, are outside the scope of this chapter, although the emerging practice of uterine transplantation is covered briefly. Cosmetic genitoplasty and gender confirmation procedures are addressed elsewhere in this volume.

OVERVIEW OF GYNECOLOGIC SURGERY

Hysterectomy, the surgical removal of the uterus, is the most common non-obstetric major surgical procedure among women of childbearing age in the United States (Cohen et al., 2014). Hysterectomy is performed for a variety of common conditions that affect the uterus and cervix, including *uterine leiomyomas*, or fibroids; endometriosis; abnormal uterine bleeding; cancer; and precancerous conditions. Hysterectomy is not the only treatment for these conditions and, in some cases, might be considered only after a trial of a less invasive or aggressive therapy. During a simple hysterectomy for benign diseases, the uterus and cervix are removed after detaching them from the ligaments and other tissues that support these organs in the pelvis. A *radical hysterectomy*, typically performed in the case of cancer, removes other structure surrounding the uterus and cervix, including the supporting ligaments and the upper portion of the vagina.

Recent decades have seen a trend toward more conversative surgeries that spare the pelvic organs as alternatives to hysterectomy. For example, surgery to repair *pelvic organ prolapse*, the protrusion of pelvic organs into the vagina, may be performed while sparing the uterus and other organs. First-line treatment for uterine fibroids, endometriosis, and other benign diseases increasingly focuses on medical management or surgical removal of abnormal lesions while leaving the uterus and other organs intact to the extent possible. Candidates for hysterectomy for benign conditions often have had a trial of at least one conservative treatment that has failed to adequately resolve pain or other bothersome symptoms (Nguyen et al., 2019).

Salpingo-oophorectomy may be performed at the time of hysterectomy or may be performed without hysterectomy for other indications. Whereas bilateral salpingo-oophorectomy (BSO) was once commonly performed at the time of hysterectomy to reduce risk of ovarian cancer, more recent research suggests that the long-term health risks of oophorectomy (especially before natural menopause) outweigh the benefits for women at average risk of ovarian cancer (Evans et al., 2016). However, risk-reducing BSO is increasingly offered to women with high-risk genetic mutations that increase the risk of ovarian cancer (e.g., *BRCA1* and *BRCA2* mutations, Lynch syndrome). In premenopausal women, BSO induces "surgical menopause," which may be managed with hormone replacement therapy (Kingsberg et al., 2020). *Salpingectomy*, the removal of the fallopian tubes alone, can be performed at the time of hysterectomy or another surgery and provides an irreversible method of sterilization. Salpingectomy also reduces risk for ovarian cancer (Hanley et al., 2022), which often originates in the fallopian tubes.

Women with advanced cancers may undergo more extensive surgery that involves the removal of organs and tissues beyond the reproductive tract. In general, more radical pelvic surgeries for gynecologic malignancies, although less common, are associated with greater functional impairment and psychosocial morbidity. For example, *pelvic exenteration* is a radical procedure involving the removal of all pelvic organs, usually including the bladder and rectum. It is a potentially curative treatment for a subset of patients with locally advanced and recurrent cervical and endometrial cancers. However, morbidity associated with pelvic exenteration is extensive, and long-term survival after the procedure is relatively low. Not surprisingly, women who have undergone pelvic exenteration have lasting decrements in quality of life, mood, body image, and sexual dysfunction (Harji et al., 2016). Treatment of advanced vulvar cancer often involves surgical removal of all or a portion of the vulva, called a *vulvectomy*, and this is also associated with reduced quality of life and negative changes in sexual function (Günther et al., 2014; Janda et al., 2004; Likes et al., 2007). Patients who are planning a radical pelvic surgery are likely to benefit from proactive PPA and counseling, given the extremely stressful and possibly traumatic nature of these procedures.

Uterine transplant is a recently developed procedure that offers a novel treatment option for women who have had a hysterectomy or who have uterine factor infertility. The donated uterus can be harvested from a living or deceased donor. This procedure has a high complication rate (Ricci et al., 2021). As with other solid organ transplants, recipients must take immunosuppressant medication to prevent rejection of the transplanted uterus. Pregnancy must be achieved by implantation of an embryo into the transplanted uterus, and once the recipient has completed childbearing, the donated uterus is removed via hysterectomy.

GENERAL APPROACH TO ASSESSMENT

For most gynecologic surgeries, PPA is not routine, and thus psychologists and mental health professionals are likely to be consulted only as needed, typically for assessment of patients who are known or suspected to have risk factors for psychological maladjustment. However, psychologists and mental health professionals may be more closely involved in teams caring for patients undergoing high-risk and high-morbidity procedures. The sections that follow outline general considerations for conducting PPA in the gynecologic surgery setting.

Patient Selection Criteria

The main reason for PPA is to identify patients who might benefit from psychological intervention before or after surgery. Because most patients adjust well to surgery without intervention, PPA may not be routine in many average-risk settings. Rather, patients may be referred for assessment based on a positive screen for psychological distress (e.g., a high score on a depression screening tool), clinician observations that raise concern for psychological comorbidity, potential for adverse outcomes (e.g., undesired loss of fertility), or the patient's expressed need for psychological support.

Data Gathering

A clinical interview that focuses on the presenting problem or referral question is recommended as the primary data gathering modality, supplemented with chart review. Patient-reported outcome instruments should be used selectively to the extent that more detailed information will meaningfully inform the assessment or monitor treatment outcomes. The use of lengthier personality assessment instruments in gynecologic disease populations have seldom been discussed in the literature, and, at present, there is no clear advantage of using these tools in PPA.

The interviewer should take care to inform the patient of the nature and purpose of the interview and to provide reassurance that responses will not be used to withhold medical treatment. Patients may fear that their physical symptoms will be interpreted as psychogenic, and these concerns should be addressed proactively and with sensitivity. It is often worthwhile to begin by inquiring about the patient's health status and somatic symptoms as well as any functional or role limitations imposed by their illness. This allows the patient to share the narrative and important aspects of their illness and is often a helpful segue to discussing the patient's distress, coping, and expectations for surgery. Questions about sexuality and other sensitive topics should be presented in a manner that normalizes these concerns and invites frank discussion. An example of such an interview question is, "Many women who have this surgery wonder how it will affect their sex lives. What questions or concerns do you have?"

In the case of uterine transplantation, PPA serves to aid in the selection of living donors and transplant recipients as well as help prepare surgical candidates. Important domains of assessment include psychological distress, coping skills, uncontrolled psychiatric conditions, substance use, social support, interpersonal conflict pertinent to the procedure, and the recipient's expectations and understanding of risks and benefits. Järvholm et al. (2018) have published a suggested framework for PPA of uterine transplant candidates, which is subject to further research and development given increased use of this surgery.

Assessment as an Opportunity for Brief Intervention and Referral

Unmet psychoeducational needs, which are not consistently addressed during preoperative clinic visits, may be feasible to address during PPA. Presurgical interventions developed in other settings to improve postoperative pain management (e.g., Darnall et al., 2019) may be adapted for use in patients undergoing gynecologic surgery, which may be of special significance in candidates with more severe pro-operative mood or anxiety symptoms (Benlolo et al., 2021; Carey et al., 2021).

PPA also presents an opportunity to introduce the idea of psychological support after surgery and establish the expectation for monitoring not only physical recovery and outcomes, but also psychological outcomes. There is no evidence to suggest that routine gynecologic surgery should be delayed on the basis of psychological risk factors (a high risk of harm to self or others is a clear exception). However, it may be appropriate to arrange a priority follow-up visit or make a referral for treatment if there is evidence of clinically significant distress or psychiatric symptoms (e.g., mood disturbance, anxiety, traumatic stress symptoms).

Collaboration With the Surgical Team

The success of collaboration with the gynecologic care team hinges on effective communication. The psychologist/mental health professional's role and scope of practice should be made clear as early as possible to all parties directly involved in the consultation or referral process. Because many PPAs will involve patients with complex psychosocial histories, psychologists and mental health professionals may find themselves advocating for "difficult" patients whose treatment needs extend beyond the surgery team. Ensuring role clarity and expectations can help prevent or mitigate these conflicts.

Timely feedback to the referring provider, whether formal or informal, is necessary to effectively to "close the communication loop" and is an essential skill for collaborative practice. Feedback can also present an opportunity to orient providers to potentially appropriate interventions and refine misconceptions about psychogenesis.

PSYCHOLOGICAL FACTORS AND GYNECOLOGIC SURGERY OUTCOMES

The following sections describe common outcomes of interest in the gynecologic surgery setting and psychological risk factors for suboptimal outcomes. Each of these domains should be assessed through a clinical interview with or without the addition of domain-specific, patient-reported outcome measures noted. Screening for trauma and other adverse experiences (e.g., housing, food insecurity) is also recommended, and for more extensive assessment, consider a structured instrument, such as the Childhood Trauma Questionnaire (Bernstein et al., 1994); Trauma History Questionnaire (Green, 1996); Accountable Health Communities Screening Tool (Billioux et al., 2017); or Extended-Hurt, Insult, Threaten, Scream Questionnaire (Portnoy et al., 2018).

Depressed Mood and Anxiety

Studies of women before hysterectomy suggest a higher than average rate of depression in women with benign gynecologic disorders (e.g., Estes et al., 2021; Leithner et al., 2009). Shared risk factors for depression and benign gynecologic diseases, and for depression and chronic pain, have been hypothesized as possible explanations for this observation (Chiuve et al., 2022). Prospective studies of patient-reported outcomes conducted in the United States and Europe suggest that hysterectomy reduces the burden of mood symptoms in this population (Farquhar et al., 2006; Persson et al., 2010; Theunissen et al., 2017). However, case-control studies based on medical claims data sets from Taiwan, South Korea, and the United States have found that hysterectomy is associated with an increased risk of depression, especially in women under age 50 (Chiuve et al., 2022; Choi et al., 2020; Chou et al., 2015). Factors related to persistence of depressive symptoms after hysterectomy include baseline pain, depression, anxiety, and other psychiatric conditions (Chiuve et al., 2022; Theunissen et al., 2017; Vandyk et al., 2011; Yen et al., 2008). Persistence of pain and surgical complications are risk factors for depression up to 1 year after hysterectomy (Theunissen et al., 2017). The course of mood symptoms and well-being after hysterectomy, therefore, is associated to some extent with improvement or deterioration in health status.

Women with a high risk of ovarian cancer because of genetic factors have a higher burden of depression and anxiety than in the general population. Typically, they are advised to undergo regular ovarian screening and eventually undergo risk-reducing BSO after completing desired childbearing. Each individual's decision making and timing for these preventive measures are complex and often highly influenced by anxiety about developing a lethal disease. Women with high-risk genetic mutations who undergo BSO report less cancer-specific worry and distress compared with those who opt for close gynecologic screening as a preventive measure (Madalinska et al., 2005; Mai et al., 2020), but outcomes for depression and anxiety in general are similar between groups (Mai et al., 2020). Younger and nulliparous women may benefit from psychological intervention to manage uncertainty and cope with cancer-related worry.

A number of standardized instruments for assessing mood and anxiety symptoms have been used extensively in the gynecologic setting. They include the Patient Health Questionnaire–9 (Kroenke & Spitzer, 2002), Generalized Anxiety Disorder 7-Item Scale (Spitzer et al., 2006), Hospital Anxiety and Depression Scale (Zigmond & Snaith, 1983), and Patient-Reported Outcomes Measurement Information System (PROMIS; Cella et al., 2007) negative affect measures (Schalet et al., 2016).

Pain

Pain frequently accompanies benign gynecologic diseases, such as uterine fibroids, ovarian cysts, pelvic inflammatory disease, and endometriosis, and is highly prevalent in women who are candidates for hysterectomy. Prospective studies indicate that both hysterectomy and more conservative surgery improve pelvic pain symptoms in the majority of women, including many women with no identifiable pathology (Allaire et al., 2018; Humalajärvi et al., 2014; Tay & Bromwich, 1998). However, up to 36% of women with preoperative pain report some degree of residual pain up to 3 years after hysterectomy (Farquhar et al., 2006; Hillis et al., 1995; Pokkinen et al., 2015; Tay & Bromwich, 1998).

Women at elevated risk for persistent pelvic pain after hysterectomy include those with no identifiable pelvic pathology, those with coexisting pain conditions elsewhere, and those for whom pain is the primary indication for surgery (Brandsborg et al., 2007, 2009; Hillis et al., 1995). Higher levels of pain in the acute postoperative period are also linked to persistence of pain up to 5 years after surgery (Brandsborg et al., 2009; Lunde et al., 2020; Pinto et al., 2018; Pokkinen et al., 2015). Behavioral risk factors for persistent posthysterectomy pain should be assessed and include pre- and postoperative anxiety, pain catastrophizing (Benlolo et al., 2021; Pinto et al., 2018), and tobacco smoking (Pokkinen et al., 2015). Interestingly, preoperative depression has not been reliably shown to influence pain outcomes in prospective studies of hysterectomy (Learman et al., 2011; Pinto et al., 2018).

Chronic pelvic pain can be assessed using general self-report instruments for pain severity, such as the McGill Pain Questionnaire (Melzack, 1975) and the Brief Pain Inventory (Cleeland & Ryan, 1994), although if pain is localized to one area, a visual analog scale is a reasonable alternative. In addition to assessment of pain severity, the Pain Catastrophizing Scale (Sullivan et al., 1995) can provide additional insight into maladaptive pain behaviors. Consider also a general measure of somatization, such as the Patient Health Questionnaire–15 (Kroenke et al., 2002), particularly if the patient is experiencing multiple somatic symptoms and comorbid pain syndromes.

Chronic pelvic pain and chronic postsurgical pain result from numerous etiologies and may be present without an identifiable underlying pathology. Women with chronic pelvic pain frequently experience other chronic conditions associated with abdominal or pelvic organ pain, such as irritable bowel syndrome, interstitial cystitis, and vulvodynia. Chronic pelvic pain has been conceptualized as a central nervous system–mediated disorder with alterations in functioning of the autonomic nervous system and the hypothalamic–pituitary–adrenal axis (Brawn et al., 2014; Heim et al., 1998; Ortiz et al., 2020). As such, a pattern of worsening with psychological stress is often present. Psychosocial risk factors for chronic pelvic pain include a prior history of both childhood and adult adversity and trauma, military sexual trauma, psychiatric comorbidity, and sexual dysfunction (Cichowski et al., 2017; Fuentes & Christianson, 2018; Latthe et al., 2006).

Sexual Function

Concerns about sexual function after gynecologic surgery are common, particularly among younger women and women who are currently sexually active. Prospective studies suggest that sexual function is either unchanged or improves for most women after hysterectomy (Dedden et al., 2020; Flory et al., 2006; Radosa et al., 2014; Rhodes et al., 1999). Similarly, after pelvic organ prolapse repair, sexual function tends to improve, and de novo sexual pain appears uncommon (Lukacz et al., 2016). However, a small proportion of women have poorer sexual function following hysterectomy, and risk factors for poorer sexual adjustment include preexisting sexual problems (Dedden et al., 2020; Rhodes et al., 1999) and depression before hysterectomy (Rhodes et al., 1999).

The quality of the partner relationship is also an important but often overlooked factor in predicting sexual adjustment after hysterectomy (Helström et al., 1995; Rhodes et al., 1999; Zobbe et al., 2004) and should be assessed. Validated self-report instruments, such as the Female Sexual Function Index (Rosen et al., 2000) and the PROMIS Sexual Function and Satisfaction Brief Profile (Flynn et al., 2013), measure sexual function in multiple domains (e.g., sexual desire, orgasmic function, sexual pain).

The influence of BSO on sexual function is somewhat controversial. Prospective studies do not necessarily reveal an effect of BSO (vs. ovarian preservation) on sexual outcomes in the short term (Farquhar et al., 2006; Teplin et al., 2007). However, risk-reducing BSO, especially in premenopausal women, is associated with reduced pleasure and greater discomfort with sexual activity compared to presurgical levels (Hall et al., 2019). In women at high risk for ovarian cancer, those who opt for risk-reducing BSO report poorer sexual function after 1 year compared with those who opt for screening only (Mai et al., 2020). Vaginal dryness and vulvovaginal atrophy resulting from the loss of ovarian estrogens lead to discomfort during sexual activity and are prevalent in both surgically and naturally menopausal women. However, relationship satisfaction also influences sexual adjustment after risk-reducing BSO and is a stronger predictor of continuing regular sexual activity than depression or anxiety symptoms (Lorenz et al., 2014). Women at risk for sexual problems after risk-reducing BSO may benefit from a multidisciplinary approach that includes psychoeducational, behavioral, and hormonal interventions.

The effects of radical hysterectomy and other invasive procedures for gynecologic cancer are difficult to separate from the effects of cancer itself and from the effects of additional treatments, such as chemotherapy, radiation, and endocrine therapy. Hypothetically, radical hysterectomy also has a greater potential to cause damage to nerves and blood vessels that regulate sexual response. However, studies of sexual adjustment suggest that a large proportion of women eventually return to near-baseline levels of sexual function after undergoing radical hysterectomy (Frumovitz et al., 2005; Jongpipan & Charoenkwan, 2007), and outcomes are comparable to those of simple hysterectomy (Plotti et al., 2011). Alternative treatment options, such as radiation therapy, have been associated with comparatively more long-term problems with sexual dysfunction (Frumovitz et al., 2005; Greimel et al., 2009; Jensen et al., 2003).

In the presurgical setting, women can be counseled on how different treatment approaches can potentially affect sexual function. This is also an opportunity to share potential treatments and resources (e.g., Bober et al., 2018; see also Brotto et al., 2010). PPA of sexual function in candidates for radical pelvic surgery should include a discussion of expectations for vaginal reconstruction and significant changes in the body's appearance and function.

Fertility-Related Distress

Treatment-related infertility appears to have a long-term effect on emotional well-being and quality of life in women treated for gynecologic diseases. In a prospective study of more than 1,000 premenopausal women who underwent hysterectomy for benign conditions, 14% of women indicated that they might have liked or definitely would have liked to have had a child or another child at the time of their treatment. This subgroup of women tended to be younger and nulliparous at the time of hysterectomy (Leppert et al., 2007). At a 2-year follow-up, women who had expressed an interest in childbearing at the time of hysterectomy also reported more symptoms of depression and reported pelvic pain to be more of a problem than women who were not interested in further childbearing (Leppert et al.).

Women who undergo elective hysterectomy may postpone treatment because of concerns about fertility. Delayed treatment is less often a viable option for women with malignant disease. Studies of cancer survivors with treatment-related infertility suggest that distress about interrupted childbearing may persist for years after treatment and is associated with lower overall quality of life (Canada & Schover, 2012; Wenzel et al., 2005). Fertility preservation, if discussed in a timely manner, can potentially spare survivors some of the distress of permanent infertility after cancer treatment (Floyd et al., 2021). Potential roles for the psychologist/mental health professional in the oncology setting include enhancing providers' awareness of the effect of infertility on patients' quality of life, helping patients cope with actual or potential loss of fertility, and assisting patients in decision making about assisted reproduction and other alternatives for family building. Standardized self-report measures for fertility-related distress include the Fertility Quality of Life tool (Boivin et al., 2011) and, for cancer survivors, the Reproductive Concerns Scale (Wenzel et al., 2005).

FUTURE DIRECTIONS

Research has established multiple psychological risk factors that are associated with short- and long-term adjustment to gynecologic surgery. However, assessment of these risk factors in routine clinical practice is limited. Trends toward increasing behavioral health integration will present opportunities to optimize the use of psychological assessment to improve care and outcomes in this setting.

Best Practices for Screening

The literature on psychosocial outcomes of gynecologic surgery has clarified that individual psychosocial factors are often more influential than specific clinical factors (e.g., route of surgery, use of hormone replacement) in predicting postoperative psychological adjustment. However, there is very little literature to inform best practices for psychological screening and assessment of women undergoing gynecologic procedures.

The recommendations provided in this chapter reflect what is known about risk factors for poorer psychosocial adjustment after gynecologic surgery. However, screening and assessment practices vary widely across clinical care settings, and the effects of screening for these risk factors are largely unknown. Controlled trials of screening, assessment, and referral processes are needed to determine whether routine identification of psychologically vulnerable patients results in better health and quality-of-life outcomes postsurgery.

Social Inequities in Surgery and Surgery Outcomes

Minoritized social groups are inadequately represented in the gynecology literature, not only in terms of proportional representation but also in terms how they are conceptualized in research. Race and other demographic categories have been inadequate proxies for the constellation of social and environmental exposures that may underlie health inequities. For instance, Black women are disproportionately burdened by uterine fibroids, are less likely than White women to undergo minimally invasive hysterectomy (McClurg et al., 2020), and express greater interest in fertility-sparing surgery than White women (Marsh et al., 2018).

Despite broad consensus on these inequities, they remain poorly explained through existing measures and models. Emerging measures aim to improve assessment of systemic racism and other factors that contribute to health inequities (Alson et al., 2021).

CONCLUSION

Because gynecologic conditions are associated with some degree of psychiatric morbidity that is not entirely relieved by treatment, psychologists and mental health professionals have a meaningful role to play in the gynecologic care setting. Unlike psychological services in other areas of surgical practice, to date, there are few clear guidelines for early screening and assessment of gynecologic surgery patients with the greatest psychosocial needs. However, based on what is known currently, psychologists and mental health professionals nonetheless can be an asset to the surgery team by educating patients and providers about psychological risk factors and informing the team's plan for treatment and surveillance.

REFERENCES

Allaire, C., Williams, C., Bodmer-Roy, S., Zhu, S., Arion, K., Ambacher, K., Wu, J., Yosef, A., Wong, F., Noga, H., Britnell, S., Yager, H., Bedaiwy, M. A., Albert, A. Y., Lisonkova, S., & Yong, P. J. (2018). Chronic pelvic pain in an interdisciplinary setting: 1-year prospective cohort. *American Journal of Obstetrics & Gynecology, 218*(1), 114.e1–114.e12. https://doi.org/10.1016/j.ajog.2017.10.002

Alson, J. G., Robinson, W. R., Pittman, L., & Doll, K. M. (2021). Incorporating measures of structural racism into population studies of reproductive health in the United States: A narrative review. *Health Equity, 5*(1), 49–58. https://doi.org/10.1089/heq.2020.0081

Benlolo, S., Hanlon, J. G., Shirreff, L., Lefebvre, G., Husslein, H., & Shore, E. M. (2021). Predictors of persistent postsurgical pain after hysterectomy—A prospective cohort study. *Journal of Minimally Invasive Gynecology, 28*(12), 2036–2046.e1. https://doi.org/10.1016/j.jmig.2021.05.017

Bernstein, D. P., Fink, L., Handelsman, L., Foote, J., Lovejoy, M., Wenzel, K., Sapareto, E., & Ruggiero, J. (1994). Initial reliability and validity of a new retrospective measure of child abuse and neglect. *The American Journal of Psychiatry, 151*(8), 1132–1136. https://doi.org/10.1176/ajp.151.8.1132

Billioux, A., Verlander, K., Anthony, S., & Alley, D. (2017). *Standardized screening for health-related social needs in clinical settings: The Accountable Health Communities Screening Tool* [Discussion paper]. National Academy of Medicine. https://doi.org/10.31478/201705b

Bober, S. L., Recklitis, C. J., Michaud, A. L., & Wright, A. A. (2018). Improvement in sexual function after ovarian cancer: Effects of sexual therapy and rehabilitation after treatment for ovarian cancer. *Cancer*, *124*(1), 176–182. https://doi.org/10.1002/cncr.30976

Boivin, J., Takefman, J., & Braverman, A. (2011). The Fertility Quality of Life (FertiQoL) tool: Development and general psychometric properties. *Fertility and Sterility*, *96*(2), 409–415.e3. https://doi.org/10.1016/j.fertnstert.2011.02.046

Brandsborg, B., Dueholm, M., Nikolajsen, L., Kehlet, H., & Jensen, T. S. (2009). A prospective study of risk factors for pain persisting 4 months after hysterectomy. *The Clinical Journal of Pain*, *25*(4), 263–268. https://doi.org/10.1097/AJP.0b013e31819655ca

Brandsborg, B., Nikolajsen, L., Hansen, C. T., Kehlet, H., & Jensen, T. S. (2007). Risk factors for chronic pain after hysterectomy: A nationwide questionnaire and database study. *Anesthesiology*, *106*(5), 1003–1012. https://doi.org/10.1097/01.anes.0000265161.39932.e8

Brawn, J., Morotti, M., Zondervan, K. T., Becker, C. M., & Vincent, K. (2014). Central changes associated with chronic pelvic pain and endometriosis. *Human Reproduction Update*, *20*(5), 737–747. https://doi.org/10.1093/humupd/dmu025

Brotto, L. A., Yule, M., & Breckon, E. (2010). Psychological interventions for the sexual sequelae of cancer: A review of the literature. *Journal of Cancer Survivorship: Research and Practice*, *4*(4), 346–360. https://doi.org/10.1007/s11764-010-0132-z

Canada, A. L., & Schover, L. R. (2012). The psychosocial impact of interrupted childbearing in long-term female cancer survivors. *Psycho-Oncology*, *21*(2), 134–143. https://doi.org/10.1002/pon.1875

Carey, E. T., Moore, K. J., Young, J. C., Bhattacharya, M., Schiff, L. D., Louie, M. Y., Park, J., & Strassle, P. D. (2021). Association of preoperative depression and anxiety with long-term opioid use after hysterectomy for benign indications. *Obstetrics & Gynecology*, *138*(5), 715–724. https://doi.org/10.1097/AOG.0000000000004568

Carter, J., Rowland, K., Chi, D., Brown, C., Abu-Rustum, N., Castiel, M., & Barakat, R. (2005). Gynecologic cancer treatment and the impact of cancer-related infertility. *Gynecologic Oncology*, *97*(1), 90–95. https://doi.org/10.1016/j.ygyno.2004.12.019

Cella, D., Yount, S., Rothrock, N., Gershon, R., Cook, K., Reeve, B., Ader, D., Fries, J. F., Bruce, B., & Rose, M. (2007). The Patient-Reported Outcomes Measurement Information System (PROMIS): Progress of an NIH roadmap cooperative group during its first two years. *Medical Care*, *45*(5, Suppl. 1), S3–S11. https://doi.org/10.1097/01.mlr.0000258615.42478.55

Chiuve, S. E., Huisingh, C., Petruski-Ivleva, N., Owens, C., Kuohung, W., & Wise, L. A. (2022). Uterine fibroids and incidence of depression, anxiety and self-directed violence: A cohort study. *Journal of Epidemiology and Community Health*, *76*(1), 92–99. https://doi.org/10.1136/jech-2020-214565

Choi, H. G., Rhim, C. C., Yoon, J. Y., & Lee, S. W. (2020). Association between hysterectomy and depression: A longitudinal follow-up study using a national sample cohort. *Menopause*, *27*(5), 543–549. https://doi.org/10.1097/GME.0000000000001505

Chou, P.-H., Lin, C.-H., Cheng, C., Chang, C.-L., Tsai, C.-J., Tsai, C.-P., Lan, T. H., & Chan, C.-H. (2015). Risk of depressive disorders in women undergoing hysterectomy: A population-based follow-up study. *Journal of Psychiatric Research*, *68*, 186–191. https://doi.org/10.1016/j.jpsychires.2015.06.017

Cichowski, S. B., Rogers, R. G., Clark, E. A., Murata, E., Murata, A., & Murata, G. (2017). Military sexual trauma in female veterans is associated with chronic pain conditions. *Military Medicine*, *182*(9), e1895–e1899. https://doi.org/10.7205/MILMED-D-16-00393

Cleeland, C. S., & Ryan, K. M. (1994). Pain assessment: Global use of the Brief Pain Inventory. *Annals of the Academy of Medicine, Singapore*, *23*(2), 129–138.

Cohen, S. L., Vitonis, A. F., & Einarsson, J. I. (2014). Updated hysterectomy surveillance and factors associated with minimally invasive hysterectomy. *Journal of The Society of Laparoscopic & Robotic Surgeons*, *18*(3), Article e2014.00096. https://doi.org/10.4293%2FJSLS.2014.00096

Darnall, B. D., Ziadni, M. S., Krishnamurthy, P., Flood, P., Heathcote, L. C., Mackey, I. G., Taub, C. J., & Wheeler, A. (2019). "My surgical success": Effect of a digital behavioral pain medicine intervention on time to opioid cessation after breast cancer surgery—A pilot randomized controlled clinical trial. *Pain Medicine*, *20*(11), 2228–2237. https://doi.org/10.1093/pm/pnz094

Dedden, S. J., van Ditshuizen, M. A. E., Theunissen, M., & Maas, J. W. M. (2020). Hysterectomy and sexual (dys)function: An analysis of sexual dysfunction after hysterectomy and a search for predictive factors. *European Journal of Obstetrics & Gynecology and Reproductive Biology*, *247*, 80–84. https://doi.org/10.1016/j.ejogrb.2020.01.047

Estes, S. J., Huisingh, C. E., Chiuve, S. E., Petruski-Ivleva, N., & Missmer, S. A. (2021). Depression, anxiety, and self-directed violence in women with endometriosis: A retrospective matched-cohort study. *American Journal of Epidemiology*, *190*(5), 843–852. https://doi.org/10.1093/aje/kwaa249

Evans, E. C., Matteson, K. A., Orejuela, F. J., Alperin, M., Balk, E. M., El-Nashar, S., Gleason, J. L., Grimes, C., Jeppson, P., Mathews, C., Wheeler, T. L., Murphy, M., & the Society of Gynecologic Surgeons Systematic Review Group. (2016). Salpingo-oophorectomy at the time of benign hysterectomy: A systematic review. *Obstetrics & Gynecology*, *128*(3), 476–485. https://doi.org/10.1097/AOG.0000000000001592

Farquhar, C. M., Harvey, S. A., Yu, Y., Sadler, L., & Stewart, A. W. (2006). A prospective study of 3 years of outcomes after hysterectomy with and without oophorectomy. *American Journal of Obstetrics & Gynecology*, *194*(3), 711–717. https://doi.org/10.1016/j.ajog.2005.08.066

Flory, N., Bissonnette, F., Amsel, R. T., & Binik, Y. M. (2006). The psychosocial outcomes of total and subtotal hysterectomy: A randomized controlled trial. *The Journal of Sexual Medicine*, *3*(3), 483–491. https://doi.org/10.1111/j.1743-6109.2006.00229.x

Floyd, J. L., Campbell, S., Rauh-Hain, J. A., & Woodard, T. (2021). Fertility preservation in women with early-stage gynecologic cancer: Optimizing oncologic and reproductive outcomes. *International Journal of Gynecological Cancer*, *31*(3), 345–351. https://doi.org/10.1136/ijgc-2020-001328

Flynn, K. E., Lin, L., Cyranowski, J. M., Reeve, B. B., Reese, J. B., Jeffery, D. D., Smith, A. W., Porter, L. S., Dombeck, C. B., Bruner, D. W., Keefe, F. J., & Weinfurt, K. P. (2013). Development of the NIH PROMIS® Sexual Function and Satisfaction measures in patients with cancer. *The Journal of Sexual Medicine, 10*(Suppl. 1), 43–52. https://doi.org/10.1111/j.1743-6109.2012.02995.x

Frumovitz, M., Sun, C. C., Schover, L. R., Munsell, M. F., Jhingran, A., Wharton, J. T., Eifel, P., Bevers, T. B., Levenback, C. F., Gershenson, D. M., & Bodurka, D. C. (2005). Quality of life and sexual functioning in cervical cancer survivors. *Journal of Clinical Oncology, 23*(30), 7428–7436. https://doi.org/10.1200/JCO.2004.00.3996

Fuentes, I. M., & Christianson, J. A. (2018). The influence of early life experience on visceral pain. *Frontiers in Systems Neuroscience, 12*, Article 2. https://doi.org/10.3389/fnsys.2018.00002

Green, B. L. (1996). Psychometric review of Trauma History Questionnaire (self-report). In B. H. Stamm (Ed.), *Measurement of stress, trauma, and adaptation* (pp. 366–369). The Sidran Press.

Greimel, E. R., Winter, R., Kapp, K. S., & Haas, J. (2009). Quality of life and sexual functioning after cervical cancer treatment: A long-term follow-up study. *Psycho-Oncology, 18*(5), 476–482. https://doi.org/10.1002/pon.1426

Günther, V., Malchow, B., Schubert, M., Andresen, L., Jochens, A., Jonat, W., Mundhenke, C., & Alkatout, I. (2014). Impact of radical operative treatment on the quality of life in women with vulvar cancer—A retrospective study. *European Journal of Surgical Oncology, 40*(7), 875–882. https://doi.org/10.1016/j.ejso.2014.03.027

Hall, E., Finch, A., Jacobson, M., Rosen, B., Metcalfe, K., Sun, P., Narod, S. A., & Kotsopoulos, J. (2019). Effects of bilateral salpingo-oophorectomy on menopausal symptoms and sexual functioning among women with a *BRCA1* or *BRCA2* mutation. *Gynecologic Oncology, 152*(1), 145–150. https://doi.org/10.1016/j.ygyno.2018.10.040

Hanley, G. E., Pearce, C. L., Talhouk, A., Kwon, J. S., Finlayson, S. J., McAlpine, J. N., Huntsman, D. G., & Miller, D. (2022). Outcomes from opportunistic salpingectomy for ovarian cancer prevention. *JAMA Network Open, 5*(2), Article e2147343. https://doi.org/10.1001/jamanetworkopen.2021.47343

Harji, D. P., Griffiths, B., Velikova, G., Sagar, P. M., & Brown, J. (2016). Systematic review of health-related quality of life in patients undergoing pelvic exenteration. *European Journal of Surgical Oncology, 42*(8), 1132–1145. https://doi.org/10.1016/j.ejso.2016.01.007

Heim, C., Ehlert, U., Hanker, J. P., & Hellhammer, D. H. (1998). Abuse-related posttraumatic stress disorder and alterations of the hypothalamic–pituitary–adrenal axis in women with chronic pelvic pain. *Psychosomatic Medicine, 60*(3), 309–318. https://doi.org/10.1097/00006842-199805000-00017

Helström, L., Sörbom, D., & Bäckström, T. (1995). Influence of partner relationship on sexuality after subtotal hysterectomy. *Acta Obstetricia et Gynecologica Scandinavica, 74*(2), 142–146. https://doi.org/10.3109/00016349509008924

Hillis, S. D., Marchbanks, P. A., & Peterson, H. B. (1995). The effectiveness of hysterectomy for chronic pelvic pain. *Obstetrics & Gynecology, 86*(6), 941–945. https://doi.org/10.1016/0029-7844(95)00304-A

Humalajärvi, N., Aukee, P., Kairaluoma, M. V., Stach-Lempinen, B., Stinonen, H., Valpas, A., & Heinonen, P. K. (2014). Quality of life and pelvic floor dysfunction symptoms after hysterectomy with or without pelvic organ prolapse. *European Journal of Obstetrics & Gynecology and Reproductive Biology, 182*, 16–21. https://doi.org/10.1016/j.ejogrb.2014.08.032

Janda, M., Obermair, A., Cella, D., Crandon, A. J., & Trimmel, M. (2004). Vulvar cancer patients' quality of life: A qualitative assessment. *International Journal of Gynecological Cancer*, *14*(5), 875–881. https://doi.org/10.1136/ijgc-00009577-200409000-00021

Järvholm, S., Warren, A. M., Jalmbrant, M., Kvarnström, N., Testa, G., & Johannesson, L. (2018). Preoperative psychological evaluation of uterus transplant recipients, partners, and living donors: Suggested framework. *American Journal of Transplantation*, *18*(11), 2641–2646. https://doi.org/10.1111/ajt.15039

Jensen, P. T., Groenvold, M., Klee, M. C., Thranov, I., Petersen, M. A., & Machin, D. (2003). Longitudinal study of sexual function and vaginal changes after radiotherapy for cervical cancer. *International Journal of Radiation Oncology, Biology, Physics*, *56*(4), 937–949. https://doi.org/10.1016/S0360-3016(03)00362-6

Jongpipan, J., & Charoenkwan, K. (2007). Sexual function after radical hysterectomy for early-stage cervical cancer. *The Journal of Sexual Medicine*, *4*(6), 1659–1665. https://doi.org/10.1111/j.1743-6109.2007.00454.x

Kingsberg, S. A., Larkin, L. C., & Liu, J. H. (2020). Clinical effects of early or surgical menopause. *Obstetrics & Gynecology*, *135*(4), 853–868. https://doi.org/10.1097/AOG.0000000000003729

Kroenke, K., & Spitzer, R. L. (2002). The PHQ-9: A new depression diagnostic and severity measure. *Psychiatric Annals*, *32*(9), 509–515. https://doi.org/10.3928/0048-5713-20020901-06

Kroenke, K., Spitzer, R. L., & Williams, J. B. W. (2002). The PHQ-15: Validity of a new measure for evaluating the severity of somatic symptoms. *Psychosomatic Medicine*, *64*(2), 258–266. https://doi.org/10.1097/00006842-200203000-00008

Latthe, P., Mignini, L., Gray, R., Hills, R., & Khan, K. (2006). Factors predisposing women to chronic pelvic pain: Systematic review. *BMJ*, *332*(7544), 749–755. https://doi.org/10.1136/bmj.38748.697465.55

Learman, L. A., Gregorich, S. E., Schembri, M., Jacoby, A., Jackson, R. A., & Kuppermann, M. (2011). Symptom resolution after hysterectomy and alternative treatments for chronic pelvic pain: Does depression make a difference? *American Journal of Obstetrics & Gynecology*, *204*(3), 269.e1–269.e9. https://doi.org/10.1016/j.ajog.2010.12.051

Leithner, K., Assem-Hilger, E., Fischer-Kern, M., Loeffler-Stastka, H., Sam, C., & Ponocny-Seliger, E. (2009). Psychiatric morbidity in gynecological and otorhinolaryngological outpatients: A comparative study. *General Hospital Psychiatry*, *31*(3), 233–239. https://doi.org/10.1016/j.genhosppsych.2008.12.007

Leppert, P. C., Legro, R. S., & Kjerulff, K. H. (2007). Hysterectomy and loss of fertility: Implications for women's mental health. *Journal of Psychosomatic Research*, *63*(3), 269–274. https://doi.org/10.1016/j.jpsychores.2007.03.018

Likes, W. M., Stegbauer, C., Tillmanns, T., & Pruett, J. (2007). Correlates of sexual function following vulvar excision. *Gynecologic Oncology*, *105*(3), 600–603. https://doi.org/10.1016/j.ygyno.2007.01.027

Lorenz, T., McGregor, B., & Swisher, E. (2014). Relationship satisfaction predicts sexual activity following risk-reducing salpingo-oophorectomy. *Journal of Psychosomatic Obstetrics & Gynecology*, *35*(2), 62–68. https://doi.org/10.3109/0167482X.2014.899577

Lukacz, E. S., Warren, L. K., Richter, H. E., Brubaker, L., Barber, M. D., Norton, P., Weidner, A. C., Nguyen, J. N., & Gantz, M. G. (2016). Quality of life and sexual function 2 years after vaginal surgery for prolapse. *Obstetrics & Gynecology, 127*(6), 1071–1079. https://doi.org/10.1097/AOG.0000000000001442

Lunde, S., Petersen, K. K., Søgaard-Andersen, E., & Arendt-Nielsen, L. (2020). Preoperative quantitative sensory testing and robot-assisted laparoscopic hysterectomy for endometrial cancer: Can chronic postoperative pain be predicted? *Scandinavian Journal of Pain, 20*(4), 693–705. https://doi.org/10.1515/sjpain-2020-0030

Madalinska, J. B., Hollenstein, J., Bleiker, E., van Beurden, M., Valdimarsdottir, H. B., Massuger, L. F., Gaarenstroom, K. N., Mourits, M. J. E., Verheijen, R. H. M., van Dorst, E. B. K., van der Putten, H., van der Velden, K., Boonstra, H., & Aaronson, N. K. (2005). Quality-of-life effects of prophylactic salpingo-oophorectomy versus gynecologic screening among women at increased risk of hereditary ovarian cancer. *Journal of Clinical Oncology, 23*(28), 6890–6898. https://doi.org/10.1200/JCO.2005.02.626

Mai, P. L., Huang, H. Q., Wenzel, L. B., Han, P. K., Moser, R. P., Rodriguez, G. C., Boggess, J., Rutherford, T. J., Cohn, D. E., Kauff, N. D., Phillips, K.-A., Wilkinson, K., Wenham, R. M., Hamilton, C., Powell, M. A., Walker, J. L., Greene, M. H., & Hensley, M. L. (2020). Prospective follow-up of quality of life for participants undergoing risk-reducing salpingo-oophorectomy or ovarian cancer screening in GOG-0199: An NRG Oncology/GOG study. *Gynecologic Oncology, 156*(1), 131–139. https://doi.org/10.1016/j.ygyno.2019.10.026

Marsh, E. E., Al-Hendy, A., Kappus, D., Galitsky, A., Stewart, E. A., & Kerolous, M. (2018). Burden, prevalence, and treatment of uterine fibroids: A survey of U.S. women. *Journal of Women's Health, 27*(11), 1359–1367. https://doi.org/10.1089/jwh.2018.7076

McClurg, A., Wong, J., & Louie, M. (2020). The impact of race on hysterectomy for benign indications. *Current Opinion in Obstetrics & Gynecology, 32*(4), 263–268. https://doi.org/10.1097/GCO.0000000000000633

Melzack, R. (1975). The McGill Pain Questionnaire: Major properties and scoring methods. *Pain, 1*(3), 277–299. https://doi.org/10.1016/0304-3959(75)90044-5

Nguyen, N. T., Merchant, M., Ritterman Weintraub, M. L., Salyer, C., Poceta, J., Diaz, L., & Zaritsky, E. F. (2019). Alternative treatment utilization before hysterectomy for benign gynecologic conditions at a large integrated health system. *Journal of Minimally Invasive Gynecology, 26*(5), 847–855.

Nnoaham, K. E., Hummelshoj, L., Webster, P., d'Hooghe, T., de Cicco Nardone, F., de Cicco Nardone, C., Jenkinson, C., Kennedy, S. H., Zondervan, K. T., & the World Endometriosis Research Foundation Global Study of Women's Health Consortium. (2011). Impact of endometriosis on quality of life and work productivity: A multicenter study across ten countries. *Fertility and Sterility, 96*(2), 366–373.e8. https://doi.org/10.1016/j.fertnstert.2011.05.090

Ortiz, R., Gemmill, J. A. L., Sinaii, N., Stegmann, B., Khachikyan, I., Chrousos, G., Segars, J., & Stratton, P. (2020). Hypothalamic–pituitary–adrenal axis responses in women with endometriosis-related chronic pelvic pain. *Reproductive Sciences, 27*(10), 1839–1847. https://doi.org/10.1007/s43032-020-00201-x

Persson, P., Brynhildsen, J., Kjølhede, P., & the Hysterectomy Multicentre Study Group in South-East Sweden. (2010). A 1-year follow up of psychological wellbeing after subtotal and total hysterectomy—A randomised study. *BJOG, 117*(4), 479–487. https://doi.org/10.1111/j.1471-0528.2009.02467.x

Pinto, P. R., McIntyre, T., Araújo-Soares, V., Almeida, A., & Costa, P. (2018). Psychological factors predict an unfavorable pain trajectory after hysterectomy: A prospective cohort study on chronic postsurgical pain. *Pain*, *159*(5), 956–967. https://doi.org/10.1097/j.pain.0000000000001170

Plotti, F., Sansone, M., Di Donato, V., Antonelli, E., Altavilla, T., Angioli, R., & Panici, P. B. (2011). Quality of life and sexual function after type c2/type III radical hysterectomy for locally advanced cervical cancer: A prospective study. *The Journal of Sexual Medicine*, *8*(3), 894–904. https://doi.org/10.1111/j.1743-6109.2010.02133.x

Pokkinen, S. M., Nieminen, K., Yli-Hankala, A., & Kalliomäki, M. L. (2015). Persistent posthysterectomy pain: A prospective, observational study. *European Journal of Anaesthesiology*, *32*(10), 718–724. https://doi.org/10.1097/EJA.0000000000000318

Portnoy, G. A., Haskell, S. G., King, M. W., Maskin, R., Gerber, M. R., & Iverson, K. M. (2018). Accuracy and acceptability of a screening tool for identifying intimate partner violence perpetration among women veterans: A pre-implementation evaluation. *Women's Health Issues*, *28*(5), 439–445. https://doi.org/10.1016/j.whi.2018.04.003

Pynnä, K., Räsänen, P., Sintonen, H., Roine, R. P., & Vuorela, P. (2021). The health-related quality of life of patients with a benign gynecological condition: A 2-year follow-up. *Journal of Comparative Effectiveness Research*, *10*(8), 685–695. https://doi.org/10.2217/cer-2020-0243

Radosa, J. C., Meyberg-Solomayer, G., Kastl, C., Radosa, C. G., Mavrova, R., Gräber, S., Baum, S., & Radosa, M. P. (2014). Influences of different hysterectomy techniques on patients' postoperative sexual function and quality of life. *The Journal of Sexual Medicine*, *11*(9), 2342–2350. https://doi.org/10.1111/jsm.12623

Rhodes, J. C., Kjerulff, K. H., Langenberg, P. W., & Guzinski, G. M. (1999). Hysterectomy and sexual functioning. *JAMA*, *282*(20), 1934–1941. https://doi.org/10.1001/jama.282.20.1934

Ricci, S., Bennett, C., & Falcone, T. (2021). Uterine transplantation: Evolving data, success, and clinical importance. *Journal of Minimally Invasive Gynecology*, *28*(3), 502–512. https://doi.org/10.1016/j.jmig.2020.12.015

Rosen, R., Brown, C., Heiman, J., Leiblum, S., Meston, C., Shabsigh, R., Ferguson, D., & D'Agostino, R., Jr. (2000). The Female Sexual Function Index (FSFI): A multidimensional self-report instrument for the assessment of female sexual function. *Journal of Sex & Marital Therapy*, *26*(2), 191–208. https://doi.org/10.1080/009262300278597

Schalet, B. D., Pilkonis, P. A., Yu, L., Dodds, N., Johnston, K. L., Yount, S., Riley, W., & Cella, D. (2016). Clinical validity of PROMIS Depression, Anxiety, and Anger across diverse clinical samples. *Journal of Clinical Epidemiology*, *73*, 119–127. https://doi.org/10.1016/j.jclinepi.2015.08.036

Spitzer, R. L., Kroenke, K., Williams, J. B. W., & Löwe, B. (2006). A brief measure for assessing generalized anxiety disorder: The GAD-7. *Archives of Internal Medicine*, *166*(10), 1092–1097. https://doi.org/10.1001/archinte.166.10.1092

Sullivan, M. J. L., Bishop, S. R., & Pivik, J. (1995). The Pain Catastrophizing Scale: Development and validation. *Psychological Assessment*, *7*(4), 524–532. https://doi.org/10.1037/1040-3590.7.4.524

Tay, S. K., & Bromwich, N. (1998). Outcome of hysterectomy for pelvic pain in premenopausal women. *Australian and New Zealand Journal of Obstetrics and Gynaecology, 38*(1), 72–76. https://doi.org/10.1111/j.1479-828X.1998.tb02963.x

Teplin, V., Vittinghoff, E., Lin, F., Learman, L. A., Richter, H. E., & Kuppermann, M. (2007). Oophorectomy in premenopausal women: Health-related quality of life and sexual functioning. *Obstetrics & Gynecology, 109*(2, Pt. 1), 347–354. https://doi.org/10.1097/01.AOG.0000252700.03133.8b

Theunissen, M., Peters, M. L., Schepers, J., Schoot, D. C., Gramke, H.-F., & Marcus, M. A. (2017). Prevalence and predictors of depression and well-being after hysterectomy: An observational study. *European Journal of Obstetrics & Gynecology and Reproductive Biology, 217*, 94–100. https://doi.org/10.1016/j.ejogrb.2017.08.017

Vandyk, A. D., Brenner, I., Tranmer, J., & Van Den Kerkhof, E. (2011). Depressive symptoms before and after elective hysterectomy. *Journal of Obstetric, Gynecologic, & Neonatal Nursing, 40*(5), 566–576. https://doi.org/10.1111/j.1552-6909.2011.01278.x

Wenzel, L., Dogan-Ates, A., Habbal, R., Berkowitz, R., Goldstein, D. P., Bernstein, M., Kluhsman, B. C., Osann, K., Newlands, E., Seckl, M. J., Hancock, B., & Cella, D. (2005). Defining and measuring reproductive concerns of female cancer survivors. *JNCI Monographs, 2005*(34), 94–98. https://doi.org/10.1093/jncimonographs/lgi017

Yen, J.-Y., Chen, Y.-H., Long, C.-Y., Chang, Y., Yen, C.-F., Chen, C.-C., & Ko, C.-H. (2008). Risk factors for major depressive disorder and the psychological impact of hysterectomy: A prospective investigation. *Psychosomatics, 49*(2), 137–142. https://doi.org/10.1176/appi.psy.49.2.137

Zigmond, A. S., & Snaith, R. P. (1983). The Hospital Anxiety and Depression Scale. *Acta Psychiatrica Scandinavica, 67*(6), 361–370. https://doi.org/10.1111/j.1600-0447.1983.tb09716.x

Zobbe, V., Gimbel, H., Andersen, B. M., Filtenborg, T., Jakobsen, K., Sørensen, H. C., Toftager-Larsen, K., Sidenius, K., Møller, N., Madsen, E. M., Vejtorp, M., Clausen, H., Rosgaard, A., Gluud, C., Ottesen, B. S., & Tabor, A. (2004). Sexuality after total vs. subtotal hysterectomy. *Acta Obstetricia et Gynecologica Scandinavica, 83*(2), 191–196. https://doi.org/10.1111/j.0001-6349.2004.00311.x

11 SURGICAL TREATMENT OF TEMPORAL LOBE EPILEPSY

GENEVIEVE RAYNER, HONOR COLEMAN, EMILY COCKLE, ANDREW NEAL, AND CHARLES MALPAS

For the 30% of people with temporal lobe epilepsy (TLE) whose seizures cannot be controlled with medication, a well-established neurosurgical procedure known as anterior temporal lobectomy (ATL) renders approximately 70% of these patients seizure free (Barba et al., 2021; Wiebe et al., 2001). Epilepsy surgery, however, is not without cognitive and psychological risks that require careful assessment and management as part of routine multidisciplinary care.

A core part of the presurgical workup is systematic clinical and psychometric neuropsychological examination (Baxendale et al., 2019). Its chief purpose is to assess what the cognitive risks of a proposed resection might be; for people with TLE, these risks commonly take the form of memory and language deficits. The findings inform presurgical patient counseling so that the patient can decide whether any cognitive risks of the intervention outweigh the potential health and lifestyle benefits of being seizure free.

In parallel, careful psychiatric and psychological examination before epilepsy surgery informs counseling sessions that aim to best prepare people with TLE and their families to adapt to the life that typically accompanies ATL.

https://doi.org/10.1037/0000346-012
Psychological Assessment of Surgical Candidates: Evidence-Based Procedures and Practices, R. J. Marek and A. R. Block (Editors)

For many patients, the newfound seizure freedom often conferred by epilepsy surgery represents the first time in many years that their lives are no longer limited by a chronic illness. Although many individuals relish this opportunity to pursue a "normal" life, others can struggle to shrug off the sick role (S. J. Wilson et al., 2007). This chapter covers psychological assessment techniques for navigating this major life transition with adult patients.

SURGICAL TREATMENTS FOR TLE

Epilepsy is a noncommunicable neurological disease affecting more than 50 million people worldwide, making it one of the most common and burdensome neurological diseases globally (World Health Organization, 2022). It is characterized by paroxysmal and recurrent seizures, which are caused by hypersynchronous electrical activity spreading along well-organized brain networks. *Focal seizures* are defined as originating within networks limited to one hemisphere of the brain and can be either discretely localized, more widely distributed, or multifocal (Fisher et al., 2017).

TLE is the most common type of focal epilepsy (Semah et al., 1998). It is defined by seizures arising from a temporal lobe network, regardless of etiology. Various subtypes of TLE have been described depending on the location of the *epileptogenic zone* (EZ), which is defined as the region of the brain from which the patient's seizures are thought to generate from. One subtype is *mesial TLE*, which typically involves the hippocampus, amygdala, and rhinal cortex. The *lateral TLE* subtype involves any part of outer cortical structures from the basal temporal region to Wernicke's area. And *temporal pole epilepsy* or *anterior TLE* broadly refers to the mesial, polar, and lateral structures in the anterior part of the temporal lobe. The normal organization of cognitive networks can be disrupted in TLE and indexed using functional magnetic resonance imaging (fMRI). This has contributed to the contemporary view that seizures propagate along established neurocognitive pathways, with cognitive dysfunction providing a marker of the underlying seizure network in epilepsy (Rayner & Tailby, 2017); commonly in TLE, this is memory or language dysfunction.

Hippocampal sclerosis (i.e., scarring of the hippocampus) is the most frequent histopathology encountered in people with TLE, found in between 25% and 70% of cases (Blümcke et al., 2013), but other lesion types in TLE include focal cortical dysplasia, dysembryoplastic neuroepithelial tumor, and encephalocele. Around 20% to 30% of individuals with TLE have no lesion resolvable on current magnetic resonance imaging (MRI) technologies (Muhlhofer et al., 2017).

Psychologists and mental health professionals in the epilepsy team can often have more overt input around the surgical approach than is typically seen in the other surgical contexts outlined in this book. Findings from the neuropsychological assessments can provide the team with confirming (or disconfirming) data in terms of the likely location of the epilepsy surgery site, and they also can provide opinion around what the extent of the surgical resection should be to balance the likelihood of seizure freedom against the likelihood of poor cognitive outcomes.

Presurgical Epileptological Evaluation

The goal of the presurgical evaluation is to formulate an accurate hypothesis of the EZ and determine the risks and benefits of its resection—that is, which brain region is primarily responsible for generating seizures and what deficits can be expected from a resection of this area. Most comprehensive epilepsy centers take a multimodal approach to the surgical evaluation, which encompasses clinical, electroencephalography (EEG), neuroimaging, and neuropsychological assessments.

Patients should be assessed for surgery when at least two appropriate antiseizure medications cannot control their seizures (i.e., meeting criteria for drug resistant epilepsy; Kwan et al., 2011). All patients undergo at least a week of inpatient video-EEG monitoring to record seizures and examine the clinical and electrographic pattern of the seizure. The collection of clinical signs and symptoms produced during a seizure are known as the *semiology*, which is the dynamic clinical expression of the seizure and can be used to localize the epileptic network. It is the result of changes to network dynamics as the seizure propagates through both physiological and pathological brain networks (McGonigal et al., 2021). For instance, mesial TLE commonly begins with an aura of déjà vu or an epigastric viscerosensory sensation that the patient can describe before losing awareness. In contrast, lateral TLE with seizures arising from the posterior superior temporal gyrus can begin with auditory hallucinations and vertigo (Barba et al., 2016).

By combining semiological and EEG information, anatomical electro-clinical correlations are used to formulate hypotheses of the EZ. These hypotheses are modified by neuroimaging, including MRI or positron emission tomography; the neuropsychological evaluation; and a variety of additional assessments, such as magnetoencephalography; ictal single-photon emission computed tomography; fMRI; EEG recorded simultaneously with fMRI (EEG–fMRI); and intracranial EEG. The decision to proceed with resective surgery is most straightforward when there is an epileptogenic lesion on

MRI that is situated in parts of the brain that do not directly control function and whose removal will not result in major neurological or neurocognitive impairment. In contrast, EZs that are located in eloquent cortex that *does* control important function require extremely close multidisciplinary consideration to avoid leaving the patient physically or cognitively disabled after surgery; these include regions such as the left mesial temporal lobe (verbal memory), Broca's area (speech), and motor cortices (movement). Other factors are key determinants in whether someone is considered for epilepsy surgery, however, including the team's confidence in localizing a nonlesional epilepsy as well as the severity of the seizure disorder, its refractoriness to other treatment options, and its effect on the patient's quality of life.

Anterior Temporal Lobectomy

The most common surgical treatment for anterior TLE is the ATL. Measuring from the most anterior point of the middle cranial fossa, ATL typically comprises resection of 6.0 cm to 7.0 cm of the anterior lateral nondominant temporal lobe, or 4.0 cm to 4.5 cm of the language dominant temporal lobe (sparing the language-crucial superior temporal gyrus). The mesial resection is maximized based on what is safety feasible and typically includes the amygdala and, at a minimum, the anterior 1.0 cm to 3.0 cm of the hippocampus (most commonly, 4.0 cm) together with the parahippocampal gyrus (Wiebe et al., 2001).

In the landmark Class 1 randomized clinical trial of the procedure (Wiebe et al., 2001), ATL was found to be superior to ongoing medical therapy for people with drug-resistant TLE of heterogenous cause. At 1 year following randomization, 64% of patients who underwent surgery were free of focal impaired awareness seizures compared with only 8% in the medical group ($p < .001$). These findings were expanded by a later randomized clinical trial, showing that in a relatively homogenous sample of people with recent-onset mesial TLE, 85% of those who had surgery were seizure free 2 years later versus none of the patients who continued with medical therapy (Engel et al., 2012). These findings indicated that ATL was a feasible, efficacious, and relatively safe procedure.

Amygdalohippocampectomy and Other Circumscribed Resections

Advancements in neuroimaging has also seen an increased detection of more circumscribed pathologies associated with TLE, such as focal cortical dysplasia and encephalocele. These abnormalities tend to be neocortically based and can often be resected or disconnected in small, targeted procedures rather than the traditional en bloc ATL (Panov et al., 2016).

A desire to preserve ipsilateral memory function when possible also saw increased uses of more circumscribed amygdalohippocampectomies (i.e., removal of the hippocampus and amygdala) for the treatment of drug-resistant ATL. Comparisons between ATL versus selective amygdalohippocampectomy indicated that patients in the ATL group were more likely to be seizure free (Xu et al., 2020). Moreover, left lateralized ATL actually resulted in *better* memory outcomes after surgery for people with drug-resistant TLE, indicating that the selective procedure might only have cognitive advantages in right TLE (Helmstaedter et al., 2008).

Minimally Invasive Ablative Techniques

In recent years, several new, more targeted surgical treatments have been developed to ablate the EZ for the purposes of controlling seizures, including laser interstitial thermal therapy, stereotactic radiosurgery, and radio-frequency thermo-coagulation. These techniques have garnered particular interest given that they aim to surgically ablate a highly focalized EZ relative to larger ATL resections, potentially minimizing cognitive deficits by avoiding the removal of functional tissue outside of the EZ. Further research is required, however, to determine if these targeted treatments do indeed preserve neurocognitive function while also providing long-term seizure control.

HOLISTIC PRESURGICAL PSYCHOLOGICAL ASSESSMENT

Stemming from a series of TLE patients rendered catastrophically amnestic from bitemporal epilepsy surgery in the 1950s, clinical neuropsychologists figure as key players in the modern epilepsy team. Precise predictions of cognitive risk provided by neuropsychologists with expertise in epilepsy can lend support to the putative location or hemisphere of the patient's EZ and help the team and patient decide whether any potential postoperative cognitive deficits are tolerable, weighted against the possible benefits of improved seizure control (Baxendale et al., 2019).

Beyond providing crucial diagnostic opinions, the modern epilepsy psychologist/neuropsychologist also plays a central role in providing prospective patient-centered counseling and prehabilitation in the lead-up to surgery. Their aim is to ensure that the patient is making an informed decision and has appropriate psychological tools for navigating the adjustment processes inherent to epilepsy surgery (S. J. Wilson et al., 2007).

The Neurocognitive Evaluation

The presurgical neurocognitive evaluation is a broad clinical activity that includes taking a cognitive history, directly observing the patient, performing a neurobehavioral examination, and administering formal psychometric tests. The aims of the neurocognitive evaluation are to

- produce a coherent formulation of the patient's cognitive status and
- offer cognitive prognostication under different surgical scenarios.

The guiding principle of cognitive prognostication is one of "congruence" among (a) the specific cognitive impairments identified, (b) the presumed epileptic lesion, and (c) the extent and nature of the planned surgical intervention (Saling & Wilson, 2011). The risk of persistent postsurgical cognitive impairment is lowest when the observed impairments are congruent with the presumed lesion location and the planned surgical margins. As described later in the section Formal Psychometric Examination, in TLE, these impairments typically include verbal memory encoding disorders and dysnomias commensurate with disease in the mesial and lateral temporal lobes. The risk of cognitive impairment is elevated when the planned surgical intervention will disrupt tissue that is still supporting functional cognitive networks. This risk is often indicated by the absence of cognitive impairment or the presence of a specific cognitive impairments that are incongruent with the location of the presumed epileptic lesion.

Neuropsychological History

As with all areas of clinical practice, time spent taking a detailed history is often more fruitful than time spent on formal examination. The neuropsychological history should cover neurodevelopmental milestones, educational attainment, occupation, psychiatric symptomatology, and medical conditions across the life span. A spontaneous cognitive complaint, if present, should be addressed first because this will often frame subsequent discussions with the patient. Care should be taken to then elicit specific details of the cognitive complaint. These details will facilitate the formation of cognitive hypotheses for later investigation. For example, a generalized spontaneous complaint of poor memory is common in patients with TLE. The elicitation of specific details will permit differentiation of primary memory impairments from secondary impairments resulting from impaired attention, language, or other cognitive functions. Taking a detailed neuropsychological history also allows the clinician to directly observe key cognitive functions, such as memory, language, processing speed, and attention. Severe impairments in these functions can often be identified at the conversational level during history taking.

As with seizures themselves, the semiology of the cognitive complaint can be particularly instructive. For example, a patient who provides a strident complaint of severe memory impairment yet can describe recent episodes of memory loss with highly specific detail is less likely to have a major memory impairment. A patient who offers little in the way of spontaneous memory complaint yet is unable to provide details of their medical and personal history and defers to a family member on questioning is at higher risk of having an underlying memory impairment. Careful consideration of the semiology of the cognitive complaint, rather than the content of complaint in isolation, has been highly profitable in other areas of neuropsychological diagnostics, such as dementia and functional cognitive disorders (Buckley et al., 2015; Poole et al., 2019).

Neurobehavioral Examination

The neurobehavioral examination involves the investigation of functions that sit between the neurological examination and the formal psychometric examination. Traditionally, this involves examining for such things as hemispatial neglect, ideomotor apraxia, impaired motor sequencing, apraxia of speech, dysarthria, dyslexia, dysgraphia, left–right disorientation, graphaesthesia, and motoric disinhibition.

Basic investigation of audition and visual acuity should also be performed because impairments in these areas can affect formal psychometric examination. Although the neurobehavioral examination is often unremarkable in patients with TLE, it is good practice to routinely examine for these impairments because doing so will occasionally reveal an unexpected finding that warrants further formal investigation.

Formal Psychometric Examination

Impairments of language and memory loom large in TLE and should therefore guide a hypothesis-driven approach to formal psychometric examination (Reyes et al., 2020). Memory has received great attention in TLE surgery, owing to rare cases of catastrophic memory impairment following respective surgery. Postresection studies led to the development of the *material-specificity hypothesis*, which postulates that verbal memory functions depend on left (dominant) hemisphere structures, whereas visuospatial memory functions depend on right (nondominant) hemisphere structures. Although elegant in its simplicity, this model assumes that verbal and nonverbal memory are unitary and homogenous constructs that are supported by independent and perfectly lateralized networks (Saling, 2009). More recently, the *task-specificity model* has emerged, which accounts for the fact that only a subset of verbal memory tasks is sensitive to lateralized pathology in TLE (Saling, 2005). Rather than separating tasks along the material-specific lines of verbal and visual information, the task-specificity model separates tasks along a spectrum of semantic-arbitrary association (Saling, 2009).

Verbal memory tasks that rely on forming associations between semantically unrelated items function as proximal neurocognitive markers of dominant mesial temporal pathology. Verbal memory tasks that rely on preexisting semantic associations are of least lateralizing specificity. The "hard" pairs from the Verbal Paired Associates test of the Wechsler Memory Scale (Wechsler, 2009) are examples of arbitrary (unrelated) verbal associative learning tasks (e.g., cabbage–pen), whereas the "easy" pairs exemplify semantic associative learning tasks (e.g., sky–cloud). Other commonly used memory tests, such as Logical Memory from the Wechsler Memory Scale (Wechsler, 2009), require the patient to remember a paragraph of narrative text. Successful performance on this task requires the use of logicosemantic associations, which minimizes dependence on arbitrary associative learning. Supraspan word list learning tasks, such as the California Verbal Learning Test (Delis et al., 2000) invoke an explicit semantic structure (via grouping of items), whereas tests such as Rey Auditory–Verbal Learning Test (Strauss et al., 2006) have an implicit semantic structure that can be imposed by examinees and observed in the order of spontaneous recall (e.g., turkey → farmer → hat; Saling & Wilson, 2011).

Taken together, the hypothesis-driven examination of memory in TLE should include measures of arbitrary associative learning, semantic associative learning, and verbal supraspan list learning. The Verbal Paired Associates subtest of the Wechsler Memory Scale (Wechsler, 2009) as well as the Rey Auditory–Verbal Learning Test (Strauss et al., 2006) serve well in this regard. In dominant hemisphere TLE, impairments in verbal arbitrary associative learning are typical, whereas normal performances are often observed on tests of verbal semantic associative learning, especially when accounting for the effects of language impairments. The examination of figural, visuospatial, or "nonverbal" memory should also be performed. The Rey Complex Figure Test (Strauss et al., 2006) delay trial is often sufficient; however, it does not allow the interrogation of learning over trials. The Brief Visuospatial Memory Test–Revised (Benedict, 1997) is a useful adjunct that includes multiple learning trials and recognition condition.

The examination of certain aspects of language function should also feature in the presurgical examination. Visual confrontation naming tests, such as the Boston Naming Test (Goodglass et al., 2001), are useful to identify impairments in word retrieval. Although patients with TLE will not usually present with a clinically apparent dysnomia, subtle impairments on visual confrontation naming are commonly observed. These are more common in TLE of the dominant hemisphere but are also observed in some nondominant hemisphere cases. Recently, auditory confrontation naming tasks have been investigated and show promising sensitivity to dominant hemisphere pathology.

Although the examination of memory and language functions form the core of the hypothesis-driven approach to presurgical diagnostics in TLE, other cognitive systems should be routinely examined. For example, it is important to examine for basic attention, higher order attention, working memory, processing speed, and executive function, which can be examined by analyzing relevant subtest and index scores from batteries like the Wechsler Adult Intelligence Scale–Fourth Edition (Wechsler, 2008) and other tests (for suggestions, see Otfried Spreen and Esther Strauss's *A Compendium of Neuropsychological Tests: Administration, Norms, and Commentary* [Strauss et al., 2006] or Muriel Lezak's, 2004, *Neuropsychological Assessment*). These impairments can provide localizing information in their own right and can also affect the interpretation of other aspects of the cognitive examination. This is especially true in patients with high seizure burden or on high-dose polytherapy.

Stereo-EEG and Other Intracerebral Approaches

For a proportion of people with drug-resistant focal epilepsy, findings from noninvasive investigations are inconclusive, and intracranial methods are required to determine whether a surgical resection of the EZ is possible. *Stereo-EEG,* the most commonly used procedure, involves implantation of electrodes through burr holes into the brain parenchyma, with the location and number of electrodes dependent on the hypothesized EZ. Each electrode contains a number of EEG contacts, enabling a 3-dimensional representation of seizures and their propagation (Isnard et al., 2018).

Cortical stimulation is a key component of stereo-EEG and involves an electrical signal delivered between two adjacent contacts on an electrode (Trébuchon & Chauvel, 2016). The two main objectives of cortical stimulation are (a) identification of an area where stimulation elicits a habitual seizure; and (b) more relevant to this chapter, functional mapping of eloquent cortex.

In terms of functional mapping, cortical stimulation causes a temporary interruption to the brain tissue surrounding the electrode, allowing an opportunity to interrogate the function of the region. Cognitive paradigms administered during cortical stimulation must be carefully selected based on a theoretical understanding of the underlying cognitive network (Trébuchon & Chauvel, 2016). For instance, tasks such as visual confrontation naming as well as spontaneous speech are often used to map language functions typically focalized to the left angular gyrus. A further challenge for neuropsychological assessment during cortical stimulation is time restraints, with high frequency stimulation used for cognitive mapping typically only delivered for around 5 seconds.

Findings from functional mapping often provide an opportunity for tailored resections that aim to spare eloquent cortex to minimize the likelihood of cognitive deficits. Conversely, proposed resection boundaries may overlap with sites observed to cause a cognitive or functional deficit during stimulation—for example, naming deficits within language areas typically resected in ATL. In the case of naming deficits arising from cortical stimulation within language areas, information obtained from cortical stimulation provides an opportunity to individualize neuropsychological counseling so the patient can weigh the benefits of a resection with better chances of seizure control against the risks of a persisting (language) deficit.

Cognitive Prehabilitation

A need has been identified for routine *prehabilitation*—that is, cognitive and psychosocial rehabilitation *before* undergoing surgery (Baxendale & Thompson, 2018). It has the advantage of using cognitive functions before they are lost to establish the compensatory cognitive strategies and routines that the patient will need after surgery to minimize the day-to-day effects of cognitive decrement (Baxendale, 2020).

Cognitive prehabilitation programs should be individualized based on the formulation of anticipated cognitive decline and the patient's strengths. A detailed discussion with the patient about the formulation and the practical implications that cognitive decline may have across all aspects of their life, including work, social, and domestic areas, is essential to facilitate engagement in the prehabilitation process. The clinician and patient can then work together to develop an individualized package of strategies. For instances, using external memory aids, such as diaries and written instructions for newly learned tasks, will help provide support for the memory system after ATL in the language-dominant hemisphere (typically, left). Fundamental to the success of prehabilitation is practicing these cognitive strategies preoperatively so they are well consolidated and seamlessly embedded into the person's typical day-to-day routine.

Prehabilitation can also include broader social skills training (Hum et al., 2010). Poor social cognition has increasingly been recognized as a comorbidity of TLE, with patients reporting ongoing social skills deficits, such as difficulty making "small talk," up to 20 years after ATL (Coleman et al., 2019). Early social skills training may therefore be an important aspect of supporting patients toward achieving some of their psychosocial expectations, such as improved job opportunities and social connection.

Psychological Assessment and Psychosocial Evaluation

A detailed psychological and psychosocial assessment is key to gauging an individual's vulnerability to poor psychosocial and psychiatric outcomes after surgery. This should involve a comprehensive semistructured interview canvassing epilepsy history and its effect on their life to date; family and other forms of socioemotional supports; psychological history and extant strategies for dealing with adversity; the degree to which epilepsy forms a part of their self-concept; understanding and expectations for epilepsy surgery; and psychometric personality assessment in some cases, using tools such as the Personality Assessment Inventory for *DSM-5* (Morey, 2007; see also 5th ed.; *DSM-5*; American Psychiatric Association, 2013) or Personality Inventory for *DSM-5* (Krueger et al., 2011). The presence of red flags or warning signs for poor adjustment does not preclude surgery but may highlight a need for close postoperative monitoring in some patients. These warning signs are outlined in more detail in the following section "Expectations for Surgery" but include unrealistic expectations or ulterior motives for surgery, premorbid psychiatric illness, low extraversion/high neuroticism, limited or maladaptive social supports, and a poorly developed sense of self. Therapeutic techniques for addressing these red flags and minimizing their effects are suggested.

Expectations for Surgery

Canvassing the patient's expectations around the short- and long-term psychosocial changes that can accompany seizure freedom is a key component of the presurgical assessment. Commonly reported expectations reflect hopes for increased employment opportunities, driving, increased independence and autonomy, and better health-related quality of life as well as intrinsic expectations that may be less easily achieved, such as feeling happier and more in control and being more interesting (S. J. Wilson et al., 1999). At the extreme, some patients' expectations may reflect hidden agendas, such as becoming more independent so that they can leave their partner. Research has consistently revealed the powerful role of patient expectations because expectations can provide a clear benchmark by which patients judge the success of surgery, with flow-on effects for well-being and health-related quality of life (S. J. Wilson et al., 1999). Patients with more realistic expectations, such as a return to driving, have been found to report greater health-related quality of life postsurgery compared with those who demonstrate inflated, unrealistic, or abstract expectations, such as "to become happier."

Current and Lifetime Psychiatric Assessment

More than half of people with a focal epilepsy experience clinically significant depression or anxiety at some point in their lives (Kanner et al., 2010; Rayner et al., 2016). Epilepsy surgery can be a trigger for the emergence or recurrence of psychiatric disorders. In the 12 months following ATL, 22% to 37% of patients experience depression, with the majority (70%) diagnosed in the first 3 months. In 65% of cases, depression persists for at least 6 months (Wrench et al., 2011).

A history of depression is the strongest predictor of depression after surgery and should be carefully interrogated before surgery (Wrench et al., 2011). Other studies have also noted that resection of the language-dominant temporal lobe and being a younger age may elevate the risk of developing postoperative depression (Doherty et al., 2021). TLE patients with a mesial temporal lobe focus seem particularly vulnerable to the development of de novo depression after surgery (Wrench et al., 2009) and may need watchful monitoring.

The Burden of Normality

ATL patients may also need support before surgery so they can be equipped to adjust to the experience of seizure freedom. Much of the framework for our understanding of this adjustment process was first formally outlined in the seminal work of epileptologist Peter Bladin and neuropsychologist Sarah Wilson (S. Wilson et al., 2001). That work revealed a complex and paradoxical process of psychosocial adjustment undergone by many patients with an objectively good surgical outcome (i.e., rendered seizure free). Termed the *burden of normality*, this adjustment process reflects a complex process of identity reconceptualization as the person moves from being chronically ill to suddenly well.

For some patients, this adjustment process can enhance their well-being and quality of life because they view it as an opportunity for personal transformation: "I'm like a new person!" Although this mindset is mostly to the benefit of the patient, it can lead to psychosocial disruption when this newfound confidence challenges long-standing social roles or relationship dynamics ("I don't need you to look after me anymore") or leads to risky behaviors, such as excessive activity or increased drug and alcohol use ("I need to make up for lost time!"), including when the person views themselves as "cured" and ceases antiseizure medications earlier than recommended.

For others, however, the challenges inherent in discarding the sick role and facing the newfound responsibilities associated with being "normal"—for instance, increased employment, domestic contributions, or social engagement—can prove overwhelming and lead to a decrement in mood (S. J. Wilson et al., 2007). Features of the burden of normality have been found to be more common in patients with TLE compared with *extra-TLE*—that is, focal epilepsies originating outside of the temporal lobes—perhaps as a result of the improved seizure outcomes following surgery for TLE (McIntosh et al., 2004; Wrench et al., 2011). As such, interrogation before surgery of the degree to which the patient integrated their epilepsy—and specifically, their disablement from epilepsy—as part of their self-concept provides crucial insights into the patient that may need additional psychological input.

Family Dynamics and Social Supports

Family dynamics may be disrupted by epilepsy in different ways, depending on whether the family unit formed around an individual with a preexisting diagnosis—referred to as a *nesting family*—or if the family unit was established before the onset of epilepsy—referred to as a *crisis family*. Nesting families form rituals and routines around the person with epilepsy, "protecting" them from making major decisions or taking on too much responsibility. In contrast, for a crisis family, the onset of epilepsy can result in a major upheaval to already established family dynamics and routines (Seaburn & Erba, 2003). The onset of epilepsy and this relationship disruption, though, are not always viewed in a negative light, with some patients reporting enriched friendships and partnerships following their epilepsy diagnosis and a heightened sense of closeness among family members (Chew et al., 2019; Thompson et al., 2014; Yennadiou & Wolverson, 2017).

Postoperatively, patients in a crisis family are generally able to return to family roles and routines established before the onset of epilepsy. Patients from nesting families, however, report greater difficulty adjusting postsurgery (Seaburn & Erba, 2003). This is because a successful operation poses a disruption to existing family dynamics and prompts a need to develop new roles. In keeping with this, some family members express concern after surgery that the person with epilepsy has become less dependent on them as a result of a good seizure outcome (Baird et al., 2002). This points to the strongly enmeshed dynamic that likely leads to the development of "hidden agendas" and highlights the need to include family in the preoperative counseling process.

Epilepsy and Sense of Self

Restrictions imposed by epilepsy on an individual's socialization and role diversity can shape personal identity development. *Personal identity* refers to the mental representation someone holds of who they are and can include memories, self-attributions, beliefs, and motivations typically formed through social roles and interactions. Although some individuals consider their epilepsy as separate to themselves and something "other" (Yennadiou & Wolverson, 2017), some feel it becomes integrated into their sense of self—and this can be both in a negative way or in a neutral/positive way (Chew et al., 2019; Kılınç et al., 2018; Rawlings et al., 2017). As put by one of Rawlings et al.'s (2017) participants, "If I could click my fingers and make you [epilepsy] vanish for the rest of my life, I honestly don't think I would" (p. 67). This integration of epilepsy into the sense of self is often a strong indicator that the patient will have difficulty adjusting to postoperative seizure freedom because the surgery therefore not only changes their seizure frequency, but it "removes" a core part of their sense of self.

Age of epilepsy onset has consistently arisen in the literature as an important factor that can influence identity development, with onset before adolescence resulting in greater altered identity development (Allebone et al., 2015). Careful psychological assessment before surgery around the degree to which epilepsy forms a part of the patient's self-concept can give clues as to which patients may require more in-depth counseling before surgery as well as closer monitoring after the operation so that the emergence of any issues can be addressed promptly.

Minimizing the Effects of Psychosocial Risk Factors

Following on from identifying key red flags, an important aspect of the preoperative assessment is addressing and mitigating these factors when possible. First, identifying and explicitly addressing patient and family expectations and as well as working to correct or manage them, if necessary, are vitally important so that the whole treating team is working toward mutually shared goals (Baxendale & Thompson, 2018). An excellent framework for this is SMART, the goal-setting techniques often used in rehabilitation settings (B. A. Wilson et al., 2002). This process of making goals specific, measurable, attainable, realistic, and anchored in a specific time frame can assist patients to shift unrealistic or overly vague expectations for surgery (e.g., "to be happy") by challenging them to think what that goal looks like in day-to-day functioning (e.g., "to be happy" equals "to make new friends I can meet up with weekly") as well as what steps they might need to get there (e.g., practicing social skills, joining social groups to meet new people). This highly pragmatic planning can give patients the insight that there are more barriers to their goals than just their seizures as well as provide them with concrete plans to help them tackle their goals.

Epilepsy surgery represents a major life change, or turning point, that forces a reexamination of their life and relationships, with the potential to prompt positive change and growth (Rawlings et al., 2017). Promotion of positive psychological growth as well as adaptive constructs, such as self-mastery or self-efficacy, are key to helping patients mitigate the effect of premorbid risk factors for a poor postoperative outcome. Supporting patients to develop more positive self-concepts around their epilepsy before surgery often leads to better psychological outcomes (S. J. Wilson et al., 2020). Along similar lines, adopting an accepting coping strategy before surgery, being able to make the best of a situation, and seeing challenges in a positive light (cognitive reframing) have also been associated with good postoperative quality of life and psychosocial adjustment in a survey of 77 epilepsy surgery patients in the United Kingdom (Kemp et al., 2016). Together, these aspects of psychological resilience can be seen as specific targets for collaborative development with the patient in routine counseling sessions before epilepsy surgery. Clinicians could also use well-established clinical approaches, such as acceptance and commitment therapy, to help guide the process of self-reflection and reconsideration of patient values and life goals (Lundgren et al., 2008). This approach also has merits for those patients who do not experience a good surgical outcome to support acceptance of postoperative seizure recurrence.

INFORMED CONSENT TO SURGERY

In common parlance, the term *informed consent* carries an implication that merely providing an individual with information validates the consent process (Bernat, 2008). Although conveying adequate information is an important component, valid consent also requires that the patient has the (cognitive) capacity to understand and retain this information, use the information to weigh up the outlined risks and benefits, and communicate their decision. Of relevance to the current chapter, intellectually intact adults with TLE may present with a selection of cognitive and psychological vulnerabilities that typically do not undermine their ability to provide informed consent to treatment but do necessitate that the clinician take additional time in presurgery consultations to facilitate effective, patient-centered consent to care. This includes time to develop an empathic rapport, to explore the patient and family's perspective and understanding of the situation and proposed treatment, to explore the patient's cognitive capability, and to allow enough time to work together to develop a shared understanding of the risks and benefits of epilepsy surgery that is tailored to the patient's cognitive strengths and limitations (Watling & Brown, 2007). This includes canvassing the patient's ability to acknowledge and accept the chance that they might also be in the minority of cases that experience the disappointment of seizure recurrence or cognitive decrement after surgery.

In accordance with the intrinsic rights of humans to make their own decisions when possible, adults with mild to moderate intellectual disabilities should also be an integral part of the surgery decision-making process, with the content of the discussions adapted to suit their intellectual limitations whenever possible. This is facilitated through the slow development of a trusting rapport with the patient and their caregivers, the repeated delivery of intellectually appropriate information, and professional cognizance around balancing patient autonomy with potentially paternalistic attitudes to patient care from some team members.

CONCLUSION

Just as the diagnosis of epilepsy can necessitate a major psychosocial adjustment, so, too, does the potential to be rendered suddenly seizure free with epilepsy surgery after many years of living with a chronic neurological illness. Careful neurocognitive, behavioral, and psychological examination before the operation forms the basis of validly informed consent to this elective procedure and can help prepare the patient for changes to their cognitive function in some cases. It also provides vital information to the clinician for tailoring supportive psychotherapy that can help the patient and their support network successfully navigate this major life event so that they may maximally benefit from finally becoming seizure free.

REFERENCES

Allebone, J., Rayner, G., Siveges, B., & Wilson, S. J. (2015). Altered self-identity and autobiographical memory in epilepsy. *Epilepsia*, *56*(12), 1982–1991. https://doi.org/10.1111/epi.13215

American Psychiatric Association. (2013). *Diagnostic and statistical manual of mental disorders* (5th ed.). https://doi.org/10.1176/appi.books.9780890425596

Baird, A. D., Wilson, S. J., Bladin, P. F., Saling, M. M., & Reutens, D. C. (2002). Hypersexuality after temporal lobe resection. *Epilepsy & Behavior*, *3*(2), 173–181. https://doi.org/10.1006/ebeh.2002.0342

Barba, C., Cossu, M., Guerrini, R., Di Gennaro, G., Villani, F., De Palma, L., Grisotto, L., Consales, A., Battaglia, D., Zamponi, N., d'Orio, P., Revay, M., Rizzi, M., Casciato, S., Esposito, V., Quarato, P. P., Di Giacomo, R., Didato, G., Pastori, C., . . . TLE Study Group. (2021). Temporal lobe epilepsy surgery in children and adults: A multicenter study. *Epilepsia*, *62*(1), 128–142. https://doi.org/10.1111/epi.16772

Barba, C., Rheims, S., Minotti, L., Guénot, M., Hoffmann, D., Chabardès, S., Isnard, J., Kahane, P., & Ryvlin, P. (2016). Temporal plus epilepsy is a major determinant of temporal lobe surgery failures. *Brain*, *139*(2), 444–451. https://doi.org/10.1093/brain/awv372

Baxendale, S. (2020). Cognitive rehabilitation and prehabilitation in people with epilepsy. *Epilepsy & Behavior*, *106*, Article 107027. https://doi.org/10.1016/j.yebeh.2020.107027

Baxendale, S., & Thompson, P. (2018). Red flags in epilepsy surgery: Identifying the patients who pay a high cognitive price for an unsuccessful surgical outcome. *Epilepsy & Behavior*, *78*, 269–272. https://doi.org/10.1016/j.yebeh.2017.08.003

Baxendale, S., Wilson, S. J., Baker, G. A., Barr, W., Helmstaedter, C., Hermann, B. P., Langfitt, J., Reuner, G., Rzezak, P., Samson, S., & Smith, M.-L. (2019). Indications and expectations for neuropsychological assessment in epilepsy surgery in children and adults: Executive summary of the report of the ILAE Neuropsychology Task Force Diagnostic Methods Commission: 2017–2021. *Epilepsia*, *60*(9), 1794–1796. https://doi.org/10.1111/epi.16309

Benedict, R. (1997). *Brief Visuospatial Memory Test–Revised: Professional manual*. Psychological Assessment Resources.

Bernat, J. L. (2008). *Ethical issues in neurology*. Lippincott Williams & Wilkins.

Blümcke, I., Thom, M., Aronica, E., Armstrong, D. D., Bartolomei, F., Bernasconi, A., Bernasconi, N., Bien, C. G., Cendes, F., Coras, R., Cross, J. H., Jacques, T. S., Kahane, P., Mathern, G. W., Miyata, H., Moshé, S. L., Oz, B., Özkara, Ç., Perucca, E., . . . Spreafico, R. (2013). International consensus classification of hippocampal sclerosis in temporal lobe epilepsy: A Task Force report from the ILAE Commission on Diagnostic Methods. *Epilepsia*, *54*(7), 1315–1329. https://doi.org/10.1111/epi.12220

Buckley, R. F., Ellis, K. A., Ames, D., Rowe, C. C., Lautenschlager, N. T., Maruff, P., Villemagne, V. L., Macaulay, S. L., Szoeke, C., Martins, R. N., Masters, C. L., Savage, G., Rainey-Smith, S. R., Rembach, A., Saling, M. M., & the Australian Imaging Biomarkers and Lifestyle Study of Ageing (AIBL) Research Group. (2015). Phenomenological characterization of memory complaints in preclinical and prodromal Alzheimer's disease. *Neuropsychology*, *29*(4), 571–581. https://doi.org/10.1037/neu0000156

Chew, J., Carpenter, J., & Haase, A. M. (2019). Living with epilepsy in adolescence-A qualitative study of young people's experiences in Singapore: Peer socialization, autonomy, and self-esteem. *Child: Care, Health and Development*, *45*(2), 241–250. https://doi.org/10.1111/cch.12648

Coleman, H., McIntosh, A., & Wilson, S. J. (2019). Identifying the trajectory of social milestones 15–20 years after epilepsy surgery: Realistic timelines for post-surgical expectations. *Epilepsia Open*, *4*(3), 369–381. https://doi.org/10.1002/epi4.12341

Delis, D. C., Kramer, J. H., Kaplan, E., & Ober, B. A. (2000). *California Verbal Learning Test—(CVLT-II): Adult version* (manual). Psychological Corporation.

Doherty, C., Nowacki, A. S., Pat McAndrews, M., McDonald, C. R., Reyes, A., Kim, M. S., Hamberger, M., Najm, I., Bingaman, W., Jehi, L., & Busch, R. M. (2021). Predicting mood decline following temporal lobe epilepsy surgery in adults. *Epilepsia*, *62*(2), 450–459. https://doi.org/10.1111/epi.16800

Engel, J., Jr., McDermott, M. P., Wiebe, S., Langfitt, J. T., Stern, J. M., Dewar, S., Sperling, M. R., Gardiner, I., Erba, G., Fried, I., Jacobs, M., Vinters, H. V., Mintzer, S., Kieburtz, K., & the Early Randomized Surgical Epilepsy Trial (ERSET) Study Group. (2012). Early surgical therapy for drug-resistant temporal lobe epilepsy: A randomized trial. *JAMA*, *307*(9), 922–930. https://doi.org/10.1001/jama.2012.220

Fisher, R. S., Cross, J. H., French, J. A., Higurashi, N., Hirsch, E., Jansen, F. E., Lagae, L., Moshé, S. L., Peltola, J., Roulet Perez, E., Scheffer, I. E., & Zuberi, S. M. (2017). Operational classification of seizure types by the international league against epilepsy: Position paper of the ILAE commission for classification and terminology. *Epilepsia*, *58*(4), 522–530. https://doi.org/10.1111/epi.13670

Goodglass, H., Kaplan, E., & Barresi, B. (2001). *Boston Diagnostic Aphasia Examination* (3rd ed.). Pro-Ed.

Helmstaedter, C., Richter, S., Röske, S., Oltmanns, F., Schramm, J., & Lehmann, T.-N. (2008). Differential effects of temporal pole resection with amygdalohippocampectomy versus selective amygdalohippocampectomy on material-specific memory in patients with mesial temporal lobe epilepsy. *Epilepsia*, *49*(1), 88–97. https://doi.org/10.1111/j.1528-1167.2007.01386.x

Hum, K. M., Smith, M. L., Lach, L., & Elliott, I. M. (2010). Self-perceptions of social function 2 years after pediatric epilepsy surgery. *Epilepsy & Behavior*, *17*(3), 354–359. https://doi.org/10.1016/j.yebeh.2009.11.022

Isnard, J., Taussig, D., Bartolomei, F., Bourdillon, P., Catenoix, H., Chassoux, F., Chipaux, M., Clémenceau, S., Colnat-Coulbois, S., Denuelle, M., Derrey, S., Devaux, B., Dorfmüller, G., Gilard, V., Guenot, M., Job-Chapron, A.-S., Landré, E., Lebas, A., Maillard, L., . . . Sauleau, P. (2018). French guidelines on stereoelectroencephalography (SEEG). *Neurophysiologie Clinique*, *48*(1), 5–13. https://doi.org/10.1016/j.neucli.2017.11.005

Kanner, A. M., Barry, J. J., Gilliam, F., Hermann, B., & Meador, K. J. (2010). Anxiety disorders, subsyndromic depressive episodes, and major depressive episodes: Do they differ on their impact on the quality of life of patients with epilepsy? *Epilepsia*, *51*(7), 1152–1158. https://doi.org/10.1111/j.1528-1167.2010.02582.x

Kemp, S., Garlovsky, J., Reynders, H., Caswell, H., Baker, G., & Shah, E. (2016). Predicting the psychosocial outcome of epilepsy surgery: A longitudinal perspective on the "burden of normality." *Epilepsy & Behavior*, *60*, 149–152. https://doi.org/10.1016/j.yebeh.2016.04.029

Kılınç, S., Campbell, C., Guy, A., & van Wersch, A. (2018). Epilepsy, identity, and the experience of the body. *Epilepsy & Behavior*, *89*, 42–47. https://doi.org/10.1016/j.yebeh.2018.10.003

Krueger, R. F., Derringer, J., Markon, K. E., Watson, D., & Skodol, A. E. (2011). Initial construction of a maladaptive personality trait model and inventory for *DSM-5*. *Psychological Medicine*, *42*(9), 1879–1890. https://doi.org/10.1017/S0033291711002674

Kwan, P., Schachter, S. C., & Brodie, M. J. (2011). Drug-resistant epilepsy. *The New England Journal of Medicine*, *365*(10), 919–926. https://doi.org/10.1056/NEJMra1004418

Lezak, M. D., Howieson, D. B., Loring, D. W., Hannay, H. J., & Fischer, J. S. (2004). *Neuropsychological assessment* (4th ed.). Oxford University Press.

Lundgren, T., Dahl, J., & Hayes, S. C. (2008). Evaluation of mediators of change in the treatment of epilepsy with acceptance and commitment therapy. *Journal of Behavioral Medicine*, *31*(3), 225–235. https://doi.org/10.1007/s10865-008-9151-x

McGonigal, A., Bartolomei, F., & Chauvel, P. (2021). On seizure semiology. *Epilepsia*, *62*(9). Advance online publication. https://doi.org/10.1111/epi.16994

McIntosh, A. M., Kalnins, R. M., Mitchell, L. A., Fabinyi, G. C. A., Briellmann, R. S., & Berkovic, S. F. (2004). Temporal lobectomy: Long-term seizure outcome, late recurrence and risks for seizure recurrence. *Brain*, *127*(9), 2018–2030. https://doi.org/10.1093/brain/awh221

Morey, L. C. (2007). *The Personality Assessment Inventory professional manual*. Psychological Assessment Resources.

Muhlhofer, W., Tan, Y.-L., Mueller, S. G., & Knowlton, R. (2017). MRI-negative temporal lobe epilepsy—What do we know? *Epilepsia*, *58*(5), 727–742. https://doi.org/10.1111/epi.13699

Panov, F., Li, Y., Chang, E. F., Knowlton, R., & Cornes, S. B. (2016). Epilepsy with temporal encephalocele: Characteristics of electrocorticography and surgical outcome. *Epilepsia*, *57*(2), e33–e38. https://doi.org/10.1111/epi.13271

Poole, N. A., Cope, S. R., Bailey, C., & Isaacs, J. D. (2019). Functional cognitive disorders: Identification and management. *BJPsych Advances*, *25*(6), 342–350. https://doi.org/10.1192/bja.2019.38

Rawlings, G. H., Brown, I., Stone, B., & Reuber, M. (2017). Written accounts of living with epilepsy: A thematic analysis. *Epilepsy & Behavior*, *72*, 63–70. https://doi.org/10.1016/j.yebeh.2017.04.026

Rayner, G., Jackson, G. D., & Wilson, S. J. (2016). Two distinct symptom-based phenotypes of depression in epilepsy yield specific clinical and etiological insights. *Epilepsy & Behavior*, *64*, 336–344. https://doi.org/10.1016/j.yebeh.2016.06.007

Rayner, G., & Tailby, C. (2017). Current concepts of memory disorder in epilepsy: Edging towards a network account. *Current Neurology and Neuroscience Reports*, *17*(8), Article 55. https://doi.org/10.1007/s11910-017-0765-7

Reyes, A., Kaestner, E., Ferguson, L., Jones, J. E., Seidenberg, M., Barr, W. B., Busch, R. M., Hermann, B. P., & McDonald, C. R. (2020). Cognitive phenotypes in temporal lobe epilepsy utilizing data- and clinically driven approaches: Moving toward a new taxonomy. *Epilepsia*, *61*(6), 1211–1220. https://doi.org/10.1111/epi.16528

Saling, M. M. (2005). Imaging and neuropsychology. In R. I. Kuzineicky & G. D. Jackson (Eds.), *Magnetic resonance in epilepsy: Neuroimaging techniques* (2nd ed., pp. 271–280). Elsevier Academic Press.

Saling, M. M. (2009). Verbal memory in mesial temporal lobe epilepsy: Beyond material specificity. *Brain*, *132*(3), 570–582. https://doi.org/10.1093/brain/awp012

Saling, M. M., & Wilson, S. J. (2011). Presurgical diagnostics. In C. Helmstaedter, B. Hermann, M. Lassonde, P. Kahane, & A. Arizmanoglou (Eds.), *Neuropsychology in the care of people with epilepsy* (pp. 191–198). John Libbey Eurotext.

Seaburn, D. B., & Erba, G. (2003). The family experience of "sudden health": The case of intractable epilepsy. *Family Process*, *42*(4), 453–467. https://doi.org/10.1111/j.1545-5300.2003.00453.x

Semah, F., Picot, M.-C., Adam, C., Broglin, D., Arzimanoglou, A., Bazin, B., Cavalcanti, D., & Baulac, M. (1998). Is the underlying cause of epilepsy a major prognostic factor for recurrence? *Neurology*, *51*(5), 1256–1262. https://doi.org/10.1212/WNL.51.5.1256

Strauss, E., Sherman, E. M. S., & Spreen, O. (2006). *A compendium of neuropsychological tests: Administration, norms, and commentary* (3rd ed.). Oxford University Press.

Thompson, R., Kerr, M., Glynn, M., & Linehan, C. (2014). Caring for a family member with intellectual disability and epilepsy: Practical, social and emotional perspectives. *Seizure*, *23*(10), 856–863. https://doi.org/10.1016/j.seizure.2014.07.005

Trébuchon, A., & Chauvel, P. (2016). Electrical stimulation for seizure induction and functional mapping in stereoelectroencephalography. *Journal of Clinical Neurophysiology*, *33*(6), 511–521. https://doi.org/10.1097/WNP.0000000000000313

Watling, C. J., & Brown, J. B. (2007). Education research: Communication skills for neurology residents: Structured teaching and reflective practice. *Neurology*, *69*(22), E20–E26. https://doi.org/10.1212/01.wnl.0000280461.96059.44

Wechsler, D. (2008). *WAIS-IV technical and interpretative manual*. Pearson.

Wechsler, D. (2009). *Wechsler Memory Scale* (4th ed.). Pearson.

Wiebe, S., Blume, W. T., Girvin, J. P., Eliasziw, M., & the Effectiveness and Efficiency of Surgery for Temporal Lobe Epilepsy Study Group. (2001). A randomized, controlled trial of surgery for temporal-lobe epilepsy. *The New England Journal of Medicine*, *345*(5), 311–318. https://doi.org/10.1056/NEJM200108023450501

Wilson, B. A. (2002). Towards a comprehensive model of cognitive rehabilitation. *Neuropsychological Rehabilitation*, *12*(2), 97–110 https://doi.org/10.1080/09602010244000020

Wilson, S., Bladin, P., & Saling, M. (2001). The "burden of normality": Concepts of adjustment after surgery for seizures. *Journal of Neurology, Neurosurgery & Psychiatry*, *70*(5), 649–656. https://doi.org/10.1136/jnnp.70.5.649

Wilson, S. J., Bladin, P. F., & Saling, M. M. (2007). The burden of normality: A framework for rehabilitation after epilepsy surgery. *Epilepsia*, *48*(Suppl. 9), 13–16. https://doi.org/10.1111/j.1528-1167.2007.01393.x

Wilson, S. J., Rayner, G., & Pieters, J. (2020). Positive illusions determine quality of life in drug-resistant epilepsy. *Epilepsia*, *61*(3), 539–548. https://doi.org/10.1111/epi.16455

Wilson, S. J., Saling, M. M., Lawrence, J., & Bladin, P. F. (1999). Outcome of temporal lobectomy: Expectations and the prediction of perceived success. *Epilepsy Research*, *36*(1), 1–14. https://doi.org/10.1016/S0920-1211(99)00016-9

World Health Organization. (2022, February 9). *Epilepsy*. https://www.who.int/newsroom/fact-sheets/detail/epilepsy

Wrench, J. M., Rayner, G., & Wilson, S. J. (2011). Profiling the evolution of depression after epilepsy surgery. *Epilepsia*, *52*(5), 900–908. https://doi.org/10.1111/j.1528-1167.2011.03015.x

Wrench, J. M., Wilson, S. J., O'Shea, M. F., & Reutens, D. C. (2009). Characterising de novo depression after epilepsy surgery. *Epilepsy Research*, *83*(1), 81–88. https://doi.org/10.1016/j.eplepsyres.2008.09.007

Xu, K., Wang, X., Guan, Y., Zhao, M., Zhou, J., Zhai, F., Wang, M., Li, T., & Luan, G. (2020). Comparisons of the seizure-free outcome and visual field deficits between anterior temporal lobectomy and selective amygdalohippocampectomy: A systematic review and meta-analysis. *Seizure*, *81*, 228–235. https://doi.org/10.1016/j.seizure.2020.07.024

Yennadiou, H., & Wolverson, E. (2017). The experience of epilepsy in later life: A qualitative exploration of illness representations. *Epilepsy & Behavior*, *70*(Pt. A), 87–93. https://doi.org/10.1016/j.yebeh.2017.01.033

12 PRACTICAL SUGGESTIONS FOR PRESURGICAL PSYCHOLOGICAL ASSESSMENTS AND FUTURE DIRECTIONS FOR THE FIELD

ANDREW R. BLOCK

When I began assessing surgical patients more than 35 years ago, the field of presurgical psychological assessment (PPA) was in its infancy. There existed minimal research, and guidance about the goals and procedures to be included with PPA were unclear. As the chapters in this book demonstrate, the field has grown tremendously in both depth and breadth. Still, many practitioners purport to conduct PPAs but either ignore or are unaware of the empirical literature and practice principles on which such assessments should be founded. In this chapter, drawing on my experience conducting PPAs, as well as the invaluable information provided by the chapter authors of this text, I provide suggestions that should assist practitioners in their practice of PPA.

Before proceeding to practical suggestions, I want to discuss a common misunderstanding of the purpose of PPA arising from the fact that such an assessment is often required by the surgeon, or the insurance carrier, before surgery can proceed. This leads some to think that a PPA is essentially an obstacle to surgery, an unethical requirement infringing on the patient's freedom of choice. This is especially the case if the referring physician states

https://doi.org/10.1037/0000346-013
Psychological Assessment of Surgical Candidates: Evidence-Based Procedures and Practices, R. J. Marek and A. R. Block (Editors)

that the patient must "pass" the PPA to have surgery. However, the truth about PPA is far different.

PPA starts with the assumption that the patient has a medical condition for which surgery is needed and is a viable treatment option. It does not assume that the patient's condition is psychogenic, nor does it question the patient's motivation for undergoing surgery, albeit the patient's expectations about the outcome of surgery constitute one of the legitimate foci of the assessment. PPA is simply designed to maximize the likelihood that patients will have the best possible surgical outcome while avoiding worsening of their physical, emotional, or cognitive states. It provides guidance to the surgeon, allowing for individualization of treatment plans. It provides feedback to the patient on issues that could adversely affect surgical results, and it creates steps to ameliorate these. It helps the patient to identify strengths on which to draw while going through the surgical recovery process.

It is true that sometimes the information provided to the surgeon flowing out of the PPA may result in delaying surgery or even avoiding surgery altogether. However, if the information obtained in the PPA is thoroughly and sensitively discussed with the patient, the rationale for the psychologist/mental health professional's conclusions should become clear, helping the patient to recognize the value of such conclusions. In the language of ethics (see Chapter 3), the PPA involves a careful balance of autonomy (the patient's right to make decisions about their own body) against beneficence (doing good for the patient) and nonmaleficence (doing no harm). The ultimate goal of the PPA is that these three ethical principles align and the patient as well as the treatment team end up on the same page.

GETTING READY

PPA is essentially a risk-assessment procedure, one in which the psychologist/mental health professional must rely on a strong foundation of empirical data and clinical expertise to weigh the extent to which psychological vulnerabilities, balanced against strengths and mitigating factors, may affect surgical outcomes. To obtain the necessary general skill set and clinical acumen to perform a PPA, it is important first and foremost to understand the proposed surgical procedure. In addition to learning as much as possible about the actual processes involved in surgical preparation, the surgery itself, and recovery after surgery, it is helpful to spend a morning or day in the office seeing patients with a referring surgeon. Observing the types of information on which the surgeon draws to reach decisions and the interaction of surgeon and patient go a long way toward informing decision making during the PPA. In addition, discussing individual cases with the surgeon can allow one to understand the surgeon's expectations and needs in referring patients for PPA and to help surgeons recognize cases in which PPA can assist in their treatment planning. This is especially important because referring surgeons will have widely varying expectations for both the types of information provided by PPA and their reliance on the PPA in decision making. Further, observing the surgeon's activity gives one a chance to point out to the surgeon how best to frame a referral for PPA and especially to avoid telling the patient that the PPA must be "passed" before surgery can proceed. Providing surgeons with written information can help them prepare patients for the PPA (for an example, see Exhibit 12.1).

If possible, it can be especially helpful to observe a surgery (if you can stomach it), with the patient's written permission. Nothing can provide greater empathy for the patient nor more insight into the rigors of surgery than the experience of seeing, hearing, and smelling what goes on the in operating room!

As the chapters in this book attest, there exists a strong and growing empirical literature examining the relationship of psychosocial factors to surgery results. It behooves anyone conducting PPA to continuously keep aware of this literature—both its strengths and weaknesses. Conducting PPA involves tremendous responsibility because assessment results may strongly affect the surgeon's decisions about the appropriateness and timing of surgery and also affect the individualization of treatment plans. Thus, one who conducts PPA should be able to point to the empirically demonstrated bases for their determinations and make explicit which conclusions rely primarily on clinical judgment.

The effective performance of PPA, of course, relies not only on general knowledge of the proposed surgery and the specific expectations of the referring physician but also on obtaining as much information as possible about each patient. In my experience, preparing for each assessment by reviewing the patient's medical records before the interview is fundamental to process. The medical record often contains intake questionnaires that identify patient symptoms and hint at motivations and expectations. Office notes allow one to examine the referring physician's diagnostic process, indicating the extent to which symptomatology matches or is inconsistent with identified physical pathology. Records of medication use, physical therapy attendance, and patient acceptance of physician recommendations give evidence to future compliance with necessary postoperative treatments and restrictions. Patients are quite appreciative and more responsive during the interview when the evaluator can express in-depth knowledge of their cases.

EXHIBIT 12.1. Sample Presurgical Psychological Assessment

Assessment Summary for ______________________________

Patient Name ______________________________

Current Psychological Symptoms

- Depression
- Sleep disturbance
- Feelings of hopelessness/helplessness
- Crying spells
- Guilt and lowered self-esteem
- Periodic excessive alcohol consumption

Psychosocial Risk Factors for Reduced Medical/Surgical Treatment Outcome

- Depression and demoralization concerns
- Substance dependence concerns
- Compliance concerns

Positive (Mitigating) Psychosocial Factors

- Previously sought mental health treatment for depression and achieved good response to combination of psychotherapy and medication
- Supportive partner
- Strong motivation to return to work

Additional Considerations

Patient was just diagnosed with low testosterone and recently started on hormone therapy.

Recommendations for Psychological/Psychiatric Treatment

- Refer to psychiatrist for consideration of antidepressant medication.
- Begin a brief course of cognitive behavioral treatment.

Recommendations to Referring Physician

- At present, the patient has a high level of risk for reduced outcome of spine surgery related to
  - untreated depression and
  - intermittent substance abuse
- Surgical results are likely to be improved if the patient begins a course of psychotherapy and starts on psychotropic medication.
- If the need for surgery is not imminent, it would be advisable to briefly delay the surgery to begin the course of mental health intervention.

CONDUCTING THE ASSESSMENT

For many surgical candidates, the idea of a required PPA is shocking and somewhat objectionable. Thus, it becomes important early in the process to break through such resistance and establish rapport.

The Interview

I have found that it is best to begin the interview by "normalizing" the PPA, explaining to the patient that the assessment is a routine part of the surgeon's diagnostic process and does not indicate that the surgeon feels the patient's physical problems are a result of psychological difficulties. Rather, the referring doctor recognizes that having protracted medical problems, and facing surgery to correct those problems, can be very burdensome, and the PPA allows an opportunity to discuss concerns and fears. It allows for individualization of treatment plans to take into account emotional and interpersonal changes created by the medical condition. Expectations for surgical outcome are discussed, allowing the patient to clarify their own projections for their postoperative futures. Thus, the patient benefits by knowing the PPA exists as a vehicle to create a holistic treatment plan, identifying and addressing any problems that might interfere with recovery, to maximize surgical outcome while minimizing the likelihood of adverse surgical results.

As with any psychological assessment, the interview requires many skills and abilities: establishment of rapport, gathering of critical information, flexibility to pursue in-depth specific problem areas, behavioral observation, and simultaneous foci on the patient's problems and their strengths. Perhaps most important is the ability to be, at once, empathic and yet objective. I have found that following a semistructured interview format is most effective for these purposes. Such a format impels one to assess all critical problem areas, yet allows for the ability to go "off script" when the opportunity arises to probe deeply into patient concerns. Initially, questions should focus on the medical issues for which surgery is being considered, including the patient's experiences of symptoms, treatments, and understanding of their conditions. However, because surgical candidates are often not inclined to discuss emotional or interpersonal issues, if patients express language indicative of an emotional experience (e.g., "It's so frustrating," "That really made me mad"), probing more deeply into these feelings may open an otherwise unavailable window into the patient's concerns and thoughts.

The goals of PPA, as noted in Chapter 1, are different from those of a general psychological assessment. In conducting the interview, one must always keep in mind that the goal is to gather information relevant to the patient's projected responses to surgery. Given our training as clinicians, it is easy to get caught up in discussions about events or issues that may have significantly affected the patient's development but bear minimal relevance for surgical results. For example, although the patient may have experienced childhood abuse or abandonment, a topic that certainly can cause lifetime trauma, in-depth exploration of such issues goes well beyond the goals of PPA and can result in leaving little time to explore other aspects of the patient's life that might be expected to influence surgical response.

Each of the medical conditions for which surgery is contemplated carries its own symptoms and behavioral effects. The interview offers a microcosm for observation of the way patients' symptoms relate to observed behaviors. For example, patients who complain of limited tolerance for sitting but are able to sit comfortably throughout the interview may be expected to have more difficulty in the recognition of improved function as a result of surgery.

Another critical area of concern is the effect of the patient's physical condition on self-image and self-esteem. For some patients, pain, dysfunction, disfigurement, cognitive difficulties, or organ system failures may lead to feelings of worthlessness or to avoidance of social interaction. Exploring disease-specific factors that adversely affect self-esteem can go a long way toward identifying deficits in coping. On the other hand, patients bring with them to the surgical process a lifetime of having dealt with adversity and stress. Discussing with patients their reactions to such adverse events can be helpful both in identifying resilience and assisting patients to build on their normal coping mechanisms to achieve the best possible outcomes of surgery.

The interview, when possible, should include at least some time with a member of the patient's support system: a spouse, partner, children, parents, and so on. An extensive body of research demonstrates both that chronic health problems have adverse effects on support members and that social support can be critical for overcoming medical problems and improving health generally (Uchino, 2008). In some cases, the actions of significant others can work at cross-purposes to desired goals (Block, 1981). All these issues should be explored to determine the manner in which support system members are likely to assist with or impair recovery after surgery. Further, inclusion of such individuals in the assessment process can confirm, expand on, or contradict the patient's own reports of their response to, and attempts to cope with, the condition for which surgery is being contemplated.

Perhaps the most critical aspect of the interview—one that is particularly difficult to capture through questionnaires—is patient expectation for surgical results. Not only is it important that the patient have a realistic outlook but, equally important, most of the surgeries included in this volume require the patient to be actively involved in their own care after, and sometimes even before, the surgery itself. Many patients view surgery as singular event, changing their life direction with minimal engagement. However, surgical outcome may rest on alterations in exercise or diet; decreased use or cessation of alcohol or drugs; and strict compliance with medication regimens, physical therapy, or other postoperative directions. In most cases, surgery is best seen as a foundation on which general physical and even mental health can be built through active patient participation. Probing deeply into the patient's knowledge of, and plans for making, such important behavioral changes can greatly inform the recommendations flowing out of the PPA.

Psychometric Testing

Chapter 2 of this book provides in-depth discussion of the importance of psychometric testing as well as advice for choosing and using psychometrics. Despite the importance of psychometric testing, the patient may view it in the context of assessment for surgery as unnecessary and burdensome. It is enough that they must be seen by a psychologist/mental health professional, let alone complete a battery of questionnaires, many of which may seem, at face value, to bear little relationship to the surgery for which they are being assessed. Thus, many patients may be resistant to accurate completion of the tests. Validity of testing is further adversely affected if the patient has been improperly prepared by the referring physician, believing that revealing too much emotional material may result in cancellation of the surgery. I have even seen that in some online support groups of patients who have undergone a particular type of surgery, potential surgical candidates are told how to answer questionnaires so that their psychosocial concerns are minimized.

For all these reasons, I consider it essential to include within the test battery some assessment of the extent to which patients may be over- or underreporting. Most broadband tests, such as the Minnesota Multiphasic Personality Inventory (MMPI) family, the Behavioral Health Inventory–2 (Bruns & Disorbio, 2003), and the Millon Behavioral Medicine Diagnostic (Millon et al., 2001), contain scales that assess such response sets. More narrowly focused symptom validity tests may be useful when time, physical or cognitive ability, or patient reluctance make administration of broadband testing impractical (for reviews, see Lockhart & Satya-Murti, 2015; Walczyk et al., 2018). However, one must be circumspect in interpreting any of these tests because most have not been normed for surgical candidates (except for the MMPI-2–Restructured Form [Ben-Porath, 2012] and MMPI-3

[Ben-Porath & Tellegen, 2020a, 2020b] in the cases of bariatric and spine surgery). When such tests indicate underreporting, the diagnostic interview and inclusion of a significant other as part of the assessment take on increased importance. Regardless of the specific tests used, it is important to identify for the patient the rationale for the use of such tests—that is, they help to provide another window into the patient's emotional and behavioral concerns with the goal of promoting the most effective, holistic approach to treatment. Assure patients that you will review test results with them and will discuss any concerns that arise from the testing.

There are arguments to be made both for having patients complete testing before and after the interview. Of course, if completed prior, the results can be reviewed with the patient at the end of the interview. However, preinterview testing occurs before rapport has been established with patients, so patients may be less forthcoming. Conducting testing after the interview may be more valid but will require an additional session to review test results with the patient. Often, however, within the context of assessment for surgery, the patient's schedule of other medical diagnostic tests will dictate when testing is given. Regardless of when it occurs, one should make use of testing as a component of the PPA process but make certain to review the results with the patient to validate or contradict any significant findings. Also, I have learned over the course of my career that psychometric testing is most valuable when it contradicts my clinical impression of the patient. Thus, even if testing is given before the interview, I do not personally examine it until the interview is complete to minimize my preconceptions. For cases in which my impression and test results are at odds, I often have the patient return to discuss these contradictions, which invariably provides for a much greater depth of understanding of the patient's situation.

The Report

It is quite a balancing act to create a document that is, at once, useful to the surgeon, provides information that can help the patient obtain the best possible surgical outcomes, meets the requirements of the insurer (if any), and maintains patient confidentiality. I have a few suggestions to offer that may be helpful.

Surgeons do not like or need lengthy psychological assessment reports. Most just will not take the time to read them. They want a simple, nonnuanced report that provides information and recommendations that they can access quickly and easily. This kind of report cuts against the grain of the training received by most psychologists and mental health professionals. Personally,

I tend to view this need for simplicity as a positive because it allows reports to avoid in-depth discussion of psychosocial history, abuse history, social support, and so forth, thus providing maximal protection for patient confidentiality. Of course, sufficient information should be included in the report to support the report's conclusions.

I personally like to provide a one-page summary at the end of the psychological assessment report (see Exhibit 12.1 for an example of a spine surgery PPA summary) that lists the following:

- current psychological symptoms
- empirically validated psychosocial risk factors for reduced surgical outcome
- risk factors based on provider judgment but that are not empirically validated
- patient strengths and other factors that mitigate risk (see Chapter 1)
- additional factors that should be considered by the surgeon
- suggestions for necessary psychological treatment to support surgical outcome
- suggestions to assist the surgeon in individualizing the treatment plan
- overall assessment of the level of risk for reduced surgical outcome

In the preceding list, I highlight the importance of overall risk assessment because that is at once the most important to the physician and the most difficult to determine. That is why, as noted in Chapter 1, it behooves the psychologist/mental health professional to use an assessment approach that is systematic, bias free, and informed by extensive knowledge of the surgical procedure for which the patient is being considered, and that relies on objective data that have been tied empirically to the outcome of each specific surgery. Of course, provider judgment will always play a large role in determining the manner in which all the information obtained in the assessment process is translated into an overall risk assessment projection. However, reliance on a fixed, systematic approach both clarifies and minimizes the extent to which this assessment is based on facts rather than on opinions.

The PPA report will become part of the patient's medical record to be read by the referring physician, most likely just before the patient's next appointment. As such, I have a few suggestions. First, if possible, find a means to limit the number of people who can read the report. Most electronic medical record programs have a means of locking reports and only allowing access to specified individuals. Try to make use of such technology. Second, the report is just that—a report. It is like any other diagnostic tool contained in the medical record. It is a statement of facts to be considered by the surgeon in the diagnostic process and treatment planning. In deciding about how to proceed, the surgeon will need to weigh all the information contained in the medical record. In some cases, the PPA will not play a strong role in that decision, especially if the surgeon feels the operation is needed imminently despite the patient's having multiple psychosocial risk factors. This is the surgeon's decision and must be accepted by the psychologist/mental health professional who performed the PPA. However strongly felt, empirically based, and clearly stated, in the end, the PPA is a valuable but not definitive diagnostic assessment.

When surgeons order diagnostic tests, most often they do not speak with the individual physician who conducted the test but, instead, rely on reading the report. Of course, there are times when it is critical that a direct conference occur. For example, if a routine MRI is ordered, and cancer is discovered, the radiologist will, of course, call the referring physician to discuss the results. So it is with PPA. When the results of the PPA indicate that the patient has a high level of psychosocial risk for reduced outcome, the assessing psychologist/mental health professional should directly contact the referring physician and discuss how this may affect the treatment plan. This discussion may cause the physician to be more circumspect or reassess the risks versus benefits of the surgery. In the ideal situation, the surgeon and the psychologist/mental health professional can then determine next steps and especially plan for informing and including the patient in the surgical decision-making process.

INFORMING THE PATIENT

The main beneficiary of PPA is the patient because this comprehensive assessment maximizes the likelihood that proposed treatment will achieve its goals and minimizes the prospect of worsening physical, emotional, or behavioral conditions. However, most patients who undergo PPA are eager to proceed with surgery and may be loathe to hear of any issues that might delay or alter the surgical planning process. Therefore, it is critical to inform patients—in a sensitive but realistic fashion—of the assessment results: their strengths as well as psychosocial risk factors identified. From this can flow a discussion of how they can use assessment results to plan for and make decisions about treatment, anticipate problems that might arise, and determine steps they can take to overcome or reduce their risks of poor results. However, one must be careful not to indicate to patients that the results of the PPA will determine whether the surgery will proceed. This decision is up to the surgeon, who must weigh all the potential risks and benefits, both physical and psychological, that might affect surgery results.

Most often, in cases in which a high level of psychosocial risk is identified, it is valuable to have a meeting involving the surgeon, psychologist/mental health professional, patient, and, if possible, the patient's primary support person. Such a meeting helps patients to both acknowledge their problems and recognize that they may play an important role in recovery. This meeting can include shared decision making about a treatment plan that addresses risk factors and defines expectations of both the patient and providers. The meeting then provides an impetus for the patient to be actively involved in their care, from seeking information and complying with their treatment plan to addressing emotional issues that may arise. In extreme cases in which the surgeon has decided not to operate, the meeting provides an opportunity for a thorough discussion of the rationale for this decision, and the development of alternative treatment strategies can address patient needs to move forward in overcoming the medical/surgical problems that first brought them to the surgeon.

Sometimes a patient with a high level of psychosocial risk factors will not agree with or easily accept the conclusions that the surgeon and psychologist/mental health professional have reached together. A patient may feel that the PPA has placed an unnecessary barrier on their road to recovery. When this occurs (and it is a rare occurrence), the patient may become hostile, passive, or refuse to engage in shared decision making. It is then that the psychologist/mental health professional must rely on the ethical foundations of the presurgical assessment, making certain in their own mind that the need for beneficence and nonmaleficence outweigh the need for patient autonomy (right to choose desired treatments). The clinician must be confident that, together with the surgeon, a decision to delay or decline surgery is in the patient's best medical interest even though the patient does not agree, whereas proceeding with elective surgery in the face of a high level of psychosocial risk carries the likelihood of failure or worsening of patient problems.

PROVIDING TREATMENT RECOMMENDATIONS

Through the PPA process, the psychologist/mental health professional becomes aware of many psychosocial issues that may affect the outcome of the proposed surgery. Thus, the psychologist/mental health professional can be a key participant in achieving the desired surgical results. This can occur in two major ways: (a) by providing brief psychological interventions aimed at improving surgical results and (b) by offering suggestions to the surgeon to individualize medical treatment plans.

Before proceeding, I want to emphasize again that in providing such recommendations, the psychologist/mental health professional must focus the goals of PPA—that is, to help patients achieve the best possible surgical outcomes and avoid worsening of their medical and psychological states. Many PPA patients have significant psychological issues that are longer term or will not affect the effectiveness of the surgery. A few examples might include marital separation, compulsive behaviors, or trauma. When the PPA reveals such issues, the clinician should discuss this with the patient and offer a referral for treatment. I would suggest, however, that if the surgery is imminent, the patient should delay psychotherapy for such nonrelated issues until after recovering from the surgery because the initial sessions of psychotherapy can be quite stressful and thus problematic during the surgical recovery process. In addition, I would recommend that the psychologist/mental health professional who performed the PPA not provide long-term therapy for the patient. This is because the surgical recovery process is often lengthy and unpredictable. It can be quite difficult to switch between psychological interventions that support effective surgery and those that treat more general psychological issues.

Psychological Treatments to Support Surgical Results

The psychologist/mental health professional who conducted the PPA should have a strong understanding of the specific surgery for which the patient is being considered. This knowledge, together with the results of the PPA, should point to significantly helpful, brief interventions. However, here, one must rely primarily on experience and clinical judgment in proposing such interventions because, in most cases, there is minimal research on the effectiveness of psychotherapy in improving surgery results. A detailed examination of each type of suggested psychological technique is beyond the scope of this chapter, but some of the most common interventions are these:

- self-regulation strategies: mindfulness meditation, biofeedback, relaxation training, hypnotherapy
- emotional stability: cognitive behavior intervention aimed at altering maladaptive cognitions, psychotropic medications (requires referral to a psychiatrist)
- expectations and pacing: primarily an educational function, helping patients develop realistic expectations of both surgical outcome and their role in achieving the most beneficial results

- improvements in health engagement and testing motivation: instructing patients in specific behaviors that will promote surgical results, such as weight loss, smoking cessation, medication reduction before surgery, information seeking and self-advocacy
- acceptance and commitment: helping patients accept limitations, anticipate problems that may occur during recovery, recognize and commit to positive aspects of their lives (e.g., Hayes et al., 2012)

Suggestions to the Surgeon to Maximize Surgery Results

The following are suggestions to the referring surgeon that can be crafted to individual treatment plans and should be included in the assessment report:

- Shared decision making: Collaborate with the patient to understand surgical success as defined by the patient's preferences and values (see Slover et al., 2012, for a review). Help patients be clear about what can and cannot be achieved by surgery.
- Define the patient role: Help the patient understand exactly what actions will be expected to achieve best results and to view surgery as only setting the foundation for success.
- Provide clear postoperative guidelines: Inform patients of the rate at which recovery is expected and the pacing of activity resumption.
- Anticipate problems before they occur: Help patients to recognize common postoperative problems, explaining how they should view and handle them.
- Include significant others in treatment planning: The patient's support system can be critical in achieving success. Provide support members with clear information about the patient's condition, the surgery, and how they can assist in recovery. Include them in shared decision making.

FUTURE DIRECTIONS

Although the inclusion of PPA within the surgical assessment process has grown rapidly, the chapters in this book point to important issues that need to be addressed if the field is to remain viable and grow. Next, I discuss several of these areas.

First and foremost, looking across the chapters, it is clear that for many types of physical conditions, that identification of objectively measurable psychological characteristics empirically linked to surgical outcome is more a goal than a reality. This is particularly true of some of the newer areas in which PPA is being used. Along similar lines, there is a dearth of studies comparing surgical outcomes of patients who received PPA with those who did not receive such assessments. Fortunately, where such comparisons have been made, such as in screening for breast cancer surgery (see Chapter 7), it does appear that overall PPA has a beneficial effect on outcomes. Future research must explicate both the specific psychological factors affecting outcome for each surgery type and demonstrate that PPA achieves its goals of improving outcome and avoiding worsening of physical and psychological issues.

Second, PPA lacks a widely accepted standardized goal-directed approach. This is true throughout psychology because practitioners of different theoretical orientations use a wide variety of tools to assess patients with a single diagnosis. However, medicine works differently than psychology, using near universally accepted diagnostic tests for the purpose of treatment planning. The surgeon then relies on their experience and expertise to integrate and interpret these tests. The RIM model, described in Chapter 1, provides an example of a similar overall approach to PPA, bringing together the objectivity of test results and the clinician's expertise. Such an approach should lead to wider acceptance of PPA as a component of the surgical diagnostic process. An additional benefit of a generally standardized approach would be the explication and reduction of conflicting ethical issues involved in PPA. A standardized approach, of necessity, would reduce bias by providing a rationale for PPA, defining the goals of the assessment, and providing rules for reaching assessment conclusions and recommendations. Thus, providers would not be forced to make subjective decisions, as in the case of creating a "letter" to clear the patient for gender embodiment surgery (see Chapter 6).

Third, because PPA identifies issues that can affect surgery results, it should point to interventions that draw on patient strengths and reduce psychosocial risk factors, Chapter 4 admirably provides a table listing psychological interventions for improving the outcome of bariatric surgery. However, with this type of surgery, as with most others in the book, there has been a lack of research examining the ability of psychological interventions to improve surgery results. Without such research, PPA has the potential to become a mechanism for excluding patients from or delaying surgeries while leaving them adrift without any means of effectively ameliorating psychological concerns.

Fourth, studies should look at why and how surgeons include PPA within the preoperative decision-making process. How broadly is PPA used within each surgical area? What are the conditions that trigger referrals for PPA?

How does the surgeon's explanation of the need for PPA influence the results of PPA? Do surgeons actually use the information provided in PPA? And if they do not, why not?

Fifth, patient expectations for the outcome of surgery need further exploration. As many chapters in this volume discuss, patients may be unrealistic in their projections of surgical results. For example, as noted in Chapter 9, patients undergoing deep brain stimulation for Parkinson's-related movement disorders often assume that this procedure will lead to "improvement of mental state," "more socializing," or "improvement of partnership," none of which improves with deep brain stimulation. When such unrealistic patient expectations are not met, satisfaction with outcome is surely affected. It is likely, then, that motivation and emotional state would follow such unmet expectations, further reducing outcomes.

CONCLUSION

As the chapters in this book indicate, PPA is a vibrant and growing field that addresses the interface of psychological and surgical problems. Its goals are clear: to maximize the likelihood of surgical success while minimizing the chances of worsening patients' medical and psychological conditions. The level of empirical support for PPA as a predictor of surgical outcome varies widely from strong (e.g., spine surgery, bariatric surgery, organ transplant) to limited (e.g., gender embodiment surgery). From the PPA can flow treatments provided by the psychologist/mental health professional and suggestions to the surgical team that can individualize and promote best results.

Whatever the case, PPA requires working knowledge of the specific surgery for which the patient is being considered and a clear focus on surgically related psychological factors. It also requires a keen ethical focus to recognize and balance the patient's desire and need for the surgery with the need to address identified psychological barriers that can adversely affect surgical results. When conducted properly and effectively, a PPA can be critical component of the diagnostic process, greatly helping the surgeon in most effectively weighing the benefits and risks involved the decision to operate and enlisting the patient in the treatment planning process.

REFERENCES

Ben-Porath, Y. S. (2012). *Interpreting the MMPI-2-RF.* University of Minnesota Press.

Ben-Porath, Y. S., & Tellegen, A. (2020a). *The Minnesota Multiphasic Personality Inventory–3: Manual for administration, scoring, and interpretation*. University of Minnesota Press.

Ben-Porath, Y. S., & Tellegen, A. (2020b). *The Minnesota Multiphasic Personality Inventory–3: Technical manual*. University of Minnesota Press.

Block, A. R. (1981). Investigation of the response of the spouse to chronic pain behavior. *Psychosomatic Medicine*, *43*(5), 415–422. https://doi.org/10.1097/00006842-198110000-00004

Bruns, D., & Disorbio, J. M. (2003). *Battery for Health Improvement 2 manual*. Pearson.

Hayes, S. C., Strosahl, K. D., & Wilson, K. G. (2012). *Acceptance and commitment therapy: The process and practice of mindful change* (2nd ed.). Guilford Press.

Lockhart, J., & Satya-Murti, S. (2015). Symptom exaggeration and symptom validity testing in persons with medically unexplained neurologic presentations. *Neurology Clinical Practice*, *5*(1), 17–24. https://doi.org/10.1212/CPJ.0000000000000092

Millon, T., Antoni, M. H., Millon, C., Minor, S., & Grossman, S. (2001). *Millon Behavioral Medicine Diagnostic (MBMD) manual*. Pearson Assessments.

Slover, J., Shue, J., & Koenig, K. (2012). Shared decision-making in orthopaedic surgery. *Clinical Orthopaedics and Related Research*, *470*(4), 1046–1053. https://doi.org/10.1007/s11999-011-2156-8

Uchino, B. M. (2008). *Social support and physical health*. Yale University Press.

Walczyk, J. J., Sewell, N., & DiBenedetto, M. B. (2018). A review of approaches to detecting malingering in forensic contests and promising cognitive load–inducing lie detection techniques. *Frontiers in Psychiatry*, *9*, Article 700. https://doi.org/10.3389/fpsyt.2018.00700

Index

A

D

E

H

I

J

K

L

M

N

O

T

U

V

W

About the Editors

Ryan J. Marek, PhD, received his doctorate in clinical psychology with a minor in quantitative methodology from Kent State University in Kent, Ohio, in 2017. He has diverse clinical experience, including at the Cleveland Clinic in Cleveland, Ohio, and at a rural outpatient mental health facility. He finished his American Psychological Association (APA)–accredited internship in 2017 at the Medical University of South Carolina in Charleston. There, he completed numerous rotations, including weight management, behavioral medicine (e.g., presurgical psychological assessments of bariatric, spinal cord stimulator, and solid organ transplant patients; treatment of chronic pain; and the provision of general assistance to patients to help them adjust to or manage their medical diagnoses), and chronic pain. He also conducted neuropsychological assessments.

Currently, Dr. Marek is an assistant professor of clinical psychology at Sam Houston State University (SHSU) College of Osteopathic Medicine in Conroe, Texas. He teaches medical students, engages in an active program of research, and serves as associate and consulting editors for medical and psychological peer-reviewed journals. He also holds a practice at SHSU Physicians, which is an extension of the university. There, he conducts various psychological assessments (including presurgical assessments) and therapy for outpatient and health-related issues.

Dr. Marek's program of research focuses on understanding how psychological factors contribute to medical outcomes. He currently has more than 50 peer-reviewed publications that focus primarily on presurgical psychological assessments and how they predict various outcomes. He uses his research to help patients manage risk factors before and after surgery to help them achieve good outcomes.

Andrew R. Block, PhD, received his doctoral degree in 1980 from Dartmouth College in Hanover, New Hampshire, and was a National Institutes of Health postdoctoral fellow in biobehavioral science at Duke University Medical Center in Durham, North Carolina. He is a fellow of the American Psychological Association in Division 38 (Health Psychology) and is board-certified in clinical health psychology, having served for many years on the board of the American Board of Clinical Health Psychology. For more than 40 years, he has provided presurgical psychological assessments and treatment for chronic pain, initially with The Spine Institute in Indianapolis, Indiana, and, for the past 32 years, at Texas Back Institute in Plano, Texas.

Dr. Block has 50-plus peer-reviewed publications focused primarily on psychosocial influences on spine surgery outcome as well as the assessment and treatment of chronic benign pain. He developed and published an algorithm for assessing spine surgery candidates that is widely taught in clinical health psychology training programs and used by many practitioners. A recipient of multiple grants, he has examined the use of the Minnesota Multiphasic Personality Inventory–2–Restructured Form (MMPI-2-RF) and Minnesota Multiphasic Personality Inventory–3, or the MMPI-3,[1] in assessing candidates for spine surgery. He is the codeveloper, along with Yossef Ben-Porath, of the MMPI-2-RF spine surgery candidate and spinal cord stimulator candidate interpretive reports. His previous books include *Presurgical Psychological Screening in Chronic Pain Syndromes: A Guide for the Behavioral Health Practitioner* (2014); *Presurgical Psychological Screening: Understanding Patients, Improving Outcomes* (coauthored with David B. Sarwer; 2013); *The Psychology of Spine Surgery* (coauthored with Robert J. Gatchel, William W. Deardorff, and Richard D. Guyer; 2003); and *Handbook of Pain Syndromes: Biopsychosocial Perspectives* (coedited with Ephrem Fernandez and Edwin Kremer; 1998).

[1]The MMPI-2-RF is from Ben-Porath, Y. S., & Tellegen, A. (2008). *MMPI-2-RF: Manual for administration, scoring, and interpretation*. University of Minnesota Press. The MMPI-3 is from Ben-Porath, Y. S., & Tellegen, A. (2020). *Minnesota Multiphasic Personality Inventory–3 (MMPI-3): Manual for administration, scoring, and interpretation*. University of Minnesota Press.